Miami Breast Cancer Experts

Your Indispensable Guide to Breast Health

Cindy Papale-Hammontree

Sabrina Hernandez-Cano, RD, LD/N, CDE

Legal Disclaimer

Cancer is a serious medical condition. It requires professional medical care. The information in this book is presented as a guide to help in your journey.

None of the authors, contributors, Writestream Publishing or anyone associated with *MIAMI BREAST CANCER EXPERTS* or the information contained in the book aim to substitute for medical care. Use this book to help you ask questions, discuss, and become proactive together with your choice of Medical professional team.

The Authors, publisher or anyone associated with Miami Breast Cancer Experts book, website or any entity under this name are not responsible or liable for any loss or damage allegedly arising from any information or suggestion in *MIAMI BREAST CANCER EXPERTS* book.

Our purpose is to bring light and awareness to the many options available in breast cancer care and to help make the journey one filled with peace, hope and lots of love and laughter.

ISBN: 0692499393
ISBN-13: 978-0692499399
Library of Congress Control Number: 2015947905
Printed in the United States of America.

www.writestreampublishing.com

MIAMI BREAST CANCER EXPERTS

Your Indispensable Guide to Breast Health

Cindy Papale-Hammontree

Sabrina Hernandez-Cano, RD, LD/N, CDE

CONTRIBUTORS

Paul P. Slawek, M.D., Nicholas Tranakas, M.D., Donna J. Tomey, C.C.T., Alejandro Hernandez-Cano, M.D., Silvia Rotemberg, M.D., Roger Khouri, M.D., Richard Nadal, M.D., Daniel Calva, M.D., Elisa Krill-Jackson, M.D., Nicolas Kuritzky, M.D., Elizabeth Anne Ouellette, M.D., Samara Christy L.D.T/C.L.T., Dennis Patin, M.D., Khin M. Zaw, M.D., Mariana Khawand, M.D., Moises Jacobs, M.D., Alex Fagenson, Janet Villalobos, A.R.N.P., Don Torok, Ph.D./FACSM, Cristina Pozo-Kaderman, Ph.D., Sameet Kumar, Ph.D., Mary Darling Montero, Ph.D., Cynthia Dougherty, B.C.C., M.F.T., Ph.D., Michella Alva, P.T., Jonathan David, Esq., Patricia San Pedro, Nicole Eldridge Marcus, Ph.D., Astrid Nicastri, Judy Garcia

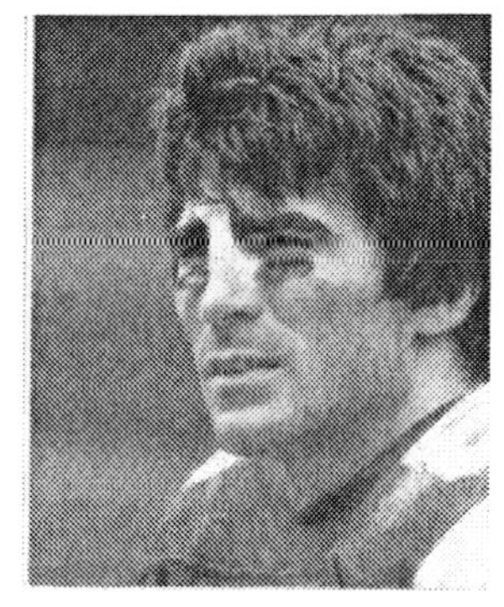

"I've been called *Invincible* but 14 years ago I nearly became invisible after learning that I had been diagnosed with colon cancer. When I think back at that moment I can't help but think of Mac Brown when he sings, *"I've got my toes in the water ... life is good today!"* And then wham, a rip current wipes you out and you reach out for somebody to save you ... anybody!

"As you read through the book *Miami Breast Cancer Experts* and experience the compelling and courageous stories of the survivors, you will certainly find out that the savior is yourself first. If these women weren't pro-active they would be not be around to share their incredible stories with us. To me invincibility is the synergy of mind, body and spirit and these women have truly proven themselves to be *Invincible*!

"As you read thru the chapters you are uplifted and exhilarated by these women's battles to refuse to be defeated by cancer. You learn to understand that it's okay to be afraid. That self-pity and "why me" is acceptable. And finally, that the reality is that you have choices and that this demon can be overcome if you so choose. Each woman's dream is to be cured, to pound her chest, and call herself a survivor. Of course, the ultimate dream for all is to find the cure for cancer. I often say, *"It takes teamwork to make the dream work!"*

"Just ask my cousin Cindy Papale-Hammontree, who shares her compelling survival story in Chapter 1 of *Miami Breast Cancer Experts*. In 2008, she released her first book, *The Empty Cup Runneth Over* (www.theemptycuprunnethover.com). She has appeared on Channel 6 South Florida Today Show and her survivor story has made the front pages of every local newspaper in Miami-Dade, Broward, and Palm Beach Counties. Cindy is also in the process of collaborating with Hollywood producers on a feature film about her breast cancer journey.

"As you follow Cindy's journey and persistence, you understand that there are so many components to the joy of becoming a survivor. Try to imagine being on a calm river watching an eight-oared boat rowing down the river in the midst of fierce competition. Every person pulling that oar has to do it in unison to get to the end of the race a winner. Each person has to dig deep and find something inside they never knew existed in order to win that battle. Imagine each oar being stroked by the uoncologist, the radiologist, the surgeon, the hospital, the caregiver, the lab tech, the nutritionist, and the fitness trainer. The 'cox' is The Family. If one oar is off cadence the entire boat rocks and the whole race is lost. In Cindy's case all was in sync and here she is 14 years later smiling and inspiring. She is truly *Invincible* and why I am so proud to be her 'Cuz.'

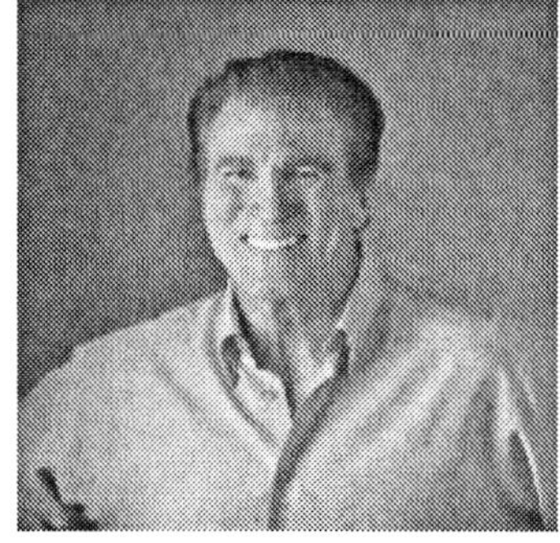

"*Miami Breast Cancer Experts* is a must read for all genders because we are all affected by cancer in some way. You will be inspired, lifted, educated while you laugh and cry at the same time. More than anything you will see that nothing overcomes the human spirit and the wonders that it brings as we overcome that rip tide called cancer."

Vince Papale
www.vincepapale.com

"This book is a smorgasbord of intelligent essays on every aspect of breast cancer. Everyone – nurses, doctors, and people dealing with the disease for the first time will find chapters of this book helpful. Breast cancer treatment in Miami seems to be at the apex of a healing mountain, there are so many highly regarded professionals working at making it not just survivable but turning it into a life challenge that can help women find enhancement for their lives beyond it. This is not a sad book, but a compilation of so much hope and possibility that you will find yourself smiling, enjoying the ride. Well worth reading!"

–Anne E. Hemingway Feuer, RN, BSN, MS (Ernest Hemingway's niece).

"From screening tests to chemotherapy, reconstruction options and more, this is a comprehensive look at breast cancer. A variety of experts share their experiences and knowledge to help guide women who are dealing with this disease. My favorite chapters are the personal stories from survivors. You'll be informed and inspired by this book."

–Diana Gonzalez, Health Producer, NBC6, Miami, Florida

"One would wrongly assume that this subject matter would conjure up images of clinical-speak and sad statistics. Wrong! What a book! "Everyone who picks up this book, will hugely benefit. It's rather unfortunate that there is no ONE person who hasn't either known someone who has battled, is battling, or has been in the ring themselves, and this book speaks to every single one of those people. These pages provide hope, inspiration, and is a true A to Z of what happens from diagnosis to remission and everything after. No topic is off limits; from alternative options, the right questions to ask, to all of those deep-seeded emotions that bubble to the surface throughout your entire journey. And this book is a journey itself, one of Love!"

–Julie Guy, Morning Personality 101.5 Lite FM

"Both Cindy and Sabrina are amazing women whose souls were brought together to save lives and share their knowledge on health and living through breast cancer. This book is a testament to God's grace, which shines in their testimonies."

-- Tracy Wilson Mourning, Founder of the Honey Shine Mentoring Program and wife to Miami Heat Player, Alonso Mourning

DEDICATION

It is with pleasure and love as a sister that I dedicate *Miami Breast Cancer Experts* to my dear brother Mike Papale, who lost his battle to colon cancer in June, 2010 at the young age of 51. Mike was an amazing, loving guy who always went out of his way to help others. We were all devastated to hear the news of his diagnosis, but Mike always remained positive. Rarely did he complain about his pain.

Because he was still a child inside a young man's body, Mike could be immature at times. I remember back to our school years when he and I had gotten pulled out of class at the same time and thought we were getting kicked out of school. I was scared; Mike was happy. Turned out, we'd been expelled from class because they found out we hadn't had our mandatory polio shots. Upon hearing the news, Mike was NO LONGER happy!

For 30 years he worked at Hollywood Memorial Hospital in the Pedi-ICU Unit, where he saved the lives of many babies. Mike was very close to his co-workers, many of whom he took under his wing. People like Jay Hill, whom he always kept laughing and De Ann Laufenberg, whom he loved like a sister (and whose family treated him as one of their own).

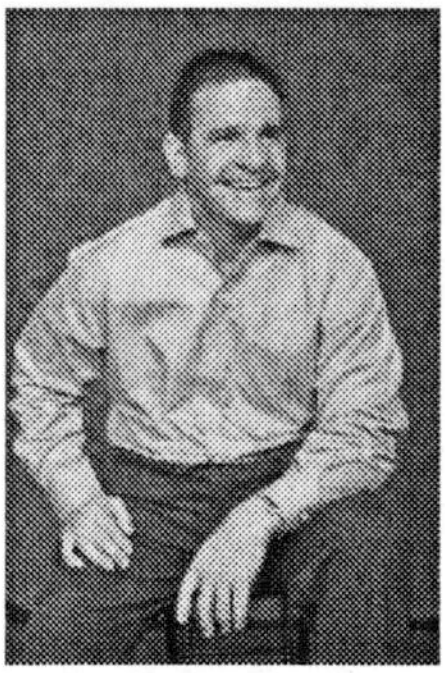

To Mike's other friends Bobbie Jones and Eileen Watkins, thank you for taking such good care of him during his final days. To his wife Debbie, know that Mike loved you more than anything in this world. He would also have been proud of his three children Debbie, Mike, and Chrissy and all eight of his grandchildren. We all miss and love Mike, and know he is resting in peace – another angel watching over our family and friends.

Much love from your sister,
Cindy Papale-Hammontree

In Loving Memory of my Business Partner, Allen Brenteson and my Brother, Ralph Lazaro Sanchez

In loving and unforgettable memory of the best business partner anyone could ask for. Allen, I know your spirit is still with me and your sky blue eyes are watching over us all.
I feel your pride and your guidance in the raising of "our baby," Hummingwell bar, our humanitarian project of love. Your passion, your words of encouragement and your business savvy linger. I think about you every day and I honor every promise I made to you before you left me. Hummingwell's commitment to St. Jude's kids will always be our first priority, while we continue to wish each and every customer wellness. I love you for all that you were during your time on earth, and everything you continue to represent: a good old-fashioned American, a Montana born-and-raised eagle.

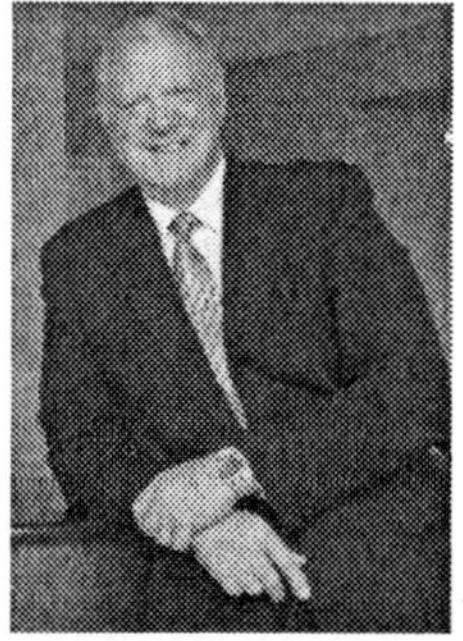

Our Humming bird is flying high; you will always be the wind beneath my wings.

I love you,
Your "best partner"
Sabrina

Allen Brenteson graduated from the Thunderbird School of Global Management. He was an International business man who joined a fortune 500 company and successfully led them through Latin America and the Caribbean. He served on the board of directors of Baptist Hospital for many years and formed the International Division at Baptist Health South Florida, where Allen and Sabrina met and worked together. In 2003, Allen and Sabrina discovered they both shared a passion for good nutrition and wellness. They founded Scientific Nutrition and developed Hummingwell wellness bars to bring to the community the message that delicious food can also be nutritionally sound. After many trials and the discovery of premium ingredients in Oregon, they took a chance and developed a bar that has all the goodness of nature with 22 vitamins and minerals. Soon after the birth of

Hummingwell bars, Allen received a devastating diagnosis: an uncommon malignant cancer called angiosarcoma on his forehead. It took his life on January 14, 2015. He leaves a legacy of leadership and friendship and his partner Sabrina to carry on the name of their little bird and message of wellness, Hummingwell.

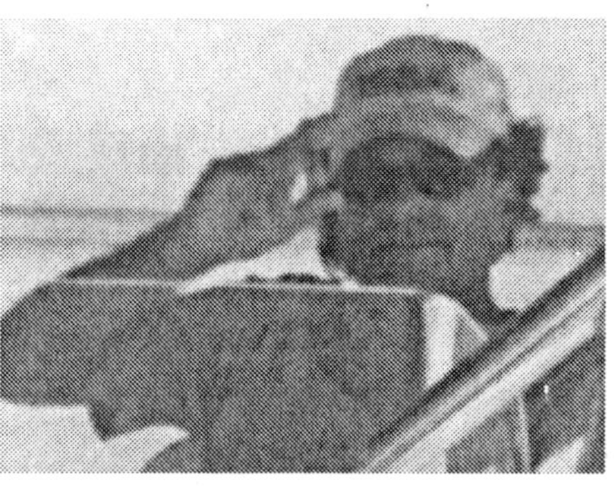

To my brother Ralph Lazaro Sanchez – a free and kindred spirit whom I lost on December 26, 2014 from metastatic prostate cancer – my brother, you absolutely rock! I'm living the life you taught me to live. Every day is a breath of fresh ocean air; every minute I hear the sound of church bells and know that your spirit is dancing in my heart.

I love and miss you, especially on every Thanksgiving Day to come.

Your sis,
Sabrina

CONTENTS

FOREWARD

Gail Ironson, M.D., Ph.D.

Cindy and Sabrina have teamed up once again to make available an outstanding book – a "must read" for anyone who has or knows anyone with breast cancer - by gathering an incredible group of experts and survivors. They have done an amazing job of making their previous book *The Empty Cup Runneth Over* even better by updating the contents and adding several chapters to provide readers with the latest treatment options.

The terrific thing about this book is that it covers multiple topics, and does so in a readable, interesting way – enabling us to be better informed about how to cope, what to expect, and how to make wise treatment decisions. It will also help you discuss options with medical personnel.

I first met Cindy over 20 years ago when she was an administrative assistant at the Psychological Services Center at the University of Miami. I was immediately impressed by her bubbly enthusiasm and her ability to make everyone who came to the Psychological Services Center feel comfortable. Her natural inclination to share and help people led to this book (and her previous one) where, in a labor of love, she has transformed her own wrenching experience with breast cancer into a vehicle to educate us about many aspects of dealing with it. She openly shares her own very personal story, from shock at the moment of diagnosis through the terror of making decisions about treatment and the fears one faces with this diagnosis. She has drawn together an amazing group of experts who write chapters on everything you would ever want to know about this illness, as well as survivors whose stories give us hope and information from the patients' view. This book takes the mystery and the fear out of breast cancer by making the diagnosis and what happens familiar.

The experts includes medical doctors, a nurse, a nutritionist, a physical therapist, and mental health professionals. In one particularly moving new chapter, oncology nurse Janet Villalobos describes the daily ups and downs of treating patients on the front lines (especially children). She also gives some useful advice to cancer patients from years of experience seeing patients go through treatment.

The medical expert coverage of different areas related to breast cancer is extensive. The book has several chapters on screening techniques and diagnosis including mammography, MRI, ultrasound, thermography, and stereotactic breast biopsies. These chapters are particularly helpful because they provide enough information to give the reader an understanding of what to expect during diagnostic procedures, what the doctors look for, and how the diagnosis is made. Thus, you do not feel that you are "in the dark." Once diagnosed, readers can learn about various treatments, including surgery (both mastectomy and lumpectomy), chemotherapy, and radiation. Of note, the chapter by Dr. Beatriz Amendola discusses new strides in breast cancer treatment, including targeted radiation. And the chapter by Dr. Nicholas Tranakas gives the latest options for lumpectomy and several types of mastectomies. Knowing what to expect during chemotherapy and radiation that the reader will gain access to in this book can help one be prepared to cope with the treatments.

After surgery, one is faced with decisions about breast reconstruction. The latest options are explored by Dr. Silvia Rotemberg in one chapter, and by doctors Khouri, Nadal and Calva in another, which includes fat grafting. The next topic covered is managing and containing two particularly troublesome symptoms including lymphedema and pain. The chapters on lymphedema from Dr. Elizabeth Anne Ouellette and Samara Christy, LDT, CLT, are especially useful in defining lymphedema and presenting an innovative approach for what to do about it. Dr. Dennis Patin's chapter on pain management provides useful information for patients and caregivers. And because this book does not hesitate to discuss difficult issues – for example, if health deteriorates significantly – it includes a thorough chapter on palliative care from Dr. Khin M. Zaw and Dr. Mariana Khawand as well as an informative legal chapter from Jonathan David, Esquire. These new chapters were added by popular request.

There are several thoughtful chapters on coping with breast cancer and maintaining emotional well-being written by mental health experts. The signature chapter in this regard is written by an experienced psycho-oncologist, Sameet Kumar, Ph.D., whom I invite every year to give a lecture in my graduate class of students training to be health psychologists . This book doesn't stop there – it provides information on deeply personal topics such as sex and sexuality from Christina Pozo-Kaderman, Ph.D., and one on mindfulness (together with a meditation exercise), self-compassion, and positive rewiring of thoughts from Cynthia Dougherty, BCC, M.F.T., Ph.D.

The survivor stories will help people with cancer to cope with and navigate this difficult illness as well. As Cindy points out, the diagnosis and treatment of breast cancer is undoubtedly difficult and often comes as a shock. Her story beautifully leads you through the series of adjustments and decisions. The interview of Astrid Nicastri illustrates resilience and maintaining a fighting spirit even in the face of multiple brain tumors and later breast cancer. Staying positive in the face of breast Cancer is also discussed by Patricia San Pedro, who wrote a book *The Cancer Dancer – Healing One Step at a Time* and is the founder of *Positively Pat* and the *Link of Hope Sistas* on Facebook. Two chapters provide a therapist's point of view with respect to breast cancer: Mary Darling Montero, Ph.D., who was diagnosed with breast cancer, and Nicole Eldridge Marcus, Ph.D., whose mother was diagnosed with breast cancer. Finally, the story of Judy Garcia, singer and songwriter, offers the perspective of someone who thought they might have breast cancer after noticing a lump in her breast.

Healthy lifestyles are another major content area with experts' chapters providing up to date information. These will be useful both for people with breast cancer and those who wish to take steps to avoid breast cancer. The chapter on nutrition, written by a nutritionist and co-editor of this book, Sabrina Hernandez-Cano, provides expanded information on healthy eating, superfoods, and supplements for cancer patients or for prevention, information on weight loss, and wonderful recipes. There is a new chapter on obesity from Dr. Moises Jacobs and Alex Fagenson which has a focus on surgical options; a chapter on exercise from Don Torok, Ph.D., FACSM; and a chapter on "nurturing moves" from physical therapist Michelle Alva, which combines physical therapy, yoga and belly dancing.

The treatment information and decisions one needs to make after being diagnosed with breast cancer can be daunting and overwhelming. This book will undoubtedly help with dealing with and making those decisions. And it will help navigate what comes after the diagnosis. It is a great service that Cindy and Sabrina have done by putting this book together and it has my enthusiastic endorsement.

Gail Ironson, M.D., Ph.D. is professor at the University of Miami specializing in Health Psychology and is a board certified Psychiatrist. She received her Ph.D. from the University of Wisconsin, and her M.D. from the University of Miami, followed by residency training in psychiatry at Stanford. She has almost 200 publications in the areas of behavioral medicine, spirituality, trauma treatment, positive psychology, and stress management and coping with chronic illness, including cancer and HIV.

Notable accomplishments include receiving a Senior Investigator Award from the Society of Behavioral Medicine in 2011 for her work on Spirituality and Health, being president of the Academy of Behavioral Medicine Research in 2002, and being awarded the Alumni Professor Award for outstanding scholarship and teaching by the University of South Florida (Tampa). She also set up and codirects the Trauma Treatment program at the University of Miami. She has been on the editorial boards of five journals (International Journal of Behavioral Medicine, AIDS and Behavior, Health Psychology, Journal of Applied Psychology, and Journal of Disaster Psychiatry).

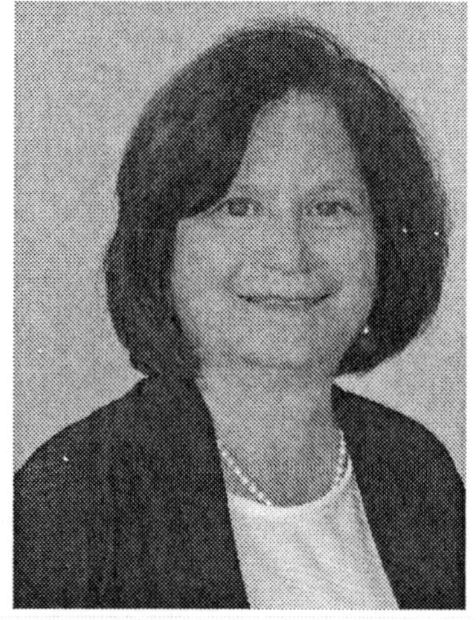

Current funded projects include an NIMH study treating trauma in people at risk for HIV, and a Templeton study examining biological mechanisms in a nationwide study of Spirituality and Health (The Landmark study), where she is one of 5 lead investigators.

INTRODUCTION

It is with great pleasure that we welcome you to *Miami Breast Cancer Experts*.

After being diagnosed in July of 2000 with a stage I, left, multifocal, invasive breast cancer, I decided that rather than have a pity party I would turn something as negative and life-threatening as breast cancer into a positive.

It was around January of 2006 when I was sitting in Dan Marino's Restaurant in south Miami, Florida and overheard a conversation Sabrina was having about breast cancer. I approached her and asked if that person was a physician I knew. She'd replied, "No, it's my business partner and dear friend Alan Brentenson." At the time they were working on a super healthy snack that today we know as Hummingwell, the wellness bar. It is available to the public through the website www.Hummingwell.com and on www.Amazon.com. Sadly, Sabrina lost her great friend Allen to an unexpected, rare form of cancer called angiosarcoma.

After that initial conversation at Dan Marino's we sat and chatted for a long time, becoming instant friends. There was something very special about Sabrina; she has an incredible passion for wellness and just from speaking with her in that short time I knew I wanted her to collaborate on my book. I invited her to one of my talks at Our Lady of Lourdes High School in Coral Gables – an invitation she graciously accepted. I wanted so much to make a difference through the writing of this book and give back as a breast cancer advocate to help educate young women and men about the disease.

A few weeks after the presentation at Our Lady of Lourdes High School, I asked Sabrina if she would be interested in collaborating with me on my book and she enthusiastically replied "yes." In 2007 we released *The Empty Cup Runneth Over*. We had an amazing book signing at Barnes and Noble in Kendall attended by over 500 people including Channel 4 and Channel 6, along with the Miami Herald. It was an incredible evening.

A few months before our book signing, my brother Mike Papale was diagnosed with an aggressive colon cancer. Tragically, he lost his battle with the disease. Mike was an awesome guy who'd worked at Joe DiMaggio Hospital where he helped save many young babies from all kinds of illnesses. His funeral was packed with people who loved him dearly. It was a huge loss in our family, something that still causes me pain whenever I think about it. Sabrina also lost her brother Ralph Lazaro Sanchez to metastatic prostate cancer – a fellow she describes as Hemmingway reincarnated. Ralph lived in the Florida Keys on his beautiful yacht, where he watched the sunset until his very last breath.

It was also during our book signing that Sabrina's mother Maribella was diagnosed with breast cancer. I was heartbroken to hear of this and instantly tried my best to be supportive. Both of us were suffering from loved ones diagnosed with cancer and could relate very much to their pain. I am happy to say that Maribella is now doing well and is a 10-year survivor.

It was during the time we were writing "Miami Breast Cancer Experts" that my own mother, Lena Papale was diagnosed with a stage IIIB breast cancer at the age of 85. I thought, "Who gets breast cancer at age 85?" I was totally shocked and began to research the best doctors for her care. We decided that due to the invasive kind of breast cancer she had my mother would move forward with a right mastectomy. She did amazing after the surgery and continues to get her Herceptin treatments. She is doing very well and living in Hollywood, Florida.

Sabrina and I stayed in touch over the years and connected again recently with the idea of writing our second book. Our first book did well, but we wanted to write another one that would be even more successful. Thus in 2014 we created *Miami Breast Cancer Experts*.

In our last book *The Empty Cup Runneth Over*, I wrote my last chapter in front of a court house. Now, with this new book *Miami Breast Cancer Experts* I sit again in front of a court house, but this time to get a marriage license to remarry my ex-husband John (more about this in my chapter "I am Cindy, From Birth,

Boobs, and Beyond").

Sabrina and I have collaborated with many special physicians over the years. It is through these collaborations that we have come together to create an indispensable new book – a treasure trove of information to help anyone who is either seeking to know more about breast cancer or has been diagnosed with breast cancer, as well as their sometimes overlooked caregivers.

Readers will be pleased with all the information in this book from experts ranging from physicians to psychologists to physical therapists. Additionally, they'll enjoy Sabrina's wonderful nutrition chapter and inspiring stories from survivors.

We would like to thank all the contributing physicians and survivors who took time out of their busy work schedules and time away from their families to help make *Miami Breast Cancer Experts* the best book available with up-to-date information.

We welcome readers to *Miami Breast Cancer Experts* and hope you will enjoy reading the comprehensive information presented throughout these pages. Many of the physicians are also available through either their own websites or hospitals they are on staff with.

NEW TO THIS EDITION

The publication of the first edition to *Miami Breast Cancer Experts* is *The Empty Cup Runneth Over*. In 2007, we set forth to accomplish one simple but important goal. Many books had been written on the subject of breast cancer but never had experts in their field come together to offer their knowledge on their particular practice. Our hope was to create greater awareness through the eyes of the survivor, along with the expertise of the medical and health care professionals who make up the wholesome care of a woman's journey through a breast cancer diagnosis. We strongly feel we accomplished our purpose. The lives of over 100,000 magnificent patients and survivors from all over the world have become informed via www.TheEmptyCupRunnethOver.com, which integrates with the new edition www.MiamiBreastCancerExperts.com

Unfortunately, cancer has affected our lives tremendously. Since our last edition, both of our mothers have been diagnosed with breast cancer. We also lost both of our brothers and dear friends to some form of cancer.

We saw very close-up and personal how critical it is to stay on top of the latest details, particulars, discoveries, and facts about surviving a cancer diagnosis. The faster the detection, the better the chances of recovery and survival.

Since the launch of our first edition, research has emerged with new scientific evidence, explanations, and perspectives on the prevention and treatment of Breast Cancer. Thus, we've added:

- New advances in the latest treatment of chemotherapy and radiation;
- The latest research and state-of-the-art techniques on topics such as plastic and reconstructive surgery;
- Key new topics such as fat grafting, thermography, pain management, and a chapter written by an indispensable part of the team, the oncology nurse;
- Delicate subjects such as money and death in response to feedback from readers of the first edition;
- The legal side of things;
- Palliative care;
- New scientific evidence on super foods in an updated nutrition chapter where we've highlighted foods that should be consumed daily due to their high anti-oxidant values and increased the color in our meal plans to increase the cancer-fighting potential in every bite;
- A Bariatric chapter to inform women about their options in the case of obesity; and
- Chapters that address the physical, emotional, and mental health of women like exercise, yoga, and mind/spirit healing.

We wish you wellness and abundant health.

It is with great honor, pride and joy that we come together to bring greater awareness with our outstanding authors who are warriors in the trenches, fighting alongside strong women in this battle we call Breast Cancer. We hope you find, knowledge, peace, and love and feel the passion and fire throughout the pages of *Miami Breast Cancer Experts*.

CHAPTER 1

Survivor, Advocate, Executive Producer:

I AM CINDY – FROM BIRTH, BOOBS, AND BEYOND

I was born on July 6, 1954 at Physicians Hospital in New York City, weighing in at five pounds, four ounces, the daughter of Joseph Papale and Lena Delsordo, who named me Asunda. However, in spite of my baptismal name (yep, we're Italian!) everyone has always called me Cindy for reasons unknown to me. I'm also the middle child and only girl, with an older (by seven years) brother, Joseph, and a younger (by three years) brother, Michael. We lived in New York City until I was five, then my family moved to Long Island where we stayed until I was seventeen. In those days, life was much simpler than it is today and I had a wonderful childhood. For example, it was OK for kids to play alone outside, there wasn't much pressure to wear designer clothing, and I wasn't spoiled by material things. I was just a kid having fun with my friends – not worrying much about anything.

Growing up in a large Italian family meant that on Sundays we all got together and enjoyed a huge family dinner. A true Italian, my dad made sure that every one of these Sundays was special. He'd see to it we had enough food and drinks to eat and savor so we could just relax and revel in the day. If not for him, I doubt my family would've been as close as we were. My mother would spend hours cooking a homemade sauce to accompany her delicious meatballs. My grandmother, Cristina, who lived with us, would get up early to help. Although she didn't speak English very well, she definitely understood it.

By noon the house would start to fill up with people; everyone would talk and laugh as the enticing aroma of food punctuated the atmosphere. My father loved to entertain by playing cards after dinner and we never knew how many guests would show up. But it was always fun and the food was amazing – somehow I stayed as thin as pencil!

As the years went by, my grandmother became very ill with severe diabetes and anemia. I remember driving back and forth to the hospital with my parents, who spoke to many doctors about her condition. I was just fifteen when she passed away in the early 1970s; I recall seeing her in her hospital bed, struggling to breathe the evening before she died. This was the first time in my life I'd witnessed anyone dying and I didn't know how to act. Her death was very traumatic for me.

Our lives changed drastically in the aftermath of her death. It was very difficult for my mother to continue living in the same home we'd all shared. I remember overhearing my parents discussing a possible move to Florida, which really upset me. I was going to be a high school senior the following year; moving at that time meant I would not be able to graduate with my friends.

In the middle of my junior year, my parents announced our impending relocation to the Sunshine State. While I can't recall if my brothers had the same reaction, I was certainly distraught. I persisted until I convinced my parents to let me stay with one of my friends to finish my junior year; after that, I had no choice but to move to Florida.

Thus I began my senior year in a new state, in a new school. It was 1972 and Florida high schools were quite different from the ones in New York – beginning with the fact that there were no windows. Back in the day, things were not discussed quite as openly as they are now. Sure, we had classes on sex education and discussions about things like teen pregnancy and venereal disease. But there was never any mention of cancer, let alone *breast cancer*, or the concept of self-examination. Growing up, I was very uncomfortable with my breasts, which were not quite as large as I would have preferred.

Although today it's almost commonplace for teens to have breast implants, the thought never occurred to me when I was a teenager. In fact, I was probably in my mid-20s before I even met someone who had them.

At home, the only time the topic of breasts came up was when my mother's sister was diagnosed with breast cancer. My mother never explained my aunt's prognosis and whether or not she would survive. It was the first time I recall even hearing the word "cancer," something people whispered with frightened expressions on their faces due to its gravely serious implications.

They might as well have been uttering the words "leprosy" or "bubonic plague," given the bleak tone of voice and lack of faith in recovery that accompanied any discussion of a cancer diagnosis. Back then, people regarded such news as an inevitable "death warrant."

Fortunately today, we have the ability to research anything – from medical information to family genealogy – on the Internet. Back then it just wasn't the same. If the information about the importance and mechanics of an effective self-breast exam was out there, we never heard about it.

Following high school graduation in 1972, I attended the University of Miami. Many teenagers find college to be stressful and I was certainly no exception. While in school I worked as both a cashier and an aerobics instructor. I went disco-dancing every weekend and had lots of friends. The 1970s was a carefree decade; bell-bottom pants were popular and I had them in many colors.

My hair was very long, straight, and parted in the middle. Whenever I look at pictures from that time period, I wonder what I was thinking; guess every generation goes through the experience of loving their particular style during its heyday only to realize its ridiculousness decades later.

At the age of twenty-four, I accepted a position as a staff associate at the University of Miami's Surgical Oncology Department, working for a cancer surgeon. As you might imagine, this was an incredibly stressful job; there were days I didn't even want to come to work.

What was the hardest part of it for me?

Having to tell a woman I needed to schedule a biopsy for her because her mammogram revealed a suspicious lesion. Hearing the distinctive fear in their voices when they asked about what to expect was more than I could handle. Some days I'd return home mentally exhausted.

During the time I worked with breast cancer patients, I began dating a gentleman who in the beginning was wonderful. He'd been previously married and the father of two children – a boy and a girl. We'd been together a year when I discovered I was pregnant. In the beginning, we were both happy about it, but when I started having difficulty carrying the baby, things changed dramatically. Unfortunately I miscarried, which was very traumatic. Not long after, we broke up and he went back to his ex-wife. Thank God I had family and friends to support me emotionally.

After my miscarriage, I asked my physician about its cause. Why did it happen? Was it something I did? He advised me I had an abnormal uterus – possibly because my mother had taken the drug DES while pregnant with me. This drug was used back in the 1950s to prevent miscarriage; today we know it has caused all kinds of abnormalities in the female offspring of the women who took it. These include: improper development of the uterus, pre-term pregnancy and increased risk of miscarriage, cancer of the cervix, and possibly an increase in the risk of breast cancer. As I recall, there was a class-action lawsuit brought against the pharmaceutical company, which my mother and I were unaware of at the time, regrettably.

Though it wasn't easy, I finally recovered medically and

emotionally from the loss of my child and moved on with my life. To this day I wonder what it would be like to have a son or daughter of my own. In spite of the fact that I sought out short-term therapy to work through these challenges, ultimately I had to help myself come to terms with losing my baby.

After twelve years of working with breast cancer patients, I was burned out and decided to make a change. After interviewing for an administrative assistant position at the University of Miami Psychological Services Center, I got the job.

Over lunch the next day, I discussed this career change with a trusted friend. As bad as I felt about the new job, I felt even worse when the topic of conversation shifted to relationships. Since breaking up with my boyfriend I'd remained single, although I enjoyed going out with my friends and going out on an occasional date when my scheduled allowed. In response, my friend encouraged me to go to a dating service with her, claiming that many professional people employed them and we should give it a try. Reluctantly, I tagged along but sat outside the office waiting for her because I was not going to pay money for a date; not only did I believe it was ridiculous, I was afraid I'd meet a weirdo!

While I sat there, an elderly woman who worked for the agency approached me and suggested I take a look at some of the resumes of the gentlemen who were interested in meeting professional women. She enticed me with the $30 special they were running that week. Well, hey, who can pass up a bargain like that! To this very day, I joke that I met my husband John at a special sale at a dating service, paying a whopping thirty dollars for him!

John and I fell in love instantly. We'd only been dating three months when he asked me to marry him. We'd met in June of 1987 and married in June of 1988. And what a beautiful wedding we had! I remember walking down the aisle as nervous as can be, with my father by my side and the smell of flowers filling the church. That day was one I'll never forget.

After the wedding it was back to reality. I returned to work at the university and John went back to his teaching position at our local high school.

Right after we celebrated our first wedding anniversary, another tragedy befell my family when my dad was diagnosed with pancreatic cancer. He passed away in June of 1990 – just two years after he'd walked me down the aisle. They say losing a child is bad but losing my father was worse for me. He was a wonderful man and I'd never met anyone who didn't like him. I know he would have been proud of me today to have successfully navigated through so many tough times.

Whenever I go in for testing I think of my dad and all of the pain and suffering he endured before his death. It was almost midnight on a hot June evening. I was with him when he drew his last breath and I remember it like it was yesterday. The days following his death were unbearable. Unsurprisingly, the funeral was packed with family and friends, thanks to Dad's gregarious nature. My father loved people and would talk to anyone who would listen – a quality I definitely share. He used to say if the wall could talk to me, I'd carry on a conversation with it!

In July of 2000 I was diagnosed with breast cancer, which changed my life forever. At 46 years-old, I was close to the age of my mother's sister when she was diagnosed, and just ten years older than my Aunt Angie, my father's sister, when she passed away at 36 years-old.

Aunt Angie had been suffering from depression since losing her husband Eddie to a heart attack on their front lawn. It's quite possible she'd had the lump for a long time prior to having it checked out. Less than a year after her diagnosis, she died of breast cancer. Did she ever examine her own breasts? I don't know. All I know is she was a truly wonderful woman.

My mother's sister Mary was diagnosed with breast cancer in the mid-1970s, although I never knew what stage she had. I was aware she had her entire breast removed and did not undergo chemotherapy. After 13 years, her cancer returned. Aunt Mary received excellent care at Memorial Sloan Kettering Cancer Center. At that time they treated her cancer with a drug called Megase. Today, we use Tamoxifen or other drugs known as Rolaxifen and Femara.

In the late 1990s, Aunt Mary was diagnosed with bone cancer. She was treated here in Miami with radiation therapy, which made her very sick. Eventually breast cancer took Aunt Mary away from us in 2005.

Because I had a family history of breast cancer and had seen countless women diagnosed with the disease, I was vigilant about getting mammograms and performing self-breast examinations. But a month before the mammogram that would change my life, my mother was diagnosed with cervical cancer – the result of having taken the drug DES. Since I wanted to be there for her, I delayed my mammogram one month, never dreaming I would be diagnosed with breast cancer.

I went to my appointment that day free of worry and anxiety; I'd been previously diagnosed ten years earlier with "fibrocystic changes" – a benign condition – but there was never any indication of cancer. As I sat in the waiting room in my gown, I noticed a young woman who looked very sad and wondered if she'd received bad news. Did she need a biopsy? Worse, had she gotten a breast cancer diagnosis? I began to feel nervous and uncomfortable.

Just as I was about to start a conversation with her, I was called in for the mammogram. After inquiring if I'd removed all my jewelry, the technician instructed me to remove the left side of my gown so she could place my left breast onto the mammogram machine.

At that moment a strange feeling overpowered me: I thought of the woman in the waiting room and suddenly my eyes began to fill with tears. The technician just advised me to hold my breath as she took the first picture of my left breast. She then turned me sideways so she could reposition the machine and before I knew it – wham! She lowered the machine onto my breast, igniting excruciating pain and making me wonder if a man invented this contraption.

As she conducted the same procedure on my right breast, I couldn't wait until it was over. I wasn't sure why, because normally I'd always been relaxed during mammograms. When it was over, the tech informed me that the radiologist, Dr. Bernard Beber, wanted to perform an ultrasound on my right breast for comparison with my mammogram the year before.

Fear shot through me as I silently prayed, "Please God, do not let me have breast cancer."

After the ultrasound, Dr. Beber advised me I needed a stereotactic biopsy of my left breast because he'd seen suspicious microcalcifications, which look like tiny white spots on a mammogram. That's when I knew my life was about to take a dramatic turn, one that would alter it forever; I was now the woman in the waiting room looking scared and worried. The stereotactic procedure was scheduled for the following week with a surgical oncologist, Dr. Fred Moffat and Dr. Bernard Beber at the University of Miami Sylvester Comprehensive Cancer Center. I had faith in both because I'd been in their care for many years.

During a stereotactic biopsy, the patient lies face-down on a table where there is a cut-out hole through which the breast hangs. What a feeling that was, to be lying down with my breast hanging through a hole and looking directly at my physician underneath!

The radiologist and the surgeon then attempt to numb the site of the suspicious lump or calcifications with lidocaine. Once the numbness sets in, a very small needle is quickly inserted and removed, extracting a tissue sample that's then sent to pathology for diagnosis. Sometimes it can take a bit more lidocaine than anticipated to fully numb the breast area. I needed four shots; nothing comes easy for me.

Several days later, my surgeon called with the news that the pathology report came back with the diagnosis of left-breast cancer. Because I had worked for a professor who had diagnosed many women with breast cancer, I knew only too well what I was in for.

Although I knew there were four stages of breast cancer, I had no idea which one applied to me. I have never felt so scared and alone as I did that day. I even flashed back to decades before when I was a 12 year-old putting on my first training bra and complaining to my mother it was too tight to wear. I informed her I *hated* having breasts. Had I known I might lose them one day, I would never have uttered such words.

How was I going to tell my husband? How was I going to tell my mother who was still recuperating from her own surgery?

Somehow I found the strength to break the news to both of them. At the time I wasn't sure what was running through my husband John's mind, but since then he's been supportive.

Having worked with breast cancer patients, I'd seen men leave their wives because they simply couldn't deal with the diagnosis and all of its ramifications. I recall one young patient in her mid-20s who was diagnosed with cancer in both breasts. On top of that, she was also pregnant. Sadly, her cancer was so aggressive (as it typically is in young women) she needed chemotherapy to shrink the large tumors in her breasts, followed by radiation therapy, then inevitably a bilateral mastectomy: the removal of both breasts. She also had to terminate her pregnancy. I will never forget that case, nor will I ever forget my shock at her young age. I wondered if she'd ever examined her breasts.

All of this was running through my head at the time of my own diagnosis. Typically calm, my husband John doesn't show much emotion. But when we got home from my first surgery – a lumpectomy – his first words were, "Just because your breast may need to be removed does not mean I will ever stop loving you." These were the most beautiful words I could have ever heard during a time when so many unsettling thoughts were running through my mind.

Two days later, after surgery, my doctor called with more bad news: the pathology report indicated I had no clear margins, which meant there was still more cancer in the remaining portion of my breast. Therefore, I had to go back to have the rest of my breast removed.

It took a while to process this news. The night before my surgery, I stood under the running water in the shower and realized this would be the last time I'd see my left breast. I gazed at it closely, wishing there was some way to take a mold of it to remember how it once looked.

The next week I was admitted for a left, modified radical mastectomy, which means the entire breast including the nipple is removed. The surgeon also removed the lymph nodes under my arm and sent them to pathology to find out if any cancer had spread to a node. Thankfully, the pathology report came back negative, confirming my nodes were free of cancer. Upon awakening after surgery, my chest felt extremely heavy. Though still groggy, I could hear the people talking around me. I was hooked up to an I.V. that contained morphine to control the pain; a cuff on each of my thighs similar to a blood pressure cuff; and a separate I.V. filled with antibiotics.

My final diagnosis was a Stage I, left multifocal (meaning more than one tumor) invasive breast cancer measuring 1.5 cm by 0.7 by 0.5 cm with 19 negative lymph nodes. Although I felt relieved that the cancer hadn't spread, knowing it was a multifocal, invasive breast cancer instilled even more anxiety and concern. Yes, my tumor was under 2 cm, but having three separate invasive ones filled me with dread.

Then there was the nagging question in spite of the fact that no lymph nodes were involved: *Had the surgeon gotten all of the cancer?*

Yet at the same time I knew that excessive worrying about something over which I had no control would only impede my recovery. Once the surgery was over and I was home convalescing, the surgeon informed me I needed to see an oncologist to determine the best course of treatment. Just what I wanted to do – make more vitally important decisions!

When I saw the oncologist the following week, she was very kind and informative, taking the time to discuss all of the different types of treatments. I could either take chemotherapy alone or accompanied by a drug called Tamoxifen, which is a hormonal treatment of choice for menopausal women. It's also an option for post-menopausal women even though it's not quite as effective for them.

If I decided to take chemotherapy with the Tamoxifen, my risk of recurrence in my opposite (right) breast would be 40 percent. I now had to face more life-altering choices.

When I left the oncologist's office with my husband, I was very depressed. I definitely did not want to take chemotherapy: I feared putting what I call the "toxic cocktail" into my body. One side effect of chemotherapy is hair loss, in addition to possible harm to internal body organs including my heart. Chemotherapy kills the good cells in the body as well as the bad. Pondering the choices my oncologist had written down just added to my distress. And no one could help me because I needed to make the decision on my own. Generally I am a very organized person, always in control of everything I do, but now I found myself in a position of having to make all of these important decisions; I was afraid I'd make the wrong one.

The next week I called my oncologist with the news that I'd decided to take the Tamoxifen treatment. Since I'd had no lymph node involvement and would possibly be having my right breast removed, I felt comfortable with this decision. The Tamoxifen protocol is five years, which I completed until cancer-free.

Approximately one year after I'd had my bilateral mastectomy I began keeping a journal in which I chronicled my thoughts and emotions. Not long after that, I was invited to speak to psychology classes at the University of Miami, where I shared my journey with breast cancer with the undergraduate students. Needless to say, these experiences were very emotional and oftentimes characterized by me struggling to hold back tears. However, I knew I had to be strong to achieve my goal of educating other young women and men about breast cancer.

During my very first lecture, I was genuinely surprised that many students didn't know much about breast cancer aside from the fact it took the lives of many women and some men every year. Yet I was gratified that they demonstrated real interest in the topic, as evidenced by their many questions and sincere attention.

From the moment I began speaking, I noticed the attentiveness on their faces; realizing they truly wanted to learn about breast cancer put me at ease as I discussed the importance of self- breast examination, awareness, and early detection in achieving a timely diagnosis and cure. I encouraged them to be proactive; if they felt something was wrong with their body to tell someone immediately.

Then I got personal, sharing the story of the loss of my child at age thirty-three, the loss of my father when I was thirty-six, and finally my third loss – the loss of my breasts at age forty-six. Upon hearing about my decision to have my right breast removed to avoid a future recurrence, the students' facial expressions were pure shock.

Days after that first lecture, many students sent emails telling me how much they enjoyed my talk and commending me for my bravery. What they didn't know was that I was petrified of keeping my opposite breast and risking a cancer recurrence, which was the ultimate motivation for having it removed. While it was difficult to arrive at such an aggressive decision, I felt more comfortable not having to live in constant fear of the cancer returning.

Soon after I completed my lectures at the University of Miami, my husband John invited me to speak to his eleventh and twelfth grade high school psychology class. I thought about it for some time before agreeing, remembering how as a teenager I believed nothing bad could happen to me – a typical attitude at that stage of life. Would these kids be able to relate to my breast cancer experience?

Despite my misgivings and a bad case of nerves on the day of the lecture, it turned out these students truly wanted to hear what I had to say. From the moment I began speaking, I was thrilled by the way in which they opened up to me. In fact, they inspired me to talk for an entire hour, sharing everything from how it felt to have a mammogram, to having a biopsy, to enduring a mastectomy.

After the lecture, one young girl approached me with questions she'd been too embarrassed to ask in front of the class. She confided that she couldn't even speak with her mother about breast cancer – something I could certainly understand. As a teen, I was also too embarrassed to discuss such sensitive topics with my mom, preferring to talk to my friends instead. Of course, they knew as much as I did about breast cancer: nothing.

After speaking at my husband's school and realizing how little these young people knew about breast cancer, I made the commitment to developing and communicating understandable and accurate information to better educate high school and college co-eds. While anyone who's been diagnosed with breast cancer can write their own story, I wanted mine to be different. That's why I kept researching and speaking in schools throughout Miami-Dade County. I wanted to discover what the students wanted to know. Along the way, I found it very interesting that in spite of the many websites dedicated to educating students about breast cancer, none of these students actually read them. I suppose school activities, sports, dating, and having fun were greater priorities, unless a student had a family member or friend with breast cancer. Thanks to over six years of lecturing, I'd discovered that students had many questions about mammograms, biopsies, the emotions involved when one is first diagnosed, the feeling of having no breasts, the process by which I made the decision to undergo breast reconstruction, and most importantly, how to examine their own breasts.

These efforts led to the publication of my first book, *The Empty Cup Runneth Over*, where I shared my personal history and interviews with several University of Miami cancer specialists who explained in detail important things like digital mammograms, biopsies, breast reconstruction, psychological ramifications of breast cancer diagnosis, chemotherapy, radiation therapy, pain therapy, the importance of nutrition, nipple tattooing, and lymphedema (swelling of the arm after the removal of lymph nodes). The book also included heart-warming stories of young women who'd been diagnosed in their early 20s.

Now my follow-up, *Miami Breast Cancer Experts*, picks up where *The Empty Cup Runneth Over* left off to bring readers up-to-date information on the latest technology and procedures employed in the battle against breast cancer. Just as with my first book, it is filled with important, accurate information written by medical doctors, nurses, psychologists, and a nutritionist. It also includes poignant, real-life stories from survivors. There are even holistic chapters on topics like thermography, yoga, and meditation in an effort to take a mind-body-soul approach to breast cancer.

Once again, my partner in this venture is Sabrina Hernandez-Cano, a licensed, registered dietician and a founder of the Hummingwell Wellness Bar. Currently in private practice, Sabrina has seen many patients with a myriad of health problems including breast cancer, diabetes, and obesity. She'll share her expertise on healthy lifestyles (diet and exercise) and medical nutrition therapy – along with several delicious recipes she's created.

With this new book, Sabrina and I worked hard to provide readers with easy-to-understand chapters – many of which are interspersed with humor – on every aspect of breast cancer. Like its predecessor, *The Empty Cup Runneth Over*, we know you'll find it informative but more than anything, we hope it will inspire you to get to know your body and become proactive about your health.

UPDATE – 2015

Fifteen years have passed since my breast cancer diagnosis. So much has happened in that time span: I went from retiring at the University of Miami School of Medicine, an institution I worked at for 27 years, to starting a new job for a plastic surgeon on Key Biscayne, Florida. During that time I got divorced and had to learn how to be single again. After having had breast cancer and losing both breasts that was not an easy task.

The last chapter in my other book, *The Empty Cup Runneth Over* was written in front of a Dade County Florida Court House as I was getting ready to file for divorce. Now I'm writing this chapter for Miami Breast Cancer Experts in front of a court house, but this time for an entirely different reason: I'm remarrying my lover, my ex-husband John. Who'd have thought that after 20 years of marriage and seven years of being divorced that we'd be marrying each other again?

Although some of my friends were shocked, most of them reacted with the comment, "It's about time." During our divorce,

John and I actually lived together. Yes, you read this right: we lived together as roommates for seven years before deciding to remarry. It was a very interesting set-up; I received alimony while we split the rent!

Over the past eight years I have met amazing people, joined a few organizations to help other breast cancer survivors, lost my younger brother Mike to colon cancer, and am now helping my mother Lena, who was recently diagnosed with Stage IIIB breast cancer at the age of 86. Needless to say, I not only have a lot of cancer in my family but hate the word "cancer" as much as ever.

In July of 2010, one month after my brother Mike passed away, I retired from the University of Miami Medical School and began to work for Dr. Roger Khouri at the Miami Breast Center on Key Biscayne, Florida. Everything around me was changing so quickly. A friend of mine told me a plastic surgeon she knew was looking for someone to hire in his practice.Dr. Roger Khouri is a renowned plastic surgeon who developed a technique to create a breast for women after a mastectomy, or even a lumpectomy by filling in areas using the Brava System prior to performing a fat transfer. The Brava is an external expander that helps create internal space to enable the fat transfer to survive (see www.miamibreastcancer.com). Dr. Roger Khouri has given many breast cancer survivors hope. While we know we'll never have the breasts we had prior to mastectomy, thanks to Dr. Khouri's technique we come pretty darn close. His book, *Your Natural Breasts* features many before and after photographs in addition to testimonials from other patients. Learn more about this remarkable doctor/medical pioneer and purchase his book at his website, www.miamibreastcancer.com. In this book, we've also included a detailed chapter on the BRAVA System and fat grafting.

After working for Dr. Khouri for five years, I decided it was my turn to have the saline implants I'd had for eight years removed and a fat transfer performed. I went for an MRI of my breasts, which confirmed that one of my implants was contracted – thus explaining why I'd been experiencing pain for several months. Many patients who receive implants are never told that they do not last forever or could rupture or contract, as mine had done. In February of 2013, I was taken into the operating room – camera crew and all – to have my implants removed and replaced with my own body fat. The post-surgery results are amazing and I am happy to have had the procedure performed. Since I went from a size four/five to a size two, I can tell you that liposuction is a nice bonus to this kind of operation!

Over these past eight years, I also developed a good friendship with Patricia San Pedro. Patricia is full of love; everyone she comes into contact with feels special after meeting her. She invited me to join "The Link of Hope Sistas," a group she created on Facebook. These amazing women support each other no matter where they are in their breast cancer journey; some are undergoing treatment and reconstruction, while others are several years out like me. Many of the women are from all over the world. The South Florida locals gather together over lunch every three to four months to catch up on our lives. If you're on Facebook, we encourage you to visit and join us if you would like.

Patricia and I are currently in the process of writing a movie script with a producer in Manhattan; we're hoping to take our audience on a roller coaster ride through this film.

I am now happily married and living with John Hammontree in South Florida, where I will continue to educate and inspire other survivors. You can find me on Facebook as Cindy Papale, on twitter @CindyPapale, and of course, working for Dr. Roger Khouri at the Miami Breast Center on Key Biscayne, Florida at (305) 365-5595.

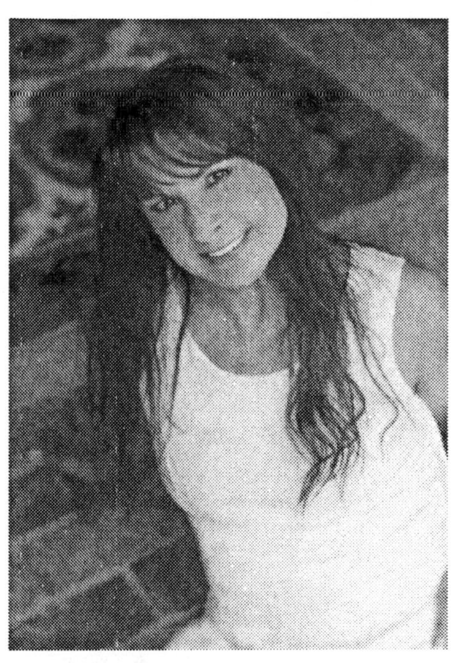

BIOGRAPHY

Cindy Papale joined the team at the Miami Breast Center as an Administrative Assistant in July of 2010. A Long Island New York native, she moved to Miami Florida in 1972, where she received a Bachelor's Degree in Business from the University of Miami. In her 27 years of working with breast cancer patients at the University of Miami School of Medicine, she's written many grants for breast cancer research. Cindy's boundless passion for helping other breast cancer survivors became even more pronounced in the aftermath of her own diagnosis and subsequent treatment in July of 2000.

In 2008, she released her first book, The Empty Cup Runneth Over (www.theemptycuprunnethover.com). She has appeared on Channel 6 South Florida Today Show and her survivor story has made the front pages of every local newspaper in Miami-Dade, Broward, and Palm each Counties. Cindy is also in the process of collaborating with Peabody Award-winning Producer Derek Britt on a feature film inspired her breast cancer journey.

This indefatigable women's champion wears many hats at the Miami Breast Center – from making appointments to coordinating surgeries – as part of her lifelong commitment to helping breast cancer patients live life to the fullest. Find her on Facebook as Cindy Papale, follow her on twitter @CindyPapale, and contact her at the Miami Breast Center at (305) 365-5595.

CHAPTER 2

MRI, Mammography, and Ultrasound

Paul Peter Slawek, M.D., J.D.

Approximately 1 in 8 women in the United States (about 12%) will develop invasive breast cancer over the course of her lifetime. What is the best protection?

Assume you are a target, become knowledgeable about the disease, and ensure that if you find a lump, you will detect the cancer at the very earliest possible moment. Early diagnosis and excellent treatment usually convert a breast cancer patient into a **"breast cancer survivor!"**

Each year, 235,000 women in the US develop invasive breast cancer and approximately 63,000 develop non-invasive breast cancer Ductal Carcinoma In-situ (DCIS). Forty thousand women die each year in the US from breast cancer. Approximately 2,360 new cases of invasive breast cancer were expected to be diagnosed in men in 2014. A woman's lifetime risk is approximately 1 in 8, or 12.4 percent.

The strongest risk factor for breast cancer is age. A woman's risk of developing this disease increases as she gets older.

Other factors that can also increase a woman's risk of developing breast cancer include:

- Inherited changes in certain genes
- Personal or family history of breast cancer
- Having dense breasts
- Starting menstruation before age 12
- Starting menopause after age 55
- Having a first full-term pregnancy after age 30
- Never having been pregnant
- Obesity after menopause

A man's lifetime risk of developing breast cancer is approximately 1 in 1,000, or 0.1 percent.

The prospects of developing breast cancer are fearful to women and their loved ones. Many see the development of breast cancer as – perhaps more than most other cancers – a life changer. This perception is partially true and partially false. The 5-year survival rate for early-diagnosed, localized breast cancer is 98%. Unfortunately, approximately 40,000 women in the US were expected to die in 2014 from breast cancer, though death rates have been decreasing since 1989—with larger decreases in women under 50. These decreases are thought to be the result of treatment advances, earlier detection through screening, and increased awareness.[1]

I must add that some in the medical profession question the true significance of 5-year survival with respect to breast cancer, which has a long natural course. We know that survival at five years consists of three groups: cured, in remission, and those with known cancer being sustained by treatment.

Surely if we had a choice, we'd opt for not having to deal with breast cancer at all but unfortunately, many of us will have to, one way or another. Some of us will be patients and others will be the

---

BREASTCANCER.ORG

family and loved ones of a breast cancer patient. Approximately 1 in 8 US women (about 12%) will develop invasive breast cancer over the course of her lifetime.

Regrettably, the occurrence of breast cancer has not responded well to the advances of modern medicine. Unlike many other forms of cancer, there are few, if any, strategies one can use to reduce the risk of developing breast cancer. For example, lung cancer occurrences have responded well to the avoidance of smoking; skin cancer occurrences have responded well to the reduction of sun exposure; and colon cancer occurrences have responded well to colonoscopy and the treatment of precancerous polyps. However, breast cancer occurrences have not responded in any significant way to lifestyle modifications.

For the most part, breast cancer occurs spontaneously, independent of lifestyle or other factors. One exception, however, has been observed. Breast cancer incidence rates in the US began decreasing mildly in the year 2000, after increasing for the previous two decades. Breast cancer occurrences dropped in 2002 to 2003. One theory is that this decrease was partially due to the reduced use of hormone replacement therapy (HRT) by women after the results of a large study, called the Women's Health Initiative, were published in 2002. These results suggested a connection between HRT and increased risk for developing breast cancer.

Other than HRT, our success with breast cancer has been primarily in early detection and better treatment, which are resulting in increased survival.

The efforts to decrease the development of new cases of breast cancer, however, have been met with little success.

A special case would be women with the genetic predisposition to develop breast cancer: BRCA1 and BRCA2 genes. Genetic counseling is advised for women who possess these genes. In appropriate circumstances, some women are electing to undergo prophylactic bilateral mastectomies.

We should all assume that we are potential victims of breast cancer and if afflicted, are determined to become breast cancer survivors. Learn the nature of this beast and commit to **EARLY DETECTION AND BEST TREATMENT**.

Knowledge of breast cancer allows you to take control and ensure that you receive the very best in early detection and treatment. Leave nothing to chance or good luck. Listen to your doctor, but be your own advocate.

EARLY DETECTION

All things considered, the detection of early small breast cancer saves lives. Smaller lesions are more likely to be successfully treated. Early lesions are less likely to spread to other areas of the body (metastasis).

When breast cancer is detected early in the localized stage, the 5-year survival rate is 98%[2]. Because early detection of breast cancer is so important, the National Breast Cancer Foundation and other organizations offer an online service that reminds women to perform a Self-Examination, and to undergo a Clinical Examination and a Screening Mammogram (www.earlydetectionplan.org).

BREAST SELF-AWARENESS

This term has replaced the older concept of "Breast Self-examination." Forty percent of all breast cancers are found by women themselves by feeling a lump. Adult women were, in the past, advised to conduct self-examinations of their breasts once a month. The "Breast Self-Awareness" concept proposes that a woman should get to know what is normal for her breasts and watch for any change from this "normal." **No time interval is associated with the concept of Breast Self-Awareness.** If a lump, area of hardness, skin thickening, redness, or tenderness is encountered, the woman MUST consult her physician. Breast nipple discharge should be further examined by a physician. A skin rash or crusting at the nipple can be a sign of breast cancer. An inversion of a nipple that develops can indicate a developing breast

[2] National Cancer Institute

cancer. A woman should be aware ON A DAILY BASIS of any change from her "normal."

CLINICAL BREAST EXAMINATION

A breast examination performed by a qualified nurse or physician. Most agree that women 40 years of age and older should have an annual clinical breast examination. It does no harm, but the effectiveness of the examination is being questioned by some. False-positive screening results are higher with Screening Mammography plus Clinical Breast Examination than with Screening Mammography alone.

SCREENING MAMMOGRAPHY

This type of mammography is generally performed annually or biannually. Opinions vary as to frequency of screening mammography because the downside of the study is radiation exposure. Radiation itself causes cancer. I decide for my patients based upon several factors, but primarily risk of neoplasm. It is clear that some women with low risk and fatty breasts can get by safely with biannual mammography. I utilize the Gail Risk protocol.

The Gail Model is a scientifically-published, nationally-accepted standard for evaluating your relative risk of developing breast cancer based on your family history. However, using the Gail Risk Model is complicated by such things as BRCA1 or BRCA2 genes.

Several other factors may also affect risk, but are not accounted for by the Gail tool. These factors include previous radiation therapy to the chest for the treatment of Hodgkin lymphoma or recent migration from a region with low breast cancer rates, such as rural China. The tool's risk calculations assume that a woman is screened for breast cancer as in the general US population. A woman who does not have mammograms will have somewhat lower chances of a diagnosis of breast cancer.

GAIL RISK PROTOCOL

1. 1. Do you have a medical history of any breast cancer or of ductal carcinoma in situ (DCIS) or lobular carcinoma in situ (LCIS)?
2. What is your age?
3. What was your age at the time of your first menstrual period?
4. What was your age at the time of your first live birth of a child?
5. How many of your first-degree relatives (mother, sisters, daughters) have had breast cancer?
6. Have you ever had a breast biopsy?
7. What is your race/ethnicity?

(From Univ. of Virginia Health Services)

THE NATIONAL CANCER INSTITUTE HAS A SIMILAR RISK ASSESSMENT PROTOCOL

1. Does the woman have a history of breast cancer, DCIS or LCIS? Has woman received radiation to chest for treatment of lymphoma?
2. Does woman have a mutation in either BRCA1 or BRCA2 gene?
3. Woman's age?
4. Woman's age at first menstrual period?
5. Woman's age at her first live birth?
6. Number of close relatives with history of breast cancer?
7. Number of prior breast biopsies?
8. Has woman had breast biopsy showing Atypical Hyperplasia?
9. What is the woman's race/ethnicity?

The Risk Calculators give a 5-year and lifetime risk of developing breast cancer, as compared with the normal population.[3]

Prior to scheduling a Screening Mammogram, a woman should make every effort to obtain prior studies. Screening Mammography is much more accurate if the radiologist has prior studies for comparison. Most mammography centers retain your mammograms for at least five years, and some longer. Make every effort to have your prior studies when you present for your mammogram.

Screening studies are performed on women with no breast symptoms. Screening mammography does not require a doctor's order. It is advisable to have a physician's name associated with all mammography, but a woman should not avoid screening mammography because she has no prescription. If a patient has a positive finding on Self-Exam or Clinical Examination, then she should have a Diagnostic Study. Digital Mammography utilizes a computer and has, for the most part, replaced Film-Screen Mammography in the US and most other developed countries. Avoid Film-Screen Mammography in favor of Digital Mammography whenever possible. The patient's experience is the same with both techniques.[4]

Mammograms involve the use of ionizing radiation to create an X-ray image of the breast in two projections: Cranial-Caudal (CC) and Medial-Lateral-Oblique (MLO).

---

[3] There are several other Risk Calculators available.

[4] Digital mammography records the images of the breast in computer format. Film-Screen (Screen-Film) records the image on x-ray film. Digital is the state-of-the-art today.

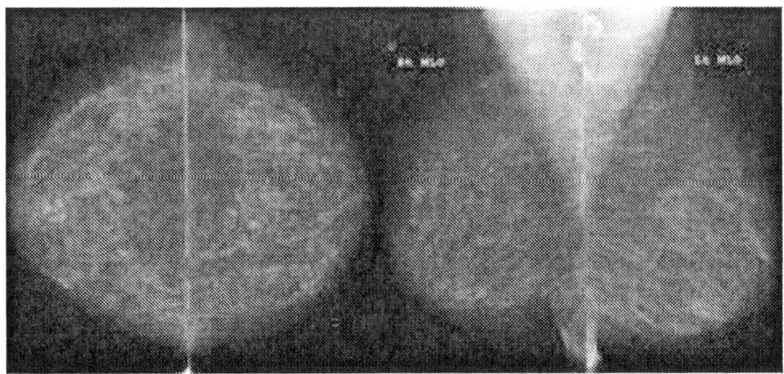

A radiologist examines the images and looks for abnormalities that may indicate breast cancer. A few of the signs of cancer include nodules, small calcifications, architectural distortion of the breast tissue, spiculation skin thickening, and nipple retraction. If an abnormality is detected, addition investigation will be ordered.

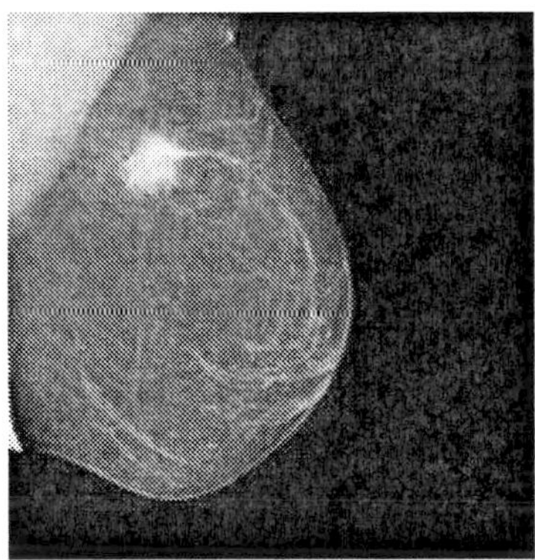

MAMMOGRAM OF BREAST CANCER IN LEFT BREAST ON LMLO VIEW

Widespread Screening Mammography has been available in the US for three decades. Over those three decades, various organizations have published guidelines for breast cancer screening (Screening Mammogram) based upon their evaluation of the available research and their understanding of the nature of breast cancer. The recommendations vary.

American College of Radiology

Over 40 years annually until life expectancy is less than 5 to 7 years.

American Cancer Society

Over 40 years annually.

U.S. Preventive Services

50 – 74 years biannually.

American College of Obstetricians and Gynecologists

Over 40 years annually.

American College of Physicians

40 to 49 years individual assessment.

Women 50 and above annually.

CAD: COMPUTER ASSISTED DIAGNOSIS

This is an assist to the radiologist in reading mammography. The computer highlights calcifications and nodules. They are marked on the images when CAD is invoked. It is not foolproof, but it does help.

BIRADS are a system of categorizing mammogram results in a uniform and easily understandable manner. They range from 1 – 6.

- BIRAD 1 Normal
- BIRAD 2 Benign
- BIRAD 3 Probably benign but short term follow-up advised.
- BIRAD 4 Suspicious findings, surgical consult and biopsy advised. (1,2,3)

- BIRAD 5 Highly suspicious, surgical consult and biopsy advised.
- BIRAD 6 Known neoplasm. Instituted appropriate therapy.

When you discuss you mammogram results with your doctor, ask questions. How dense are your breasts? What is the BIRAD Category?

How reliable is your mammogram? Would it be wise to include ultrasound in your routine screening?

Remember: if you have a palpable (able to be touched or felt) abnormality, negative mammography means very little. It is just the state of your investigation.

TOMOSYNTHESIS (3D) MAMMOGRAPHY

Good for some women, but not all. It inflicts higher radiation exposure than digital mammography.

Tomosynthesis, 3-D Mammography technology, may be an improvement over Conventional Mammography. The FDA approved it on February 11, 2011. Studies have found that adding Tomosynthesis to routine digital mammography screening of women with **dense breasts** may improve health outcomes relative to digital mammography screening alone.

Advantages of Breast Tomosynthesis include:

1. Earlier detection of breast cancers that are small and may be hidden during conventional digital mammography.
2. More accuracy in precisely locating the cancer.
3. Reduces unnecessary biopsies or additional tests.
4. Greater likelihood of detecting multiple breast tumors, which occur in 15% of breast cancer patients.
5. Better images of dense breast tissue. It allows radiologists to see through layers of tissue and see areas of concern from

multiple angles. [5]

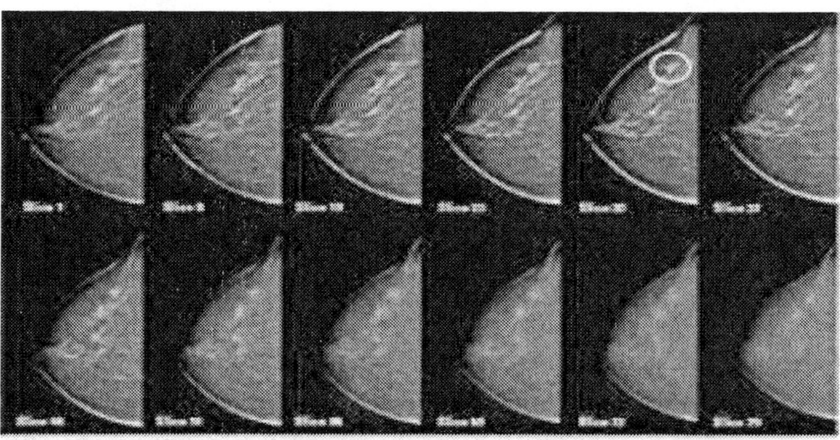

By looking at the breast slice by slice, tomosynthesis may be able to uncover hidden cancers

3D Tomosynthesis is not for everyone. If your breasts are not dense, digital mammography is just as good and delivers half the radiation exposure. It is more expensive and radiation dose is 2 Xs higher than digital mammography.

DIAGNOSTIC MAMMOGRAPHY

If a patient has a palpable nodule or other findings, the initial mammogram would be considered diagnostic, not screening.

Diagnostic Mammography would also include additional images obtained after a Screening Mammogram, requiring additional images. Usually Diagnostic is used to clarify a questionable finding on the Screening Mammogram.

Diagnostic views can be:

1. Spot Compression coned down views.
2. Magnification Spot Compression views.
3. Views of the breast from different angles.

[5] Massachusetts General Hospital (Breast Tomosynthesis)

4. Tangential views.

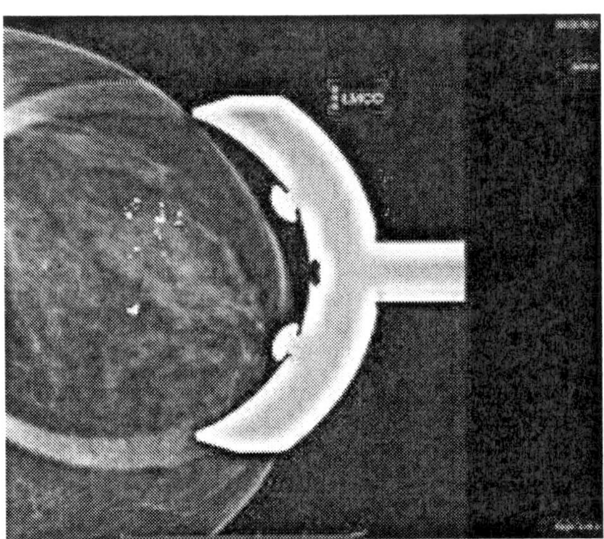

Spot Compression Diagnostic view for small calcifications

MORE ON BIRADS AND MAMMOGRAPHY REPORTING

Learn how mammography is reported. What are the BIRADS? Is your mammography a Bi-Rad 0, 1, 2, 3, 4, 5, or 6? Are your breasts dense or fatty? How does it impact upon the reliability of your mammogram? The American College of Radiology (ACR) came up with a standard way to describe mammogram findings and results. In this system, the results are sorted into categories, numbered 0 through 6. This system is called the Breast Imaging Reporting and Data System (BIRADS). Having a standard way of reporting mammogram results lets doctors use the same words and terms, which can help ensure better follow-up of suspicious findings. Here's a brief review of what the categories mean:

Results of mammography are classified according to the BIRADS.

This system is called the Breast Imaging Reporting and Data System

(BIRADS; this codification of mammography results is required by the FDA.[6]).

THE BIRADS

Category 0: Incomplete

Need additional imaging studies. This does not mean you have cancer. It only means that additional studies or views are needed to complete the evaluation. It may suggest additional mammographic views such as spot compression views, views at different angles, magnification views, ultrasound, or magnetic resonance imaging (MRI).

Category 1: Negative

There's no significant abnormality to report. The breasts look the same (they are symmetrical) with no masses (lumps), distorted structures, or suspicious calcifications. In this case, negative means nothing bad was found.

Category 2: Benign (non-cancerous) finding

This is also a negative mammogram result (there's no sign of cancer), but the reporting doctor chooses to describe a finding known to be benign, such as benign calcifications, lymph nodes in the breast, or calcified fibro adenomas. This ensures that others who look at the mammogram will not misinterpret the benign finding as suspicious. This finding is recorded in the mammogram report to help when comparing to future mammograms.

Category 3: Probably benign finding – Follow-up in a short time frame is suggested

The findings in this category have a very high chance (greater than 98%) of being benign (not cancer). The findings are not expected to change over time. But since it's not proven benign, it's

---

[6] ACR

helpful to see if the area in question does change over time. Follow-up with repeat imaging is usually done in 6 months and regularly after that until the finding is known to be stable (usually at least 2 years). This approach helps avoid unnecessary biopsies, but if the area does change over time, it still allows for early diagnosis.

Category 4: Suspicious abnormality – Biopsy should be considered

Findings do not definitely look like cancer, but could be cancer. The radiologist is concerned enough to recommend a biopsy. The findings in this category can have a wide range of suspicion levels. For this reason, some doctors divide this category further:

- **4A:** finding with a low suspicion of being cancer
- **4B**: finding with an intermediate suspicion of being cancer
- **4C**: finding of moderate concern of being cancer, but not as high as Category 5

Not all doctors use these subcategories.

Category 5: Highly suggestive of malignancy – Appropriate action should be taken. The findings look like cancer and have a high chance (at least 95%) of being cancer. Biopsy is very strongly recommended.

Category 6: Known biopsy-proven malignancy – Appropriate action should be taken.

This category is only used for findings on a mammogram that have already been shown to be cancer by a previous biopsy. Mammograms may be used in this way to see how well the cancer is responding to treatment.[7]

If your mammogram is reported to be BIRADS 0, you should comply with the suggestions for additional studies or views. If your study is

[7]From American Cancer Society.

BIRADS 1 or 2, you generally need no further studies. If your mammogram is BIRADS 3, you must return for additional imaging, such as Spot Compression Views or Ultrasound. It does not mean you have cancer. BIRADS 4 and BIRADS 5 require biopsy. This does not mean you have cancer. Approximately 25% – 30% of biopsies are positive. BIRADS 6 is only used if breast cancer has already been diagnosed.

BIRADS REPORTING FOR BREAST DENSITY

Since the density of breast tissue alters the reliability of mammography, it is now common practice to indicate the density of the breast on the mammogram report. This allows the physician to more accurately judge how much to rely upon a negative report. A negative mammogram report in very dense breast tissue may mean little. Some states now require a DENSITY CODE to be reported with all mammogram reports. Get to know the density of your breast. If your breasts are very dense, #3 or #4 diminish your reliance on mammography alone. Consider adding ultrasound or MRI to your screening program.

Mammogram reports will also include an assessment of breast density. BIRADS classifies breast density into 4 groups:

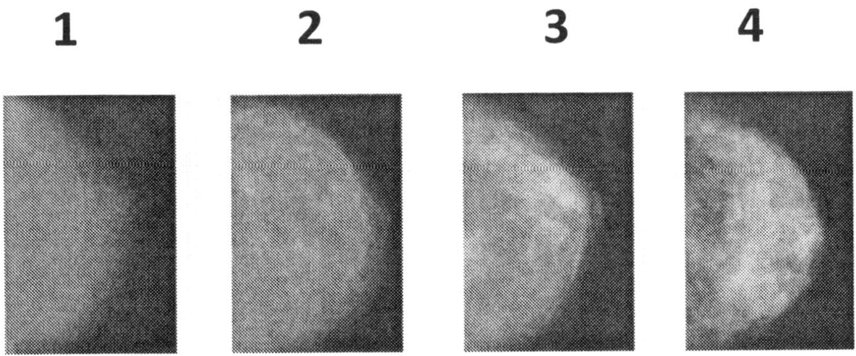

DENSITY CODE 1 - The breasts are almost entirely fatty

DENSITY CODE 2 - There are scattered areas of fibroglandular density

DENSITY CODE 3 - The breasts are heterogeneously dense, which may obscure small masses

DENSITY CODE 4 - The breasts are extremely dense, which lowers the sensitivity of mammography.

If your breasts are very dense, the reliability of mammography is reduced. It would be appropriate to discuss with your physician supplementing screening mammography with screening ultrasound or MRI.

RELIABILITY INDEX (RI)

Reliability Index is my own idea. To my knowledge, it is not used generally in mammography. I conclude all my mammogram reports with a Reliability Index from 1 - 4. Mammograms with a RI of 1 are very reliable and those with RI of 4 are very unreliable. I attempt to advise the referring physician and the patient of my assessment regarding how much reliability to place on the mammogram report.

I establish a RI by not only accessing the density of the breast, but also through several other factors. Some breasts are not so dense, but very heterogeneous in their structure, thereby reducing their reliability. Mammograms on breasts with implants would, in most cases, be reduced in reliability. Surgical changes can become a factor in establishing an RI. Prior breast reduction surgery may create changes in the breast that reduce the reliability, even though the breast may not be very dense. Multiple nodules previously assessed as benign create reduced reliability of mammography. A newly-developed nodule would easily be confused with the many benign nodules and neoplasms missed.

Reliability Code: 1. Based upon the nature of the fibroglandular elements, the reliability of this mammography is excellent.

Reliability Code: 2. Based upon the nature of the fibroglandular elements, the reliability of this mammography should be good.

Reliability Code: 3. Based upon the nature of the fibroglandular elements, the reliability of this mammography is somewhat reduced.

Reliability Code: 4. Based upon the nature of the fibroglandular elements, the sensitivity of this mammography is very significantly reduced. If questions persist clinically following mammography and ultrasound, one should resort to MRI.

ULTRASOUND (US)

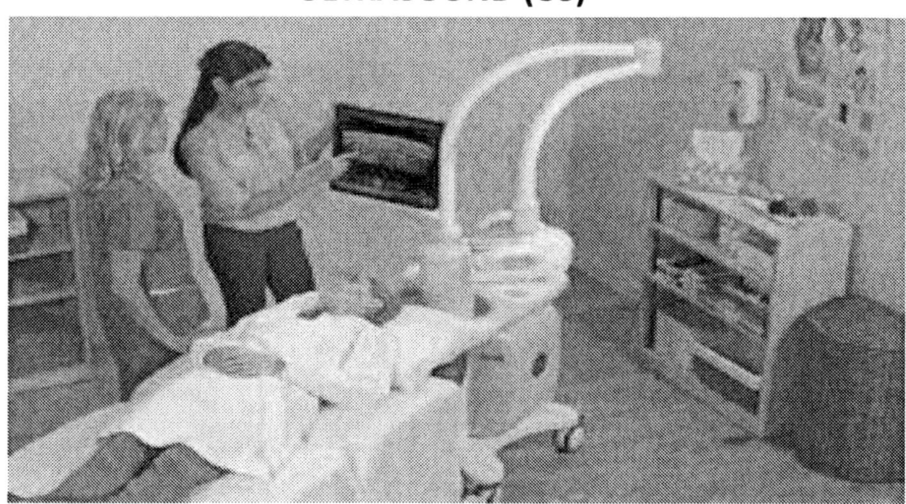

An ultrasound (US) examination of the breast involves a transducer or probe moved across the breasts by a technician looking for abnormal findings. It is not painful. Selected images are recorded for the radiologist to read. An ultrasound study is commonly performed to determine if an abnormality detected by mammography or a palpable lump is a cyst or a solid tumor (benign or malignant). Cysts are fluid-filled, whereas breast cancers are solid. Breast ultrasound may also be used to identify masses in women whose breast tissue is very dense and the sensitivity of mammography is low. Breast ultrasound does not always detect some early signs of cancer, such as micro calcifications, and is not a first-line screening procedure, like Screening Mammography.

Ultrasound may be used in some women who should avoid radiation, such as pregnant women, women younger than 25 years old, and women who are breastfeeding. The procedure may also be used to guide interventional procedures, such as breast biopsies and cyst aspiration (removal of fluid from cyst). Some doctors may order screening ultrasound with an annual mammogram, if the breasts are very dense.

The risks of breast ultrasound are few. Ultrasound emits no radiation, and, therefore, poses no risk to pregnant women and does not expose a woman to ionizing radiation. One should keep in mind that breast ultrasound may not image all small lumps that are detected with mammography. Although breast ultrasound is good, it is not a replacement for mammography, which is the gold standard.

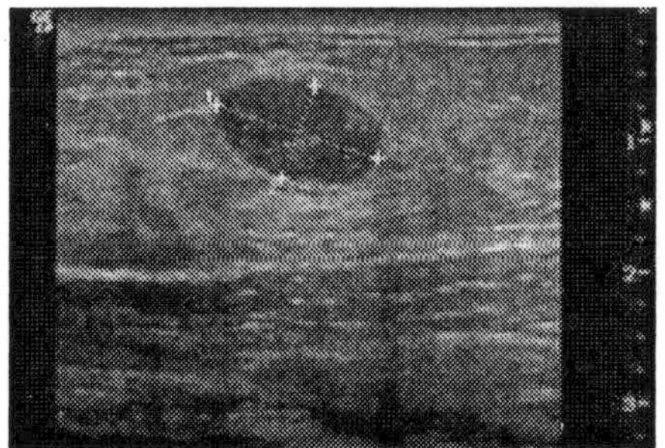

BENIGN FIBROADENOMA

BREAST CANCERS

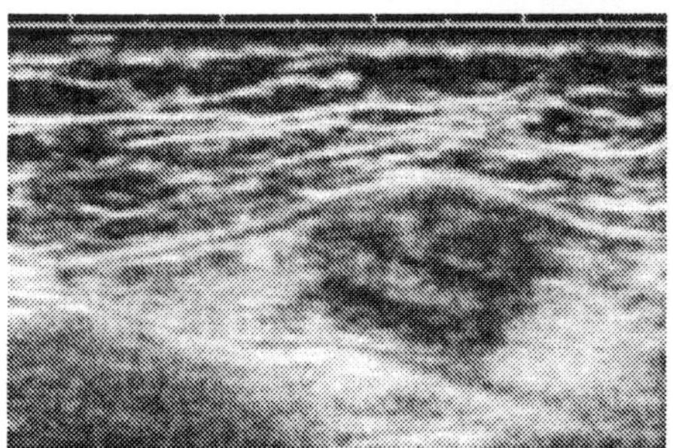

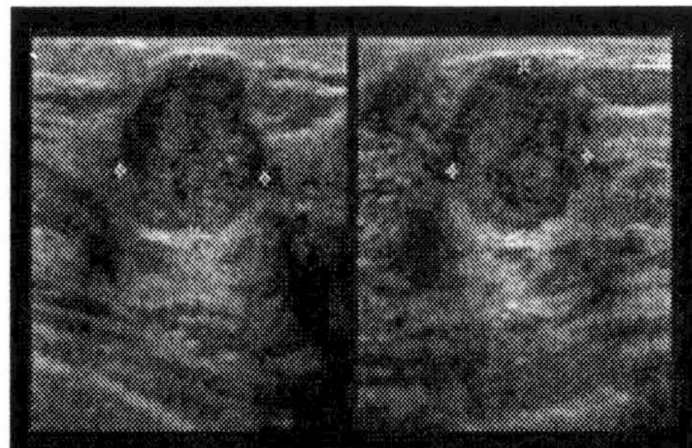

SIMPLE CYST

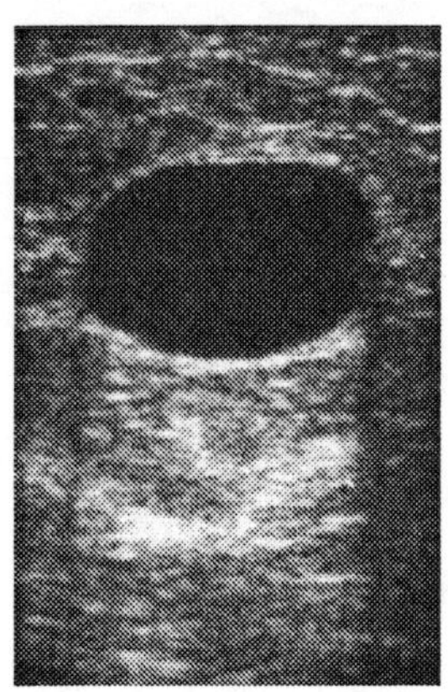

MAGNETIC RESONANCE IMAGING

BREAST MRI

Breast Magnetic Resonance Imaging (MRI) is a test that uses a large magnet, radio waves, and a computer to produce detailed images of the breast. It is the best test for breast cancer in most situations. If there are any questions after you have mammography and ultrasound you should insist upon MRI. If you have a genetic predisposition to developing breast cancer (BRCA I or II) you probably should have MRI if your breast are the least bit dense. See below for other indications for MRI of the Breasts.

The MRI machine is a large, tube-shaped machine that creates a strong magnetic field around the patient. Cross-sectional views can be obtained to reveal further details. MRI does not use radiation, mammography, or computed tomography (CT scans). There is no radiation in MRI. Radiation can provoke the development of cancer.

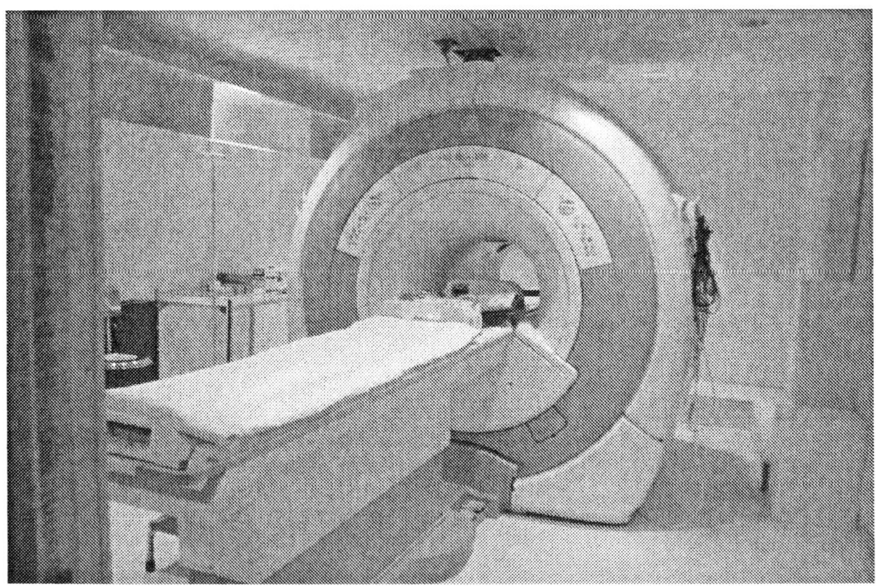

For Breast MRI, a special breast coil is utilized.

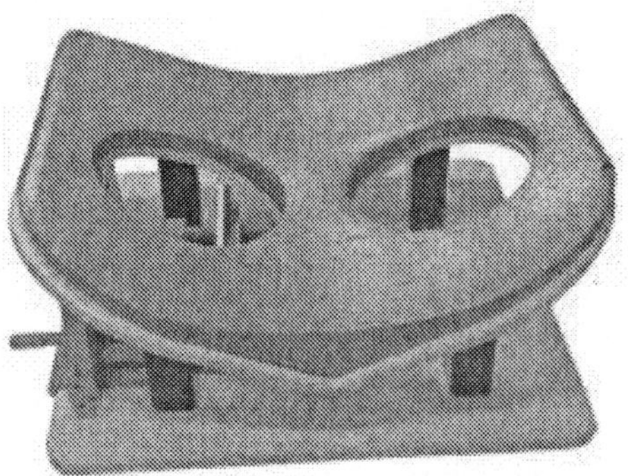

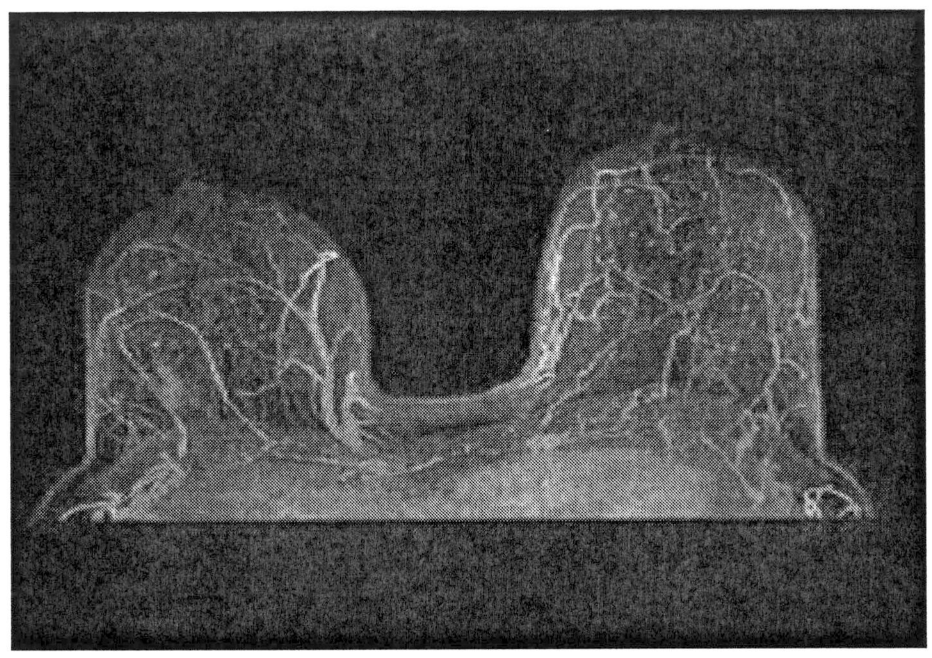

Figure 1 Normal Breast MRI

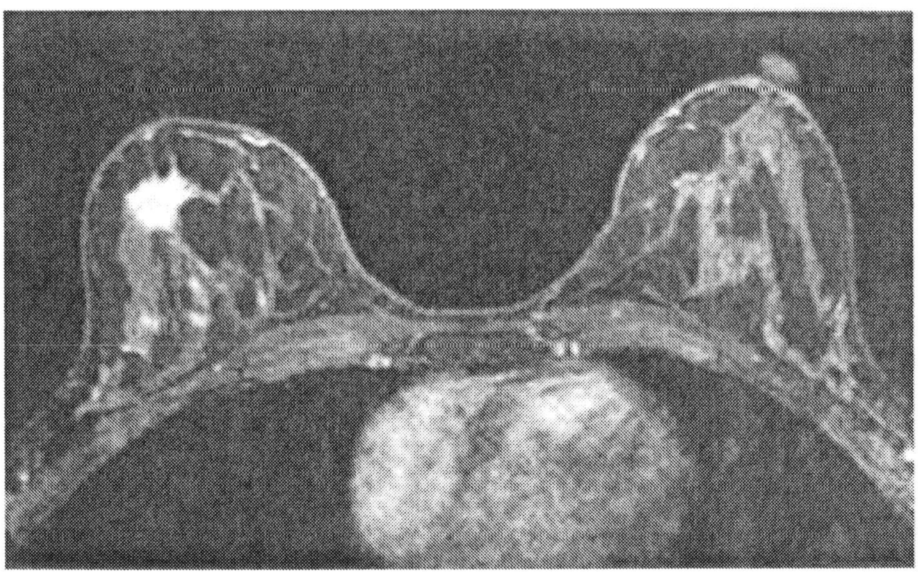

Figure 2 Right Breast Cancer MRI

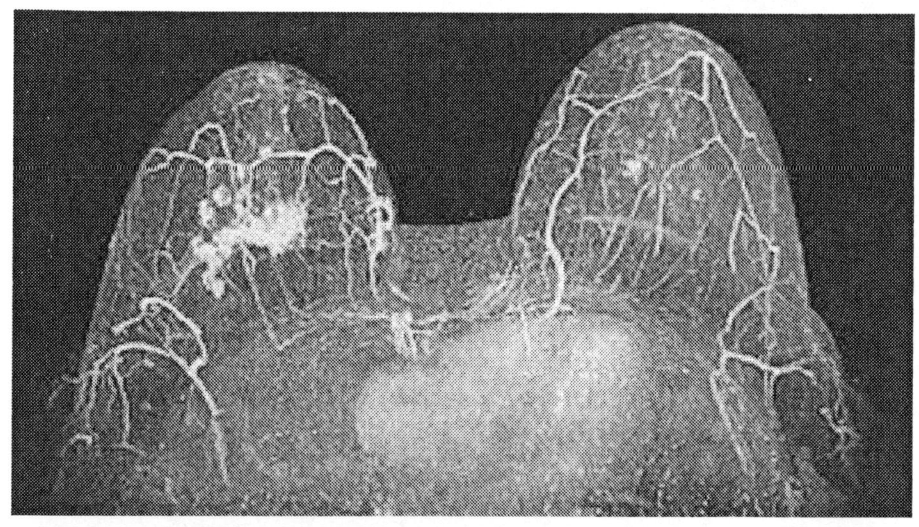

Figure 3 Right Breast Cancer MRI

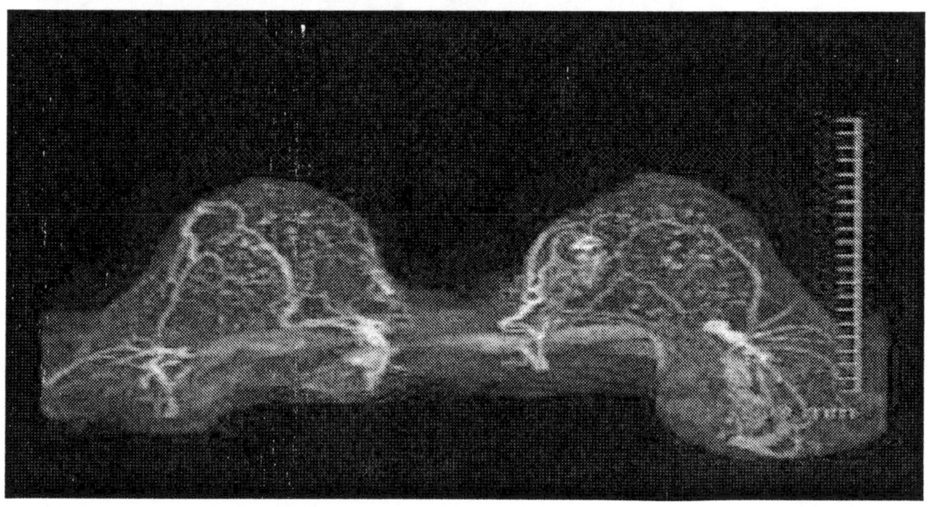

Figure 4 Normal Breast MRI

Figure 5 MRI with intramammary Lymph Nodes

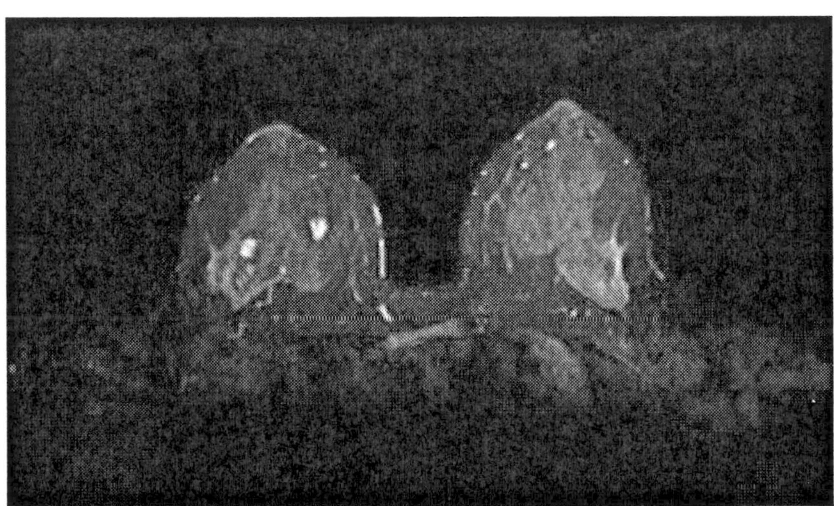

Who should get MRI of the breast? The most recent guidelines from the American Cancer Society include screening MRI with mammography for certain high-risk women. This option should be considered for the following:

•Women with BRCA1 or BRCA2 mutation (BRCA1 is a gene, which, when altered, indicates an inherited susceptibility to cancer. BRCA2 is a gene, which, when altered, indicates an inherited susceptibility to breast and/or ovarian cancer.)

•Women with a first-degree relative (mother, sister, and/or daughter) with a BRCA1 or BRCA2 mutation, if they have not yet been tested for the mutation

•Women with a 20% to 25% or greater lifetime risk of breast cancer, based on 1 of several accepted risk assessment tools that look at family history and other factors

•Women who have had radiation treatment to the chest between the ages of 10 and 30, such as for treatment of Hodgkin disease

•Women with the genetic disorders Li-Fraumeni syndrome, Cowden syndrome, or Bannayan-Riley-Ruvalcaba syndrome; or those who have a first-degree relative with the syndrome

Some common uses for breast MRI include

- Further evaluation of abnormalities detected by mammography
- Finding early breast cancers not detected by other tests, especially in women at high risk and women with dense breast tissue
- Examination for cancer in women who have implants or scar tissue that might produce an inaccurate result from a mammogram. MRI can also be helpful for women with lumpectomy scars to check for any changes.
- Detecting small abnormalities not seen with mammography or ultrasound (for example, MRI has been useful for women who have breast cancer cells present in an underarm lymph node, but do not have a lump that can be felt or can be viewed on diagnostic studies)
- Assess for leakage from a silicone gel implant
- Evaluate the size and precise location of breast cancer lesions, including the possibility that more than one area of the breast may be involved (this is helpful for cancers that spread and involve more than one area)

- Determining whether lumpectomy or mastectomy would be more effective
- Detecting changes in the other breast that have not been newly diagnosed with breast cancer (There is an approximately 10 percent chance that women with breast cancer will develop cancer in the opposite breast. A recent study indicates that breast MRI can detect cancer in the opposite breast that may be missed at the time of the first breast cancer diagnosis.)
- Detection of the spread of breast cancer into the chest wall, which may change treatment options
- Detection of breast cancer recurrence or residual tumor after lumpectomy
- Evaluation of a newly-inverted nipple change

There may be other reasons for your health care provider to recommend breast MRI[8].

PET OF BREAST: POSITRON EMISSION TOMOGRAPHY

PET uses radioactive labeled sugar to find active breast cancer. Cancers burn much more sugar than most normal tissue. The radioactive sugar is taken up by the breast cancer and the PET Machine shows the breast cancer as a bright structure because of the high sugar metabolism in the cancer.

[8] AMERICAN CANCER SOCIETY

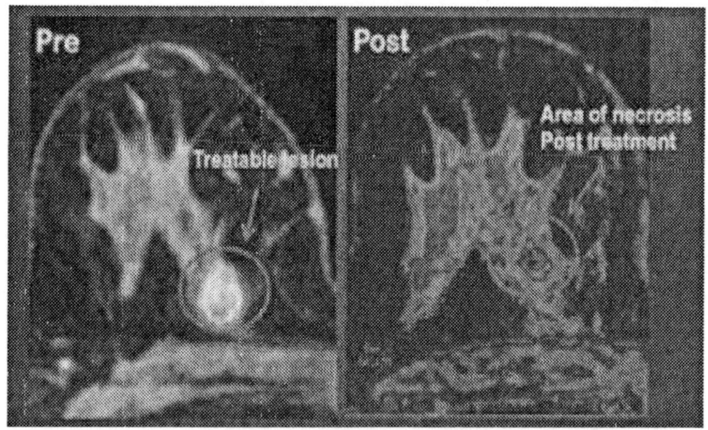

PET IMAGES - BREAST CANCER
BEFORE AND AFTER TREATMENT

BIOPSY: A piece of the suspected tumor is removed. There are several ways a physician can obtain a small piece of the nodule or calcifications. In some cases, only cells are removed (Fine Needle Aspiration).

The specimen is then examined by a pathologist and whether it is cancer or benign is determined with certainty.

Ultrasound Guided
Stereotactic Biopsy
MRI Guided Biopsy
Open Surgical Biopsy

CONCLUSION: The best self-defense is early diagnosis of small, non-invasive breast cancers and securing the best treatment possible promptly.

Learn your risks. Calculate your lifetime risk of developing breast cancer based upon Gail Protocol or one of the other reliable schemes. Know the density of your breast and the reliability of your mammography. Become self-aware of the nature of your breast. Respond immediately to any changes in the nature of your breast. If changes occur, consult your doctor immediately. Hope for the best, but assume the worst. Seek the very best medical-surgical care, if necessary.

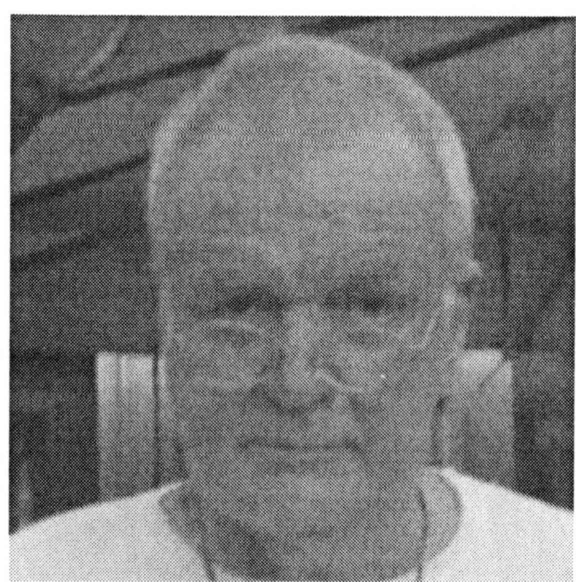

Paul P. Slawek, M.D., J.D.

is a Medical Doctor specializing in diagnostic radiology. He is an expert in breast imaging. He is an authority in MRI of the breast. He currently interprets Breast MRI for several South Florida radiology groups.

Doctor Slawek is a Diplomat of the American Board of Radiology. He is an adjunct professor at Florida Atlantic University. He currently a consulting radiologist for several imaging centers in Broward and Dade Counties. He has testified frequently as an expert in state and Federal Courts.

Dr. Slawek earned his M.D. from Thomas Jefferson University Medical College in Philadelphia, PA after earning a Bachelor of Science Degree from Drexel University in Philadelphia, PA. He also holds a Juris Doctor (J.D.) from Widener University School of Law in Wilmington, DE. He received his radiology training at Pennsylvania Medical College in Philadelphia. He can be reached via email at peteslawek@aol.com or by phone at (954) 257-5714.

CHAPTER 3

THERMOGRAPHY – AN EARLIER SCREENING OPTION

Donna J. Tomey, C.C.T.

Breast thermography is an underrated screening tool that is very different from a mammogram. However, it is incredibly useful as a preventative screening method without any of the harmful radiation or compression. Using only digital infrared thermal imaging, it is safe, non-invasive and can see what a mammogram cannot.

In 1982, thermography was FDA-cleared as an adjunct to mammography yet not surprisingly, it is still not widely accepted in mainstream medicine. One would guess this is because in order for a physician to remove an offending structure such as a tumor, it must actually be seen, which makes sense. But thermography detects more than just a tumor; it sees inflammation, active blood flow, and abnormal vascularity (angiogenesis), which every active tumor requires for growth and proliferation. It sees the pathology and process of cancer, and the physiological changes occurring in the breast to support that active tumor in the first place – in most cases, seven- to- ten years earlier than when it becomes a structure a mammogram is capable of seeing.

In the Journal of Oncology, the following chart indicates the cell replication process. Active cancer cell doubling rate is every 90 days; when those cells grow to over four-billion, it becomes a viewable structure with an X-ray or mammogram.

Is this what we consider prevention? Or is this simply detection once cancer is already there?

When you feel that lump in your breast, it is *not* the beginning of cancer. Such a discovery means you've had cancer growing inside of you for years, and the END result is the tumor.

Because of this 90-day doubling rate, it is necessary to do a 90-day comparison thermogram study with the goal of establishing a stable baseline.

Now if you have dense breasts, it is difficult to see breast tumors with a mammogram, much like "looking for a snowflake in a blizzard." In fact, 21 states have now passed the "Dense Breast Law," making it mandatory for your doctor or radiologist to inform you of other imaging options. The picture on the left is a mammogram of a dense breast. The one on the right is of a normal breast.

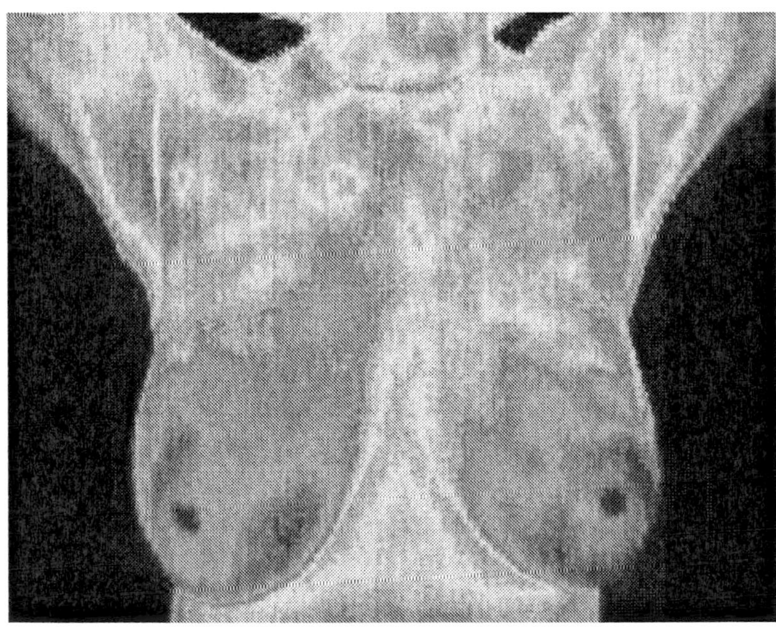

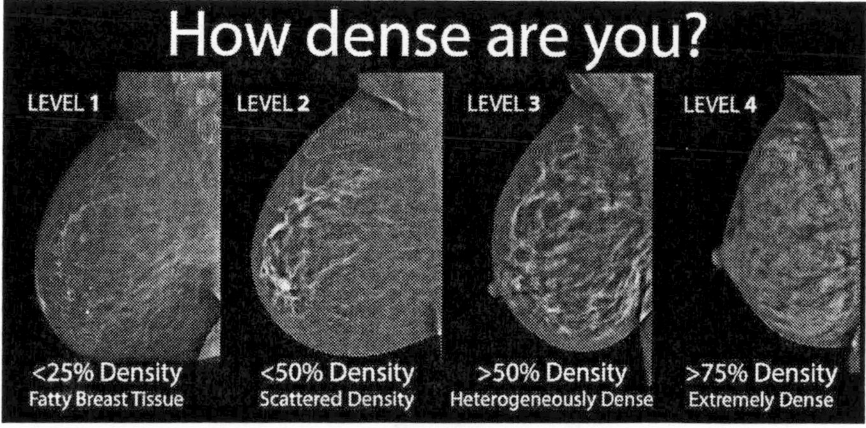

There are studies that indicate as high as a 50% false negative rate in these women (and 40% of women have dense breasts), which is why as a general rule women with dense breasts must undergo both a mammogram and an ultrasound. Keep in mind, the 3-D mammogram has twice as much radiation; therefore in many cases, you still need to do a regular mammogram, giving you a nice triple dose of radiation.

Radiation causes DNA and cellular mutation.

What is a cancer cell? A mutated cell; you do the math.

If you have a suspicious thermogram and take your report to your conventional doctor, chances are they won't know what to do with it. Since most doctors aren't trained in nutrition, they cannot offer you a protocol to start reversing those suspicious areas discovered by thermography. Since thermography only sees inflammation – which presents as vascular changes, active blood flow, pattern changes, etc., -- either a natural practitioner or a functional medicine doctor would be your new best friend. These doctors will get to the underlying cause, the root of the problem, and begin a protocol to reverse it. For me, the cause of my breast cancer was fueled by estrogen dominance – a story I will share with you a little later in this chapter.

Every woman has a unique pattern, as unique as a fingerprint, sort of like a thermal road map. Thermography monitors breast health over time, and after your two 90-day studies are compared and a baseline is established, you need only return annually. Your thermographic scan is interpreted by a thermologist, who is an M.D., certified in thermology.

INFLAMMATION: THE SILENT KILLER, THE FOUNDATION OF DISEASE

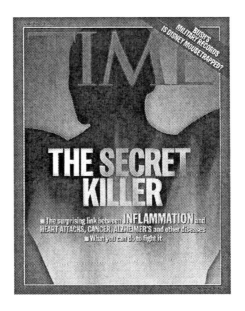

Every doctor, conventional or holistic, knows that the root of almost all disease – including cancer – starts with inflammation. If left unchecked, inflammation will manifest into a physical symptom, i.e., cancer, diabetes, heart disease, auto-immune, arthritis, etc. Thermal imaging can see the inflammation *before* there are symptoms, alerting you early enough to enable you and your doctor to then plan accordingly and lay out a careful program to further diagnose and MONITOR you during and after any treatment. Whether it's a nutritional protocol or hormone balancing, the early stages of breast cancer can potentially be reversed. It's not just for your breasts either; thermography can analyze the entire body, except for the head/brain.

On the front page of the New York Times in February, 2014, the caption read "Vast Study Casts Doubt on Value of Mammograms" The largest study ever done on the subject concluded the following:

Study Results

A large, 25-year study of Canadian women aged 40 to 59 found no benefit for women who were randomly assigned to have mammograms.

WITH MAMMOGRAMS	WITHOUT MAMMOGRAMS
44,925 women received breast exams and mammograms	**44,910 women** received breast exams
3,250 women had diagnoses with breast cancer	**3,133 women** had diagnoses with breast cancer
500 women died from breast cancer	**505 women died** from breast cancer

The death rate from breast cancer was the same in both groups, but **1 in 424 women** who had mammograms received unnecessary cancer treatment, including surgery, chemotherapy and radiation.

Source: British Medical Journal

THE TEST

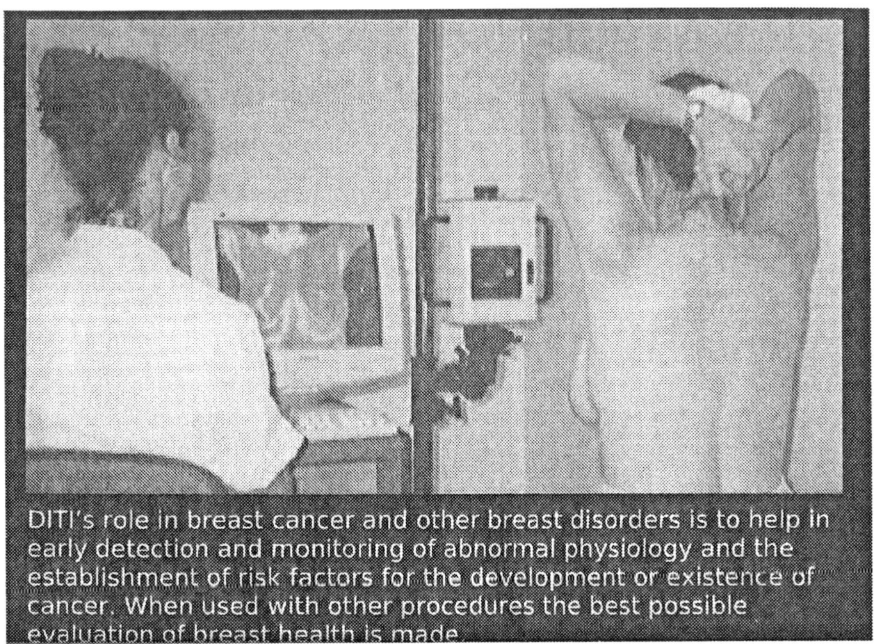

DITI's role in breast cancer and other breast disorders is to help in early detection and monitoring of abnormal physiology and the establishment of risk factors for the development or existence of cancer. When used with other procedures the best possible evaluation of breast health is made.

When you enter the room, you will find it a cool 69-71 degrees. You will first disrobe from the waist up and the fill out some paperwork while you are cooling off. There are a few instructions you will need to follow before you scan, such as no shaving under the arms, no oils or creams on the breast/chest area, no antiperspirants, no smoking at least three hours before your appointment time, etc.

After the thermographer reviews your patient form, the imaging – which only takes about five minutes – begins. Afterwards, you will be shown your images before they are sent electronically to a thermologist for interpretation. Hard copies will be mailed to you in about a week. You will need to return in three months in order to establish a stable baseline, which I discussed previously.

Thermography, an effective way to monitor breast health and the very early stages of breast disease, offers the opportunity of earlier detection of breast disease than has ever been possible through self-exams, doctor exams, or mammography alone.

MY STORY

In June 2002, I had my first thermogram at the insistence of my sister Theresa, who is an acupuncturist physician. I was in my late 30's at the time and it was almost time for me to start routine mammograms. She kept hounding me about thermography until I finally had one at her office, along with a few other women. When I received my report, it said "abnormal vascular patterns above both breasts….clinical correlation is warranted…"

I wasn't quite sure what that meant and dismissed it, never returning for my three-month follow-up. Fast forward to February, 2006...

I was sitting on the couch, just kind of poking my chest area when I noticed a lump in the outer quadrant of my right breast. It was a strange feeling, because just five days earlier my gynecologist had performed a routine breast exam during my annual check-up and hadn't felt anything.

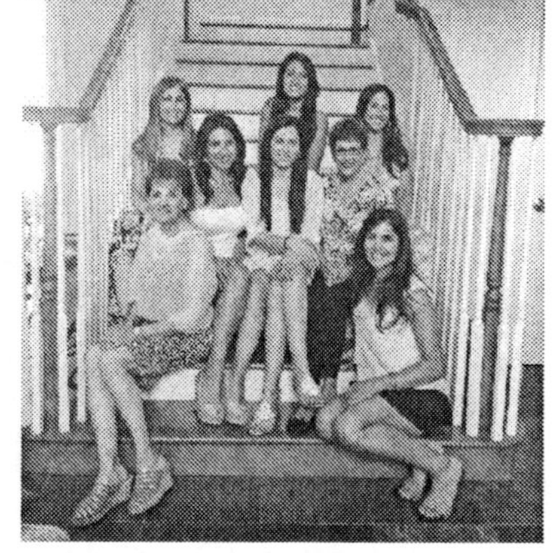

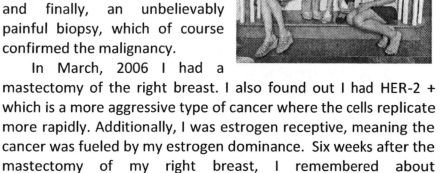

The next day I made an appointment to go back to my gynecologist, who upon feeling the lump, scheduled me for a mammogram. Since it was suspicious, we then did an ultrasound, followed by an MRI, and finally, an unbelievably painful biopsy, which of course confirmed the malignancy.

In March, 2006 I had a mastectomy of the right breast. I also found out I had HER-2 + which is a more aggressive type of cancer where the cells replicate more rapidly. Additionally, I was estrogen receptive, meaning the cancer was fueled by my estrogen dominance. Six weeks after the mastectomy of my right breast, I remembered about thermography, and decided to do another one.

Comparing the February, 2002 to the May, 2006 scan revealed

noticeable changes. Specifically, the report read "significant changes suspicious for developing pathology..." In a nutshell, I was also getting cancer in my left breast. After the hell I had just been through, I was determined to avoid an encore!

I was then introduced to Dr. Karen Corcoran, a functional medicine doctor in Fort Lauderdale, who put me on an aggressive nutritional protocol. She also did some hormonal testing, including one called "Estronex," a 24-hour urine test, to show how my estrogen was metabolizing, since it was fueling my cancer. Tests results were conclusive: estrogen was my problem and I had to get it under control. Without addressing the underlying cause, cancer would have reared its ugly head somewhere else inside of me.

During a 10-month very aggressive nutritional protocol, along with hormone balancing and constant monitoring with thermography, I was able to reverse the cancerous changes in my left breast. It was then that I realized WHY I got breast cancer: I was determined to become a thermographer and promote the "world's best breast screening tool." If it hadn't been for thermography, there's no doubt it would have only been a matter of time before I got cancer again.

I remember experiencing a full spectrum of emotions, but mostly determination and anger. Determination because if I had to have this disease, then I would do everything in my power to **never** have it again; anger because the doctors kept telling me if I didn't get chemotherapy I would die. Scared out of my mind, I succumbed to the pressure and got three rounds of chemo, but did not finish the cycle because I was just too sick. Besides, I hated those scare tactics; I wanted to hear positive things, reassuring things. So I just tuned them out and went my own way. Fortunately, my family is very much into holistic and alternative health care; everything I did, from acupuncture to herbs, to homeopathic injections, really helped repair my immune system after chemotherapy destroyed it.

I also did a lot of my own research. I have never been the type of person to just believe what anyone tells me, and this is true also with my health. I have never been much of a conformist, and have always prided myself in finding things out for myself and educating myself about a particular subject – especially when it comes to health.

I first coped by finding everything out I could about breast cancer, to really educate and arm myself with the facts. I even took a leave of absence from my job. My daughter was 16 at the time, and therefore, pretty self-sufficient. While I remained strong for her, there were times, of course, when I fell apart. However, I usually did that alone. I knew I would come through this, and there was no way in hell I was going anywhere.

People often ask me, "What was the hardest part of the entire ordeal?"

There were a few things:

- **Seeing a long diagonal scar across my chest, where my breast used to be.** That was hard because you look and feel totally disfigured. You wonder *"Who is going to love me like this?"* But then you come to your senses and thank God that you are alive.

- **Being so sick from the chemo and dealing with the pain from the surgery**. I couldn't lie down to sleep, I couldn't sneeze, cough or walk straight for weeks, and I had drains sticking out of my body. Chemo caused nosebleeds as I slept and turned my nails gray. It's incredibly painful having your breast removed. I was constantly poked with needles, and whenever they couldn't find a vein, I'd fear *"Where are they going to stick me next?"* I also developed a blood clot in my left arm where the PICC line was, which was not resolved with weeks of blood thinners such as Coumadin, and Luvenox shots in my stomach. However, after three acupuncture treatments, an ultrasound proved that the clot had dissolved.

This is going to sound a little harsh, but I think pretty much everyone is "aware" of breast cancer. Now we need to focus on PREVENTION and not so much a "cure." I doubt a cure will even be allowed in this country; think of the billions of dollars the cancer industry would lose.

If every woman got a thermogram beginning in her mid-20's, we would begin to see the end of breast cancer. I prefer to promote prevention with thermography and other alternative ways moreso than the walks, or the "Race for the Cure," because I firmly believe that prevention is the cure – not dumping millions into research or drugs.

In 2007, I was asked to be part of a "Beauty & Bravery" Calendar as Ms. February 2008. All 12 of us girls were breast cancer survivors, all featured in that calendar. To my astonishment, on October 7, 2007, my calendar picture was featured, larger-than-life, on the entire front page of the Sun-Sentinel, Lifestyle Section. Talk about a surprise!

Having cancer completely affected my outlook... I have always appreciated life, but now even more than ever. I no longer take it for granted and want to live mine to the absolute fullest. I want to be happy every day I live. Life is too short to be with anyone with whom you're not compatible or joyful. Life is too short to be unhappy, PERIOD.

I appreciate being outside more, enjoying nature, learning, educating myself about the important things in life. I have learned to grow more spiritually and to be thankful for everything I have...and everything I don't.

Truly, the fight against cancer is all about prevention. I have had more women come to me and say "something doesn't feel right, but my doctor says not to worry about it...."

Listen to your instincts. You know your body. If something feels wrong within you, chances are you're right.

I have lived through this and I am out there making a difference. I'm unbelievably passionate about what I do, and nothing is going to stop me. My life will have been worth living when I see every woman doing thermography; when I start seeing doctors recommending it to their patients before they are 40 years old; and when we can stop using radiation to detect breast cancer.

This is my mission.

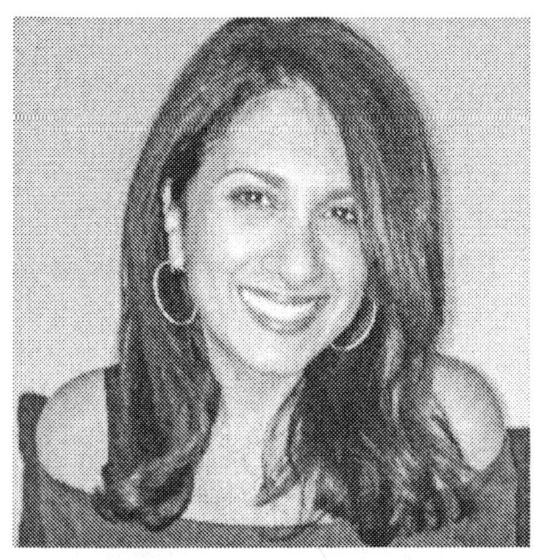

Donna J. Tomey, C.C.T.

Certified Clinical Thermographer

received her certification at Duke University under the auspices of the American College of Clinical Thermology, Inc., in Feb. 2007.

After her own experience with breast cancer in early 2006, she learned about thermography, the earliest breast cancer screening tool available. Shortly after the mastectomy of her right breast, Donna did a thermogram of her other breast and discovered significant vascular changes that put her at serious risk for a cancer recurrence. With the help of a functional medicine doctor and other alternative care, she was able to reverse these changes by making the necessary alterations to her diet and hormones.

Since then, Donna has made it her mission to educate as many people as possible about this valuable screening tool.

You can reach Donna at 954-673-2221 and via email at thermographyfirst@yahoo.com

CHAPTER 4

Surgical Oncology, Mastectomy, Lumpectomy

Nicholas Tranakas, M.D.

I remember one day early during my training waiting for the head of the Surgical Oncology Division to arrive for morning rounds. Dr. Alfred Ketcham, not only the head of the division but my mentor, arrived an hour late and was profusely apologetic. He explained to us that he had been up late the previous evening with an emergency breast consult. We all looked at each other chuckling as to what could possibly constitute as an emergency breast consult. It was many months later when I was caring for patients myself as a junior attending at the Sylvester Cancer Center that I understood what Dr. Ketcham meant. He truly is a great surgeon and mentor. I am eternally grateful for all that he taught me.

A woman who has discovered a lump in her breast or has received news of an abnormal imaging study of her breast, does indeed constitute an emergency. The prevalence of breast cancer in this country (one in eight women will develop breast cancer in their lifetime) along with the constant media attention, has brought this disease to the forefront in the minds of most people. The fear of having a breast cancer diagnosis creates such stress that it rivals other medical emergencies. We as clinicians must be aware of this fact and do everything within our power to see these patients in a timely fashion and expedite the work-up in order to alleviate some of this stress.

Once a breast cancer diagnosis has been made, it is important to note that it is no longer a death sentence. Our treatments have advanced and offer better outcomes, even for the more aggressive types of breast cancer. The first decision that needs to be made is to whether or not the cancer needs to be treated with surgery followed by additional therapy or chemotherapy followed by surgery. Most cancers diagnosed at an early stage require surgery which will usually come first. However, in cases where the cancer has spread or there is a need to shrink it in order to have a better surgical outcome, we need to give chemotherapy first.

The second decision that needs to be made is breast conservation versus mastectomy. The idea of breast conservation is a relatively new one. At the turn of the last century, very radical surgical procedures were devised in hope that they would lead to better and longer survival. This theory lasted many decades only to find that more radical surgery did not always work even for very early cancers. We were and still are at mercy of the biological behavior of the cancer. As we became more knowledgeable and our systemic therapies became better, we started focusing on less radical surgery that produced equivalent results. Thus, breast conservation was born. We went from the radical mastectomy to the modified radical mastectomy which spared the pectoralis muscles and the lymph nodes in the neck. Next came breast conservation with the introduction of the lumpectomy in the 1970s. Finally, in the 1990s we went from complete lymph node removal to the sentinel lymph node biopsy. The current option of breast conservation with radiation therapy to the remaining breast tissue versus complete mastectomy yield similar results on local recurrence.

The whole reason for breast conservation surgery however, is to preserve the overall appearance of the breast. By definition, a lumpectomy involves the removal of the cancer with enough margin of normal breast tissue surrounding it in order to be sure that the entire cancer has been eliminated. If we have to remove a significant amount of breast tissue such that the breast will be deformed, there is no advantage to breast conservation. Breast conservation requires us to add radiation treatments to the remaining breast tissue in order to minimize recurrence rates. This added treatment can further add to the deformity. Thus, the option for breast conservation is strictly a cosmetic decision. If radiation cannot be given to a patient for a variety of medical reasons, then breast conservation is also not an option. The decision, therefore for breast conservation is based on the size of the cancer in relation to the size of the women's breast and the ability to deliver radiation therapy. There are some options if the size criterion prevents breast conservation. We do have the opportunity to give chemotherapy first in the hope that we can shrink the tumor sufficiently such that a reasonable cosmetic result can be obtained with breast conservation. If however a mastectomy is required, are there choices? The answer is yes. I will now delve into the next decision making.

Before describing the various types of mastectomies, there is another question that must be answered. Do we do one side or two? If we eliminate the fear and the emotion from the decision, there are some very good and valid reasons to consider bilateral mastectomies. The most compelling reason to consider such a seemingly radical option is if a patient is a carrier of the BRCA gene. In many studies, bilateral mastectomy seems to confer the best long term results for carriers. Even with close follow up and extensive imaging with mammograms, ultrasounds and breast MRI, the long term survival in patients who are BRCA carriers seems to favor the bilateral mastectomy option.

Bilateral mastectomy may also be considered if there is size discrepancy between the affected breast and the remaining breast that would require further surgery for symmetry. If any premalignant lesions are identified on the unaffected breast, or a diagnosis of invasive lobular cancer is found that would increase the risk for cancer in the unaffected breast, would be a further consideration for removing both breasts. Finally, some women for psychological reasons may opt for removal of both breasts in order to remove the stress of diagnosing a future cancer. I would caution any woman who chooses this more radical approach however, to be sure she is 100% certain this is what she really wants. If there is any wavering, I would advise against this approach.

If a mastectomy is needed or wanted, what are the different types of mastectomies?

Modified Radical Mastectomy

A modified radical mastectomy means the removal of all the breast tissue (including the nipple and areola) along with the lymph nodes in the underarm area. Typically in this country one also removes the outer lining of the pectoralis muscle (fascia) while leaving the muscle intact. This approach removes all the breast tissue and offers the lowest recurrence risk. Normally following a mastectomy, radiation therapy is not needed unless the cancer was larger than 2 inches in diameter, margins were involved or cancer had spread to multiple lymph nodes. By leaving the pectoralis muscle intact, the plastic surgeon has better tissue coverage if reconstruction with implants is planned.

Radical Mastectomy

A radical mastectomy which was commonly practiced at the turn of the last century until the 1970s is rarely done these days. This procedure removes the breast tissue, all lymph nodes in the underarm area, as well as the pectoralis muscle. This is the most disfiguring breast operation. It also precludes implant reconstruction due to the lack of overlying tissue coverage unless the flank or abdominal muscles are used for the coverage. Again this operation is rarely used unless the cancer has directly invaded the underlying muscle. Fortunately, such advanced cancers are not commonly seen these days with increased awareness and better imaging techniques. Such advanced cancers are seen typically when patients are in denial of a breast abnormality and allow the cancer to reach a locally advanced stage.

Skin Sparing Mastectomy

Skin sparing mastectomy also removes all of the breast tissue and nipple along with the lymph node(s) while preserving as much of the skin as possible. By leaving the unaffected skin, the plastic surgeon has more tissue at their disposal for a better cosmetic result with the reconstruction. This however presupposes that an immediate reconstruction is planned at the same time as the mastectomy. If an immediate reconstruction is not planned, there is no role for skin sparing mastectomy. The reason for this is that the extra skin left for future reconstruction will ripple and scar to the point of most of it, if not all, will be useless at the time of the reconstruction.

Nipple Sparing Mastectomy

More recently the concept of nipple sparing mastectomy has come into vogue. In this type of mastectomy, all the breast skin along with nipple and areola are spared. While this procedure is acceptable for the breast that is unaffected by cancer, it is not standard therapy for a breast with breast cancer. Some clinicians however do offer nipple sparing mastectomy if the cancer is small and far away from the nipple. We do not have long term studies proving this form of mastectomy is safe. We must remember that the nipple is a collection of eight to sixteen major milk ducts. Eighty percent of breast cancers arise from the lining of the ducts of the breast tissue. By leaving the nipple intact, there is a possibility of future cancers arising in the tissue that is left behind during this procedure. So until further studies are available as to the safety of this procedure, one should proceed with caution.

Further, the whole idea of nipple sparing mastectomy is to leave the woman with an intact functional nipple. During the performance of this procedure, the surgical incision to leave the nipple intact severs potential nerve stimulation to the nipple making it insensate. Also, at times the blood supply to the nipple may be compromised which leads to necrosis and the ultimate removal of the nipple. From a cosmetic perspective, if the woman's breasts are ptotic, that is droopy, there is no way to maintain viability of the nipple while moving it in an upward location when the breast is reconstructed. After all, the reason for considering nipple sparing is for cosmesis and function. It would not be cosmetically pleasing if the nipple ends up on the bottom of the breast. Therefore, the number of occasions that all these considerations are satisfied are few. This has to do with technical reasons and not the skill set of the plastic surgeon or surgical oncologist. The ideal candidate for nipple sparing mastectomy would be woman with relatively small, non-ptotic breasts. My bias from an oncologic standpoint is to remain conservative and tend to stay away from nipple sparing mastectomy for a breast with breast cancer.

In conclusion, we have come a long way in the treatment of breast cancer. As our anesthetic agents became better, we started with very radical surgery but without necessarily better outcomes. It took a while until we realized that we were at the mercy of the biological behavior of breast cancer. It was this realization that led to less radical surgery without compromising cancer cures. As we continue to improve our targeted therapies and our surgical interventions, our patients will live longer with better chances for cures and fewer side effects while maintaining better cosmesis.

As we continue to improve our targeted therapies and our surgical interventions, our patients will live longer with better chances for cures and fewer side effects while maintaining better cosmesis. The best advice I can give anyone trying to make a decision regarding surgery for breast cancer, is to make an informed decision. We need to separate emotion from facts and to engage the medical team in making that informed decision. Seek a second opinion whenever there is any doubt or the thought crosses your mind. You need to remember that the medical team is there to serve you, not the other way around. We can help you make a decision but ultimately the decision is up to the patient taking into account the information that has been provided along with that patient's biases and past experiences. My role as a surgical oncologist is to help the patient process the facts and put them in the proper prospective. Focus on the fact that breast cancer is no longer a death sentence as it may have been in the recent past.

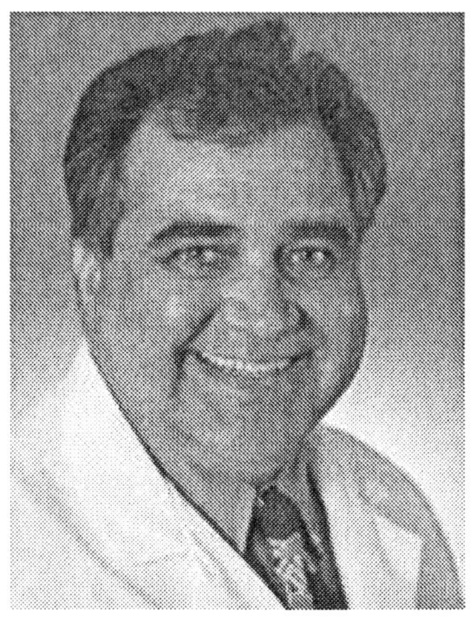

Nicholas Tranakas, MD

is the Medical Director of Cancer Services for Broward Health and of the Comprehensive Breast Center at Broward Health Medical Center.

Dr. Tranakas received his medical degree from the University of Miami School of Medicine. He completed his internship, residency and a fellowship in surgical oncology at the University of Miami School of Medicine/Jackson Memorial.

His honors and awards include the American Cancer Society Clinical Oncology Fellowship, the Doris Faircloth/Alfred Ketcham Surgical Oncology Fellow Award and recognition as Most Valuable Physician at Broward Health Medical Center.

He is a member of the Society of Laparoendoscopic Surgeons and has presented his research on cancer and laparoscopic surgery before a number of professional societies.

Dr. Tranakas is a clinical assistant professor of surgery at the University of Miami School of Medicine. He serves as a consultant in surgery for the Veterans Administration Medical Center in Miami. He is current president of the Broward County Division of the American Cancer Society and serves on the executive board of Gilda's Club of South Florida.

He frequently is asked to provide authoritative interviews for news stories about cancer.

Dr. Tranakas lives in Fort Lauderdale with his wife and three children. His hobbies include backgammon, racketball and boating.

Chapter 5

Stereotactic Breast Biopsies

Alejandro Hernandez-Cano, M.D.

In order to make a diagnosis of breast cancer, a tissue sample is needed. Many times on routine mammograms or on comparison follow-up, the radiologist reports a suspicious lesion or change that may require further diagnostic studies. For example, an ultrasound may be recommended to determine if an abnormality is solid or cystic (fluid-filled). The radiologist may also request spot compression film of the abnormality to separate the different shadows to ensure the abnormality is not an overlapping of shadows or a true lesion. At that time, a tissue sample is taken to determine whether or not this abnormality is a cancerous growth.

On these occasions, a referral is recommended to a surgeon with special interest in treating diseases of the breast to perform the biopsy – when the lesion is palpable and easily removed by an incision made into the breast. This procedure may require the patient to be under general anesthesia with intravenous sedation in the operating room. Once the tissue is removed, stitches are used to close the area and the patient will spend time in the recovery room.

In cases where the lesion is not readily palpable, needle localization may be required. This procedure requires a radiologist to locate the area in question via mammogram. A needle is passed through the breast into the lesion, followed by a thin wire guided through the needle into the breast. Once the wire is inserted, the patient is taken into the operating room, where the surgeon will remove the tissue around the wire, which is then sent to pathology for evaluation. The procedure is entirely diagnostic; further surgical intervention will be necessary if a malignancy is found.

Approximately 85 percent of these biopsies are benign (no cancer); therefore, no further surgeries are needed. However, there is a less invasive, alternative method of obtaining sufficient tissue for diagnosis without the use of an operating room and with minimal scarring.

In Sweden, the use of a stereotactic system to locate the lesion in the breast with sampling obtained by a needle was reported in the late 1970s. In the mid-1980s, Dr. Dowlatshahi established the dedicated prone stereotactic table, though at the time it was noted that only localization of the lesion excised or open biopsy was still being used. Then in 1989, Dr. Steve Parker reported the use of an automatic gun with a large bore (thick) trocar to take cores of tissue from the breast with a very high correlation to the subsequent open biopsy. Thus, the acceptance of stereotactic biopsy for on-palpable lesions of the breast became a reality.

The concept of stereotactic imaging is very similar to the phenomenon of your vision. By observing an object from two angles, its depth can be determined (this is why people who suffer from loss of sight in lack depth perception). The dedicated stereotactic mammography table is equipped with a cathode tube (the machine that makes the X-rays) that rotates 180 degrees, creating various angles, one of which will offer the best access to the lesion. Prior to undergoing stereotactic breast biopsy, the patient should not take medicine such as anticoagulants that alter coagulation including aspirin, Plavix, or Coumadin for ten days, to minimize the risk of bleeding.

The table has a bed with an opening on top. The patient lies face down with her breast protruding through the opening. The breast drops into a lateral compression plastic tray (to enable X-rays to pass through it) and no movement of the breast occurs. There is a window through which the actual cores can be taken.

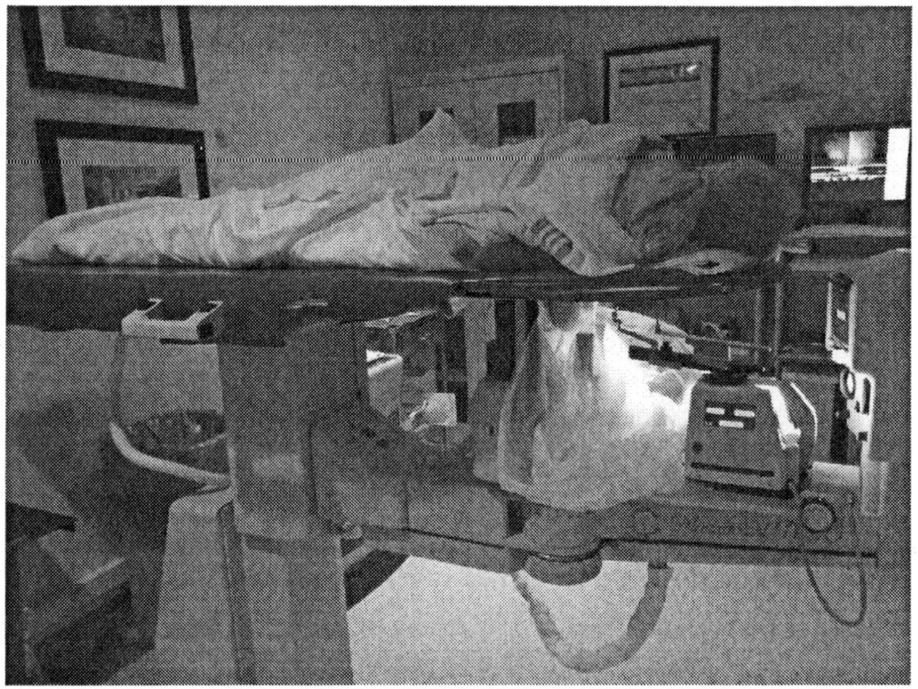

Beneath the opening is also the mammography machine, connected to a computer. Once the breast lesion is located, the mammography machine is rotated fifteen degrees to target the lesion. This information is fed to the computer, which figures the exact depth and pitch. The mammogram gun is then set to pre-fire position.

The skin overlying the lesion is cleansed with an antiseptic iodine-based solution (if a patient is allergic to iodine, she should alert her physician who will use a non-iodine cleanser). A local anesthetic (xylocaine 1-percent) is administered into the skin and deep into the tissues. Using a number 11 pointed scalpel, the surgeon makes a small nick on the skin and the trocar needle is inserted into the breast. The trocar needle is connected to the core gun and fired into the breast by a spring action mechanism that allows the trocar needle to penetrate into the breast approximately two centimeters (less than one inch) into the breast. Follow-up mammogram determines whether the trocar needle is overlying the targeted area and not accidentally displacing the lesion. Newer machines use automatic suction and sampling experience with stereotactic biopsy concepts are necessary, as errors in the X-Z coordinates have occurred. Therefore, the actual lesion may be missed. When breasts are very thin, adapters can be placed to reduce the length of the trocars sampling windows.

These are called Eviva Variance (I, II, III).

Limitations to stereotactic biopsy can occur in certain cases, for example if the lesion is too close to the skin surface or in severely obese women when the lesion is too close to the chest wall. But these situations are rare. When they do happen, open biopsy is recommended.

The trocar has a side vent that sucks part of the bulging tissue into the shaft, where a circulating rotating blade cuts and extracts it. This procedure is repeated in radial fashion (following the hands of the clock) until the desired amount of the tissue has been removed for diagnosis. Post-biopsy stereotactic mammograms are performed to confirm the removal of part or the entirety of the lesion. The removed tissue (the slivers of tissue excised) is about the size of a small olive.

In the case of clusters of micro calcifications, their absence will be noted in the post-procedure films as well as by performing a mammogram of the cassette into which the slivers of removed tissue are collected. After satisfactory removal of the desired specimens, a metal marker is placed into the biopsy site. Extremely small, this marker serves only as a reference for future mammograms so that the area in question can be seen. Some patients develop scars at the biopsy site side of the breast; the marker will allow the mammographer to interpret whether or not there are any changes in the area.

Once the procedure is finished, the patient is then positioned sitting up. Pressure is applied at the incision site and the edges are wrapped with an adhesive tape. A bandage with an ice pack is recommended for several hours to prevent swelling or bruising. There is no need for fasting before the procedure, which often takes less than 30 minutes. No narcotics are administered and if there are no complications, the patient can return to full activity.

After the tissues are removed, they are sent to the pathology department for analysis. The specimen is put into special solutions of formalin and dyed with tissue colorants. Then it is mounted into a paraffin block (similar to wax), sliced very thin, and mounted on microscope slides for cellular examination to determine the diagnosis.

As mentioned earlier, most results are benign (not cancer), and follow-up at either three-, six-, or one-year intervals will be recommended. If the biopsy is malignant, further treatment will be necessary.

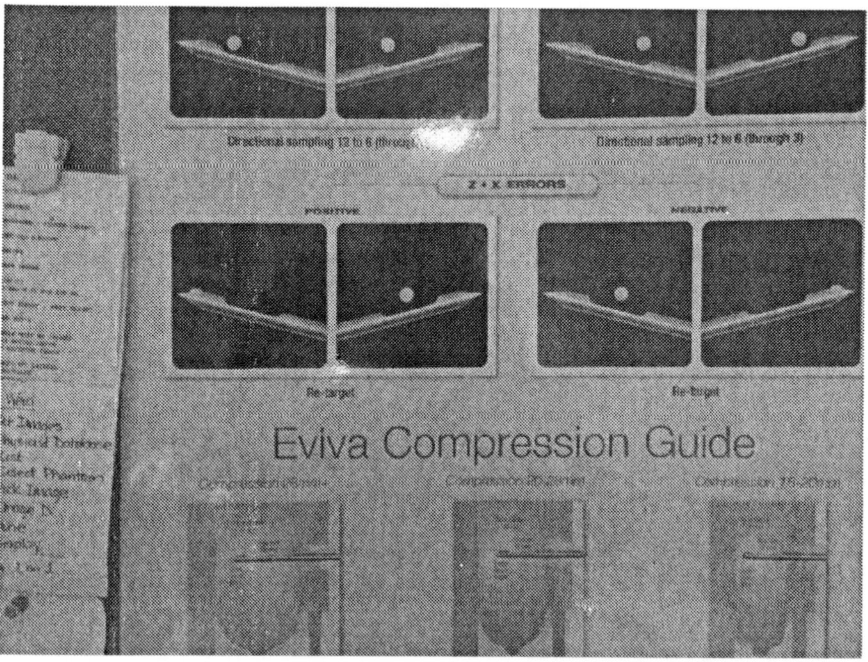
Z + X ERRORS
Re-target
Re-target
Eviva Compression Guide

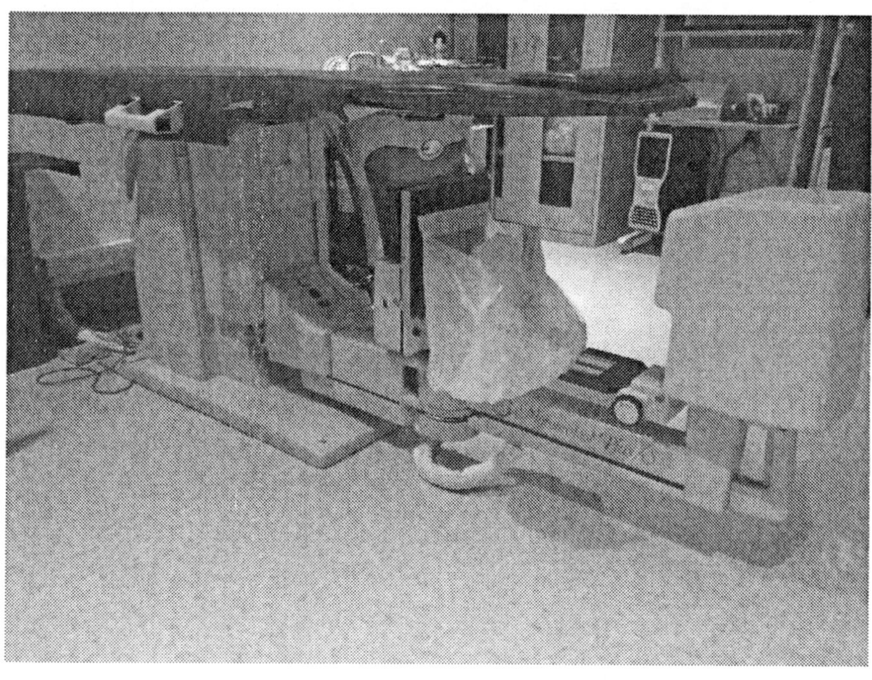

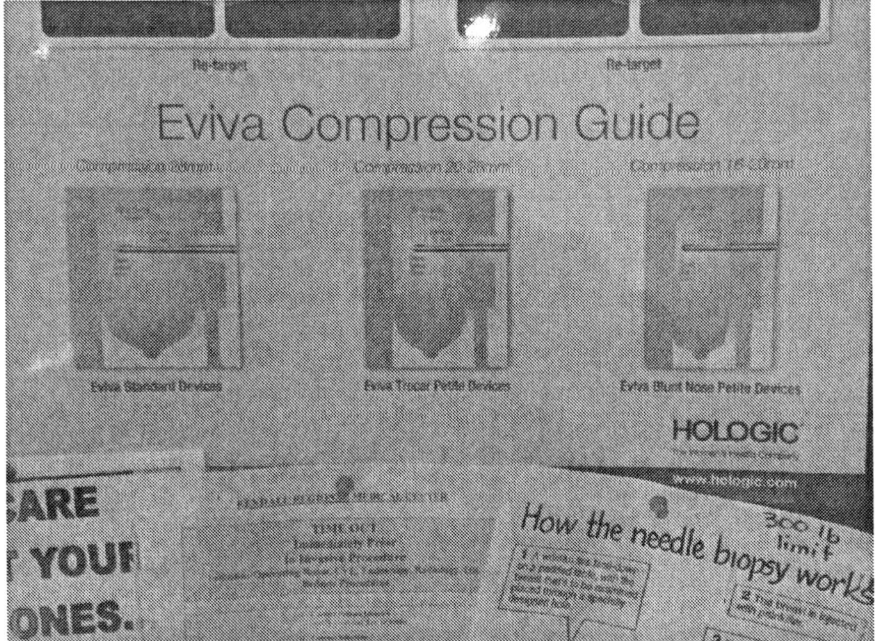
Re-target
Re-target
Eviva Compression Guide
Eviva Standard Devices
Eviva Trocar Petite Devices
Eviva Blunt Nose Petite Devices
HOLOGIC
www.hologic.com
ARE
YOUR
ONES.
TIME OUT
How the needle biopsy works
300 lb
limit

References

Stereotactic Breast Biopsy." *High-Yield Imaging: Interventional* (2010): 501-03. Print. Dowlatshahi, K., M. L. Yaremko, L. F. Kluskens, and P. M. Jokich.

"Nonpalpable Breast Lesions: Findings of Stereotaxic Needle-core Biopsy and Fine-needle Aspiration Cytology." *Radiology* 181.3 (1991): 745-50. Print.

Parker, Steve H. "Minimally Invasive Breast Biopsy." *Journal of Vascular and Interventional Radiology* 7.1 (1996): 282-85. Print.

Parker, Steve H., Terese I. Kaske, and Judy L. Chavez. "Minimally Invasive Breast Biopsy." *Early Diagnosis and Treatment of Cancer Series: Breast Cancer* (2011): 151-74. Print.

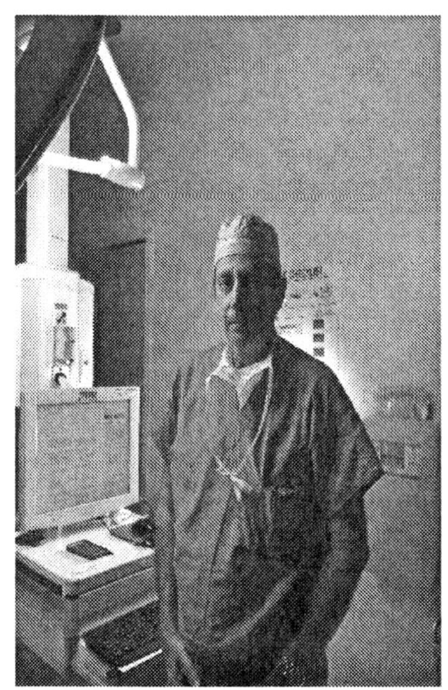

Alejandro M. Hernandez-Cano

received his medical degree at the Universidad San Carlos De Guatemala 1979. He completed his residency in general surgery at the University of Miami, Jackson Memorial Hospital in Miami, Florida. In 1984-1985 he was chief resident in general surgery, and 1985-1986 he did his fellow in Pediatrics at the university at Colorado Health Sciences Center in Denver, Colorado. He servers on many committees, and is a member of numerous professional organizations at Jackson Memorial Hospital in Miami Florida. Dr Hernandez-Cano is affiliated with Baptist Health Systems, South Miami Hospital, Kendall Medical Center and Palm Springs General Hospital. He was a Contributing Author in *The Empty Cup Runneth Over*.

Chapter 6

Breast Reconstruction After Breast Cancer Surgery

Silvia Rotemberg, M.D.

Any woman who has been told she has breast cancer knows the worry, stress, and fear that accompany the diagnosis. Once she has come to terms – at least to some degree – with the reality of having treatable breast cancer, she must then endure one or more of the following:

- Chemotherapy
- Radiation
- Surgery

Almost all breast cancer treatment plans include the removal of tumors (lumpectomy) or the entirety of one of her breasts (mastectomy). In some cases, a woman must undergo a double-mastectomy, the removal of both breasts.

Even before any surgery is performed to remove the cancer, the patient needs to consider and discuss her choices for breast reconstruction (the formation of a new breast shape) with a plastic surgeon.

Having her breast reconstructed after the grueling course of breast cancer treatment can help make a woman feel more like her former self.

Most women don't realize that they are entitled to this procedure either at the time of the initial cancer surgery – or months or even years later. A recent study indicated that less than 30% of eligible women were even told by their oncologic breast surgeon that they had a right to breast reconstruction following a mastectomy or lumpectomy.

In an attempt to rectify this terrible situation, federal and state laws were put into place to protect a woman's right to breast reconstruction.

The law requires health insurance companies including Medicare and Medicaid, to provide coverage for breast and nipple reconstruction in addition to any needed procedures on the healthy breast to improve the balance between the two. Insurance must also cover any complications arising from mastectomy or reconstruction.

In short, breast reconstruction must be covered by insurance – including Medicare and Medicaid – whether or not the surgery is performed immediately or years later.

You can decide to have immediate breast reconstruction after a mastectomy with the mandatory consent of your oncological surgeon. If your doctor recommends mastectomy without reconstruction for advanced cancer, it's better to wait one month after you complete chemotherapy and six months after your radiation, due to the potential for wound-healing problems. Over time, radiation treatments can permanently affect the skin's pigment, elasticity, and texture, which could also impact the appearance of reconstructed breasts or the lumpectomy alone.

BREAST RECONSTRUCTION IS DONE WITH ONE OF THE FOLLOWING PROCEDURES:

Implants

A breast implant is a round or teardrop-shaped silicone shell filled with either a saline solution (salt water) or silicone gel. In most cases, the first step of breast cancer reconstruction with an implant is the placement of a tissue expander. A tissue expander is a temporary implant that can be filled over the course of two- to- three months. This stretches this skin and chest muscles in preparation for the placement of the more permanent saline or silicone implant.

In a situation in which a woman has had a nipple-sparing mastectomy, there's sometimes enough remaining breast skin to forego the need for a tissue expander. Therefore, in this case an implant can be placed within the breast in an immediate reconstruction, with mastectomy and reconstruction in a single operation.

Breast implants are available with two different fillers: saline and silicone. Saline-filled breast implants consist of a silicone elastomer shell filled with saline solution.

Silicone implants have a longer history. The newer generation of silicone implants comes in different shapes and features a more cohesive gel. The thickest of these are sometimes called "gummy bear" implants. Made with highly cohesive silicone, they are more scientifically known as "form stable" implants. For many women, these are the best choice.

Surgical reconstruction with implants is shorter than autologous reconstruction; it also has a faster recovery time.

Autologous Breast Reconstruction

When a plastic surgeon uses a patient's own tissues to replace tissue lost in a lumpectomy or mastectomy, it is referred to as "autologous breast reconstruction." In such a procedure, the patient's body is both the donor and the recipient of the relocated tissue. The term autologous means "from the same individual." This procedure is also known as "tissue flap reconstruction."

During the operation, the plastic surgeon takes skin, fat,

and sometimes a "flap" of muscle from one location of the body and forms it into a breast shape. While doing so, the surgeon also ensures that the transplanted tissue retains the proper blood supply.

The most common donor sites – places from which the tissue is extracted – are the belly, back, buttocks, or inner thighs.

Autologous reconstruction includes several options based on how the surgery is performed and the location of the donor site. The initials in the terms below refer to this location:

- **TRAM Flap** – the best known of these options, in this procedure tissue is taken from the abdominal area, from which the plastic surgeon reconstructs and forms the new breast.
- **Lattissumus Dorsi Flap** – this reconstruction takes its name from the latissimus dorsi muscle, located in the upper back. During this surgery, the plastic surgeon takes muscle, fat, and skin from the upper back and uses them to create the new breast mound.
- **DIEP (Deep Inferior Epigastric Perforator)** – in this flap procedure no muscle is moved, making it essentially like a "tummy tuck." The DIEP flap takes tissues from the abdominal wall, leaving the muscles in place.
- **SGAP (Superior Gluteal Artery Perforator) Flap** – this procedure employs fat and skin from the upper buttock to recreate the breast. Most women have enough fat and other tissue in their upper gluteal area to create the new breast. If there's no sufficient tissue, a small implant can be used to help fill out the form of the new breast. This procedure is similar to that used for a buttock lift, but includes an artery and vein to supply blood to the newly transplanted tissue. No gluteal muscles are cut or moved during the operation.
- **IGAP (Inferior Gluteal Artery Perforator)** – this procedure is similar to the SGAP flap. However, the

IGAP flap uses fat and skin from the lower buttock to create the new breast. As in the case of the SGAP procedure, if there's insufficient tissue in the area, a small implant can be used to increase the size of the breast as needed. Again, this procedure is similar to the one used for a buttock lift with the important distinction of including an artery and vein to supply blood to the newly transplanted tissue. No gluteal muscles are cut or moved during the operation.

FAT TRANSFER USING FAT GRAFTING PROCEDURES

In a fat transfer reconstruction procedure, fat is taken from a donor site on the woman's own body – usually the thighs, belly, or buttocks. The tissue is then specifically prepared and processed into a liquid and transferred to the breast in order to increase volume and size. The procedure is also known as fat grafting, fat transfer, or autologous fat transfer.

First, the patient is fitted with an external tissue expander called a "Brava." Prior to the surgery, the patient will be required to wear the Brava for four to six weeks. The Brava device looks like a bra; however, it features plastic cones for cups. These cones exert suction on the breast area and expand the tissue to create a matrix into which the surgeon will inject the specifically prepared and liquefied liposuctioned fat. Studies have proven the importance of the use of this Brava device for a breast reconstructed with fat grafting to retain its size and volume.

Reconstruction of larger breasts may require multiple fat graft procedures completed over a period of months.

One of the advantages of this fat grafting technique is that the fat is removed from an area of excess on your body – in a way combining cosmetic liposuction with breast reconstruction.

Another benefit? Many women who have had their breast reconstructed using fat grafting report that it has retained some sensation, allowing it to feel much like the other unreconstructed breast.

Standard fat grafting procedures can transfer naturally present stem cells with the tissue removed from the donor site.

COMBINATION RECONSTRUCTION

Several factors can create a situation where a woman may need to have a combination of reconstructive procedures in order to achieve proper results. This is often the case when a woman's breasts are large and also in some scenarios where there's insufficient fat in any one area of the body to complete the reconstruction.

A Board Certified plastic surgeon can combine procedures to achieve the very best results possible with breast reconstruction.

MEDICAL FACTORS OF BREAST RECONSTRUCTION

Although the patient's wishes are a crucial part of the decision-making process regarding the choice of breast reconstruction procedure, the plastic surgeon will address other medical issues as well.

Each procedure has its associated benefits and risks. A technique that may be best for one patient may be less optimal for another. A Board Certified, experienced plastic surgeon can help guide you along in your decision.

Here are some of the medical factors the surgeon must take into consideration:

- The patient's current state of health (healthier individuals can tolerate longer surgeries)
- Previous medical history
- Patient weight and body mass index (BMI)
- Previous surgical history including any cosmetic procedures. Previous abdominal, back, buttock, or thigh surgery can sometimes limit the amount of tissue available for a fat transfer procedure

Ultimately, the type of reconstruction a patient received will be based first on sound medical decisions, followed by the patient's other wishes.

THE SURGERY AND HOSPITAL STAY

The preparation for a breast reconstruction surgery takes up to two hours, including the administration of the anesthesia. The actual surgery takes from one to six hours.

If implant reconstruction is being done, the time involved in the operation is far shorter than that for autologous reconstruction. Frequently, the patient undergoing reconstruction with implants will be able to go home the same day as the surgery. Otherwise the usual hospital stay is one night.

With any of the flap procedures, the surgery is longer, with a hospital stay of 3-5 days.

DOWNTIME AND RECOVERY FROM BREAST RECONSTRUCTION

The time it takes to fully recover from a breast reconstruction depends on two things: an individual's personal rate of healing and the type of reconstructive surgery they had.

Surgical procedures performed ONLY with an implant have a shorter and easier recovery time than those employing any of the flap procedures or combined procedures.

The patient may have drainage tubes for a short while following surgery. These tubes remove fluids that collect in the surgical site.

The patient will likely be tired or sore for a few weeks following surgery; therefore, the doctor may prescribe medication to control any pain. Be sure to take all pain meds exactly as directed.

Downtime and recovery with these procedures takes about two to four weeks because different people recover at different rates. One woman may get back to her usual activities within six weeks, another may take much longer. As I've mentioned previously, much depends on the individual's physical condition before the surgery and the type of surgery they have.

No matter the procedure she undergoes, it's important for the woman recovering from breast reconstruction surgery to take it easy during the recuperation period.

Although a member of the surgical team will review specific

recovery instructions with you, here are a few tips for how to take care of yourself during your recuperation:

- Take care of the surgical site and dressings as specifically instructed
- Keep all appointments with the doctor
- Move slowly, taking care to avoid reaching, pulling, or pressing movements
- Avoid raising your arm above the head or behind the back
- If told it's alright o take a shower, face away from the spray to allow it to hit the back and not the chest area
- Don't lift any heavy weight – nothing above five pounds. If uncertain about the weight of any object, err on the side of caution
- Avoid sleeping on your stomach
- Do not vacuum, sweep, or take out the garbage
- Do not drive until you receive your doctor's approval – and only if you're not taking narcotic pain medication
- Avoid physically strenuous physical activity and aerobics

After breast reconstructive surgery, you will need to do some exercises for your shoulder and arm. A nurse or physiotherapist can demonstrate exactly how to perform each exercise and for how long.

When exercising, wear a comfortable and supportive bra, free of any under wires. Front-fastening bras are easier to get on and off than those that clasp in the back. Even when not exercising, your bra can help support and mold your breast reconstruction.

TIPS TO MAXIMIZE YOUR RECOVERY

- Walk each day
- Take naps and get plenty of rest
- Catch up on your reading
- Keep in close contact with your doctor about any worries or concerns that may arise

- Keep all of your doctor appointments
- Invite friends over to chat whenever you feel up to it

PROBLEMS AND COMPLICATIONS

As with all surgeries, breast reconstruction comes with some risks and possible complications. In general, the longer and more complicated the surgical procedure, the greater the potential risks.

Some risks immediately following surgery:

Pain and Discomfort – you will usually experience some pain and discomfort following breast reconstruction. Once you leave the hospital, it can usually be managed with prescription or over-the-counter pain relievers.

Wound Infection – this is a risk with any surgery. Telltale signs of a wound infection include a fever of over 101F, while your incision may appear red, warm to the touch, and maybe even swollen. If you experience any of these, you must contact your doctor immediately. Most likely, you'll be prescribed antibiotics and instructed to rest. Typically the infection will clear up in about a week or so. In some cases, hospitalization may be necessary in order for you to receive intravenous antibiotics for three days.

Fluid Under the Wound – any surgery will produce fluid, which may collect in the wound area. Your surgeon will have placed one or more of the long, thin tubes in the wound to drain off this fluid. Notwithstanding these drains, fluid can sometimes collect under the wound. If there's only a little, it may reabsorb into the surrounding tissues. If there's too much fluid for the body to absorb on its own, your surgeon or nurse will remove it using a small needle and syringe.

Flap Failure – with autologous tissue reconstruction such as flap surgery, one risk is that the flap of tissue, once transplanted, may die due to poor circulation. If this occurs, the patient must go back into surgery during which the surgeon will try to salvage the flap. If it's unsalvageable, the flap will have to be removed.

COMPLICATIONS THAT MAY ARISE IN THE LONG RUN

- Breasts unequal in size due to weight changes in the patient
- Leaking of implant fluid
- Changing shape or hardening of the implant
- A need to change the implant in 5-10 years
- Radiation changes such as hardening and tightening of the skin

Keep in mind that breast reconstruction surgery has been successfully performed for decades. Just be sure to select a Board Certified plastic surgeon; one you trust and with whom you have a good rapport.

RECREATING THE NIPPLE AND AREOLA

Sometimes, the surgeon performing the mastectomy can preserve the areola, nipple, and skin. This is called a "nipple-sparing mastectomy." Frequently however, this cannot be done; therefore recreating the nipple after the reconstruction is the only solution. All breast reconstruction procedures create a smooth breast shape and surface with no nipple and no areola (the pigmented area surrounding the nipple).

Some women choose to have their nipples reconstructed and some don't. This remains a personal decision.

If a woman does not wish to have her nipple and areola recreated, she has several choices to consider:

Nipple Made from Her Own Body Tissue – at least three to four months after breast reconstruction surgery and evidence of full healing and settling are present, a surgeon can create a new nipple from a woman's own body tissue. This is an additional surgery and it offers the most natural-looking result of all the nipple recreation options.

This procedure is done on an outpatient basis, under local

anesthetic.

During the surgery, the surgeon reconstructs the new nipple and areola to match the position, shape, color, projection, and texture of the remaining natural one.

The tissue used to build the new nipple is taken from another area of the woman's body. Called a "donor site," this area might be the newly created breast, the nipple and areola of the natural breast, the ear, buttocks, or upper inner part of the thigh.

Since this procedure for reconstructing the nipple is considered minor surgery, most patients can return home shortly after it's completed.

Tattooing may additionally be used to match the color of the nipple and the areola of the other breast. Three-dimensional color shading of the nipple can increase the visual perception of physical depth. Frequently, medical aestheticians use the dermabrasion technique, where a high-frequency probe is used to push pigment into the skin. To achieve the best results, several sessions may be required.

Nipple Tattoo – Nipple tattoos are an option for women who do not want to undergo the surgical procedures required to achieve a nipple made from her own body tissue.

Nipple and areola tattoos have been an option with breast reconstruction for many years. This type of tattooing is very similar to any other tattoo procedure. In fact, there are tattoo artists who specialize in nipple and areola tattoos; however, most insurance will not pay for tattooing done outside the medical environment.

During the nipple and areola tattoo the doctor will match the size, shape, and color with those on the opposite breast. A skilled surgeon may be able to make the tattooed nipple appear three-dimensional, creating an even more natural look.

A tattooed nipple will not protrude or be detectable under clothing.

Latex Stick-On Nipple – if a woman doesn't want any more surgery, she may decide to have a stick-on nipple fashioned from a mold of the nipple on the other breast. To accomplish this, a mold is created. Then a technician fills the mold and creates a stick-on nipple that's a close replica of the natural nipple in shape and color.

This latex nipple can be stuck on every day and is held in place with special glue. The advantage to choosing a latex nipple? You can avoid another surgery. The disadvantages? A latex nipple must be put on every day, the glue can be messy, and the nipple may not stay in place.

Another stick-on nipple option is a self-adhesive, peel and stick nipple. These are not specifically tailored to match the natural nipple on the other breast. However, they have the advantage of being inexpensive and self-adhering.

ADDITIONAL SURGERY TO MAKE THE BREASTS MATCH

If you're having surgery performed on just one breast (after a single mastectomy), your plastic surgeon will pay particular care to match the new reconstruction with the other natural breast. However, creating a match may not be possible unless the patient undergoes surgery to the other breast as well. At least a third of all women having reconstruction to one breast will also need surgery for the other.

Surgery to the opposite breast will achieve one of the following:

1. Make the breast bigger to match the reconstructed one.
2. Make the breast smaller to create the match.
3. Tighten and lift the breast to prevent it from drooping more than the newly reconstructed breast.

Each of these surgeries involves different procedures and resulting effects, including recovery time and the location of any scars.

Making the other breast larger will usually involve the

placement of an implant and possibly some fat grafting. The resulting scar is small and difficult to detect – situated usually in the fold under the breast.

The position of the scars following surgery to either decrease the size of the breast or to make it less droopy varies depending on the technique used by your surgeon. The scar may be around the areola, in the skin fold beneath the breast, and sometimes in a vertical line joining the two.

WORKING WITH A BOARD CERTIFIED PLASTIC SURGEON

The American Board of Medical Specialties has identified 24 medical subspecialty boards offering certification.

Plastic surgery is identified as one of those 24 specialties.

Board Certification is a rigorous process involving extensive training (5-8 years in plastic surgery), written and oral examinations, adherence to a strict ethical code, and ongoing demonstration of competence.

Any licensed physician can call himself or herself a cosmetic surgeon; therefore, it's of paramount importance to find a properly trained and certified provider.

To have a safe and successful breast reconstruction, it's vital that you locate a plastic surgeon with the expertise and experience necessary for a successful procedure.

Make sure your surgeon is Board Certified in Plastic Surgery.

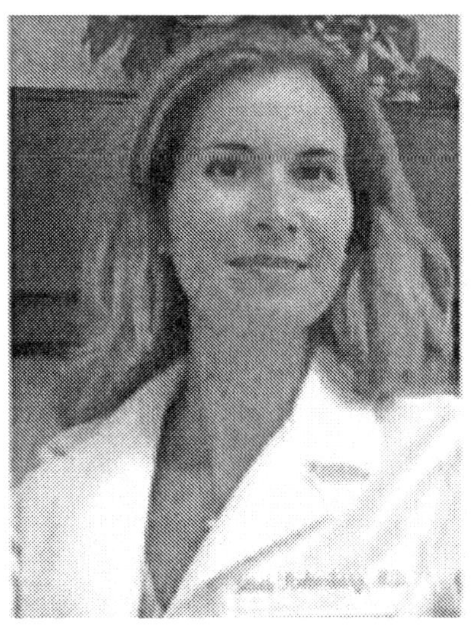

Silvia Rotemberg M.D.

is a cosmetic and reconstructive plastic surgeon in South Miami, Florida.

She is board-certified by the American Board of Plastic Surgery and is a world leader in her industry having worked at the highest levels of plastic surgery, including the world-renowned Cleveland Clinic where she practiced for many years.

Dr. Rotemberg believes plastic surgery is both a science and an art. Dr. Rotemberg's passion for aesthetics is demonstrated through her artistic eye as well as a wealth of scientific know-how.

Through her focus on individualized procedures, efficient recovery, and organic results, Dr. Rotemberg's plastic surgery South Miami office has become a highly sought-after location for tasteful cosmetic and reconstructive surgery procedures.

Visit her website: www.rotembergmd.com

Chapter 7

Fat Grafting, BRAVA, Breast Reconstruction Options

Roger Khouri M.D.,

Richard Nadal M.D., and

Daniel Calva, M.D.

Fat Grafting and Percutaneous Surgery in Breast Reconstruction

The Benefits of BRAVA and Autologous Fat Transfer (BRAVA + AFT)

"Fat grafting with percutaneous surgery is an extremely versatile departure from the traditional approach to breast reconstruction allowing a more precise method of molding the tissues while at the same time providing the flexibility to enhance specific areas

of the breast."

Introduction

The field of medicine continues to evolve, and plastic surgery is no different. Plastic surgery takes its name from the Greek word "Plastikos" which means "capable of being shaped or molded." In this chapter, we will see how advances in technology and refinements in surgical instrumentation now allow plastic surgeons to perform true tissue molding in breast reconstruction through a series of minimally invasive outpatient procedures. We will describe our experience at the Miami Breast Center with Fat Grafting, also known as autologous fat transfer (AFT), in breast reconstruction. Our protocol pays special attention to preoperative preparation and postoperative care. Active patient participation before and after the surgery is key to a successful outcome, and can help decrease the number of procedures required.

As discussed in Chapter 6, breast reconstruction is typically performed in stages. The objectives are: the creation of a breast mound, creation of a nipple-areola complex, and achieving optimal symmetry. For various reasons, we often have to manipulate the other breast with a reduction, lift, or augmentation in order to achieve proper symmetry. As we saw in that chapter, there are now many alternatives when it comes to reconstruction following any type of ablative surgery for breast cancer. There is no perfect technique and each has its advantages and disadvantages.

Why Fat?

Reconstruction of the breast mound requires the addition of volume to compensate for the volume of tissue removed. Fat is found throughout the body and can be removed from areas where it is not wanted and placed in areas where it is needed. It is harvested by low negative pressure liposuction, and injected into the breast in small volumes to create, or add volume to, the breast mound. To be successful, it is essential to respect the tissue requirements for graft survival. We accomplish this by observing meticulous technique during the harvesting, processing, and grafting procedure. With proper technique, large volume fat grafting can now be performed safely and effectively, exactly what breast reconstruction requires. Either by itself, or in combination with other procedures, fat grafting has now become a practical alternative in breast reconstruction. It also has the added benefit of improving the overall shape of the body in the areas from which the fat is taken.

History

While fat grafting to the breast has been tried since the late nineteenth century, it wasn't until the last decade that it became popularized throughout the world. The combination of mammography, breast ultrasound imaging, and MRIs make the screening and diagnosis of breast cancer more precise. Suspicious lesions can now be differentiated from artifacts, such as calcifications resulting from injected fat. Thus, major hurdles in the implementation of fat grafting have been addressed, and this procedure can now deliver consistent results with properly planned outpatient fat grafting sessions. It is now accepted as a viable alternative in breast surgery by major plastic surgery societies as a safe and effective procedure that does not increase the risk of cancer.

Theory of Fat Grafting, Tissue Molding and Percutaneous Surgery

Fat survival after grafting is essential if it is to be a reliable method of reconstruction. In other words, the grafted cells have to survive once they are placed in the recipient tissue. While normal tissue is usually quite ready to accept a modest amount of volume, previous surgery or radiation can create a more hostile environment for the survival of these delicate fat cells. The proposed recipient of the graft has to be prepared in order to provide an adequate bed much like the preparation and irrigation of arid land prior to planting a crop. This is where we need the patient's help. We utilize preoperative external tissue expansion by applying a suction cup known as BRAVA system, which we will discuss in more detail in the next section. Briefly, it applies a three dimensional pull on the tissues of surface of the chest that allows the tissues to expand; increasing the size of the recipient and improving its blood supply. We can then graft more fat with a better chance of survival.

Even so, the surgeon then has to determine the correct amount of fat to be grafted in order to avoid over-grafting. If too much fat is grafted, the pressure in the tissue will rise, compromise the capillary blood supply, and the graft fails. We use dilute fat on purpose to allow fluid absorption after surgery. Tissue pressure decreases and fat survival improves. We also depend on the BRAVA system before surgery to help by stretching the tissues before surgery. The larger space can accept more volume than could otherwise be safely grafted. In this way we can decrease the number of procedures required in the creation of a breast mound.

As always, proper instrumentation is necessary for the success of any procedure by providing efficiency, precision and safety. Specialized instruments developed at The Miami Breast Center for fat harvesting and grafting increase efficiency by economy of movement. This facilitates the procedure and allows the required precision for optimal fat graft survival. By improving efficiency, the surgeon can also save precious time under anesthesia without compromising the consistency of the results.

Special instrumentation is also required to break up deep scars and permit movement and molding of the tissue. During the grafting process deep scars are released then injected with fat so as to separate portions of the scar itself. We call this changing the cicatrix into a matrix. After a few sessions the tissue becomes softer and its quality and mobility improves. It can then be properly molded by percutaneous suturing.

Percutaneous surgery refers to surgery that is performed through the skin via needle sticks rather than typical incisions. It is a minimally invasive way to manipulate the tissues without significant scarring. Liposuction is a type of percutaneous surgery. AFT is another type of intervention that relies on percutaneous surgery. For purposes of tissue shaping we have also developed special instrumentation that allows us to mold the tissues using different suturing techniques to advance tissues percutaneously. Recruiting tissue from the upper abdomen and the side of the chest percutaneously allows us build a breast mound without major surgery or the scarring associated with other techniques. For symmetry, we can also reduce, lift and/or augment the opposite side percutaneously. Percutaneous suturing is a powerful tool in harnessing the benefits of adjacent tissue recruitment into the breast mound with less morbidity than the more traditional flaps described in Chapter 5.

Preoperative Preparation and BRAVA Protocol

Prior to AFT, a preoperative MRI is essential to evaluate the soft tissues under the mastectomy flaps, or the remaining breast gland if a partial mastectomy was performed. The MRI is a critical component not only to evaluate for any potential recurrence, but also for long term follow-up and evaluation for any potential complications. The MRI is performed with a contrast called Gadolinium, and patients are screened for any potential allergies to the contrast, for renal or liver insufficiency, and for pregnancy, which might preclude the use of the contrast. Gadolinium contrast is necessary in breast MRI since it improves the clarity of the scanned images and internal structures.

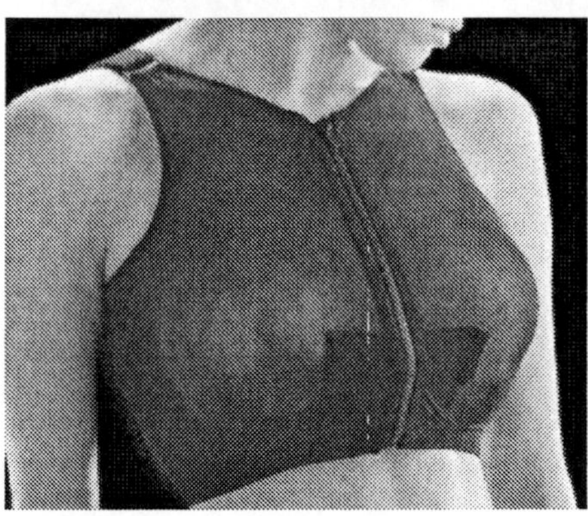

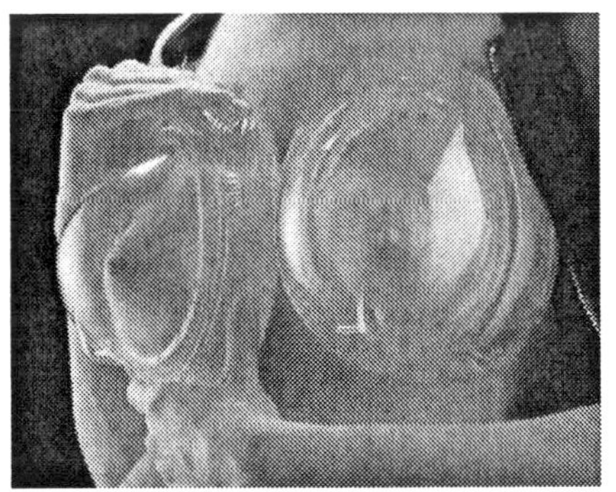

We take our time educating patients who are contemplating breast reconstruction with BRAVA assisted tissue expansion and AFT. It may take several educational sessions and emailed tutorials in order to familiarize patients on how to wear and cycle the BRAVA system. In the office, the patient will have a trial using the BRAVA device. This typically consists of a suction cycle over a 20 min period wearing the BRAVA device. The specific size of the BRAVA device will be selected depending on the patient's chest dimensions and breast size. The patient then decides if she can tolerate the cycles and wishes to proceed with BRAVA assisted tissue expansion and AFT.

BRAVA is started 3-4 weeks prior to surgery. The patients are instructed on how to apply and operate the device, and we monitor their progress during the preoperative period. Patients wear the BRAVA system for four hours the first day, adding two hours every day until they reach 14 hours per day of continuous wear. The BRAVA device is then utilized for 14 hours a day until the day of surgery. The recommended final total dose prior to AFT is 200 hours of breast expansion with the BRAVA system in the final two weeks prior to surgery.

When BRAVA is used correctly we expect to see some swelling, superficial bruising, and blistering of the expanded skin as well as small red spots on the skin known as petechiae which result from capillary rupture. These changes are temporary and resolve on their own after surgery. Their presence indicates that the soft tissues are well expanded and optimized for autologous fat grafting. Applying Opsite or Tegaderm on the skin can minimize blistering and helps prevent irritation.

We typically do not use BRAVA in patients that have implants. In this situation, the tissue simply pulls away from the implant and does not expand. Our approach is to downsize the implants and replace the implant volume with fat. The implants can eventually be removed altogether with the help of percutaneous suturing in one of the fat grafting sessions if that is the objective.

Each Patient is Different

Reconstruction with fat grafting can be performed in a complete mastectomy whether immediate or delayed, skin or nipple sparing. It has a role in reconstruction after breast conservation surgery with lumpectomy and radiation. It also gives us an additional tool as a "salvage" procedure when other techniques have failed. Fat grafting with percutaneous surgery is an extremely versatile departure from the traditional approach to breast reconstruction, allowing a more precise method of molding and shaping the tissues while at the same time providing the flexibility to enhance specific areas of the breast.

In the immediate reconstruction, the first stage is performed at the time of mastectomy. This is the perfect opportunity to add fat prior to the onset of scarring. It adds volume, minimizes the detrimental effects of postoperative scarring, and prepares the terrain for a greater volume of fat grafting in the next procedure. In many cases, immediate reconstruction with fat grafting can provide sufficient cleavage to simulate a social breast after the mastectomy. We can even perform what we call a delayed immediate reconstruction. This occurs when a patient has her mastectomy in her hometown and a few days later proceeds with fat grafting. If radiation therapy is planned postoperatively however, we prefer to preserve valuable fat until radiation has been completed.

In delayed primary reconstruction the first stage is performed several months or years after the mastectomy. The number of procedures depends on whether or not the patient has had radiation. Without radiation, breast mound reconstruction may be achieved in approximately three outpatient sessions. With radiation it may be up to six.

As discussed in chapter 4, in breast conservation surgery a lumpectomy is followed by radiation therapy. This typically preserves much of the breast tissue depending on the original size of the breast. However, the remaining breast tissue has to be radiated in order to control local disease. Radiation will then lead to local tissue scarring that is difficult to contain and difficult to reconstruct. We have found that the best time to proceed with fat grafting is immediately after the end of radiation. The swelling in the tissues can provide safe sanctuary for a fat graft and the graft can help prevent many of the changes resulting from the radiation itself. We can take advantage of this adversary and turn it into an opportunity. It is quite a change from the traditional way of thinking.

Unfortunately, there are times when other reconstructive procedures fail. It is reassuring to know that fat grafting is still available as an option to complete the breast reconstruction. With patience and dedication, the scarred tissue in these very difficult cases can be slowly softened and augmented to the point where sufficient soft tissue molding is possible. It may take some extra procedures, but a very reasonable result can usually be obtained.

Revising a previously reconstructed breast can pose significant challenges depending on the existing situation. We carefully analyze the patient needs, the amount and quality of the tissues along with residual scarring, and establish realistic objectives.

Each situation requires an individually designed plan of action. Each series of procedures is specifically tailored to address the particular needs of the patient. From our perspective, each patient is different.

Postoperative Care and Follow-Up

The follow up period and care are ongoing, and patients are followed for life. The postoperative care includes prevention of fat re-absorption, identifying possible complications, and evaluating for the need of future surgical interventions. Before surgery, BRAVA expands the soft tissue in preparation for grafting. After surgery, the BRAVA expanded tissue has been turned from a cicatrix into a matrix occupied with small droplets of fat grafts. However, the healing process can create fibrosis and cause the expanded fat grafted matrix to contract. We like to maintain the matrix as large as possible to allow the maximum amount of fat to survive. Therefore, after the first week, the patient is encouraged to wear the BRAVA device as much as possible to maintain the matrix expanded. Once the fat survives, the fat graft will maintain the matrix expanded. This will allow a greater amount of fat to be grafted in a subsequent session.

Most planed re-interventions are done within a 3-6 month period. This allows the prior fat graft to stabilize, and the inflammatory process to subside. Only after the inflammation subsides, will the surgeon know the extent of graft survival. It is at this point that the patient and surgeon will have a more accurate understanding of how much volume or shaping is still needed. The particular goals of the next procedure can then be determined. A post-operative MRI is always performed 6 months following the last procedure.

Conclusion

Fat grafting has been found to have many beneficial effects on local tissue. By breaking up the scar tissue and introducing fat we can ultimately decrease the amount of contracture and improve the overall quality and mobility of the tissue. With percutaneous surgery the tissue can then be shaped as needed. The fat is used for volume enhancement and at the same time as a glue to hold the molded tissue in its new position.

Percutaneous surgery with AFT is a twenty first century procedure, a paradigm departure from the mutilating patch-like flap reconstruction, and from the insertion of foreign body implants. It empowers women with the ability to regenerate, in situ, beautiful and sensate breasts without incisions. The process takes time. Reconstructing a new breast requires patience and compliance with BRAVA use. At the Miami Breast Center we have developed a reliable intervention that optimizes the success of each fat grafting session thereby decreasing the number of procedures required. It has many advantages over traditional methods of reconstruction. It is performed in an outpatient setting, it has less morbidity and has been shown to lower costs. With this excellent alternative, we are at the forefront of breast reconstruction.

REFERENCES

R.K. Khouri, J.M. Smit, E. Cardoso, et al. "Percutaneous aponeurotomy and lipofilling: A regenerative alternative to flap reconstruction?" *Plast Reconstr Surg.* 132.5 (2013): 1280–1290. Print.

R.K. Khouri, G. Rigotti, E. Cardoso, et al. "Megavolume Autologous Fat Transfer: Part I. Theory and Principles." *Plast Reconstr Surg.* 133.3 (2014): 550-557. Print.

R.K. Khouri, et al. "Megavolume Autologous Fat Transfer: Part II Practice and Techniques." *Plast Reconstr Surg.* 133.6 (2014): 1369-77. Print.

R.K. Khouri, G. Rigotti, et al. "Tissue-Engineered Breast Reconstruction with Brava-Assisted Fat Grafting: A 7-Year, 488-Patient, Multicenter Experience." *Plast Reconstr Surg.* 135.3 (2015): 643-658. Print.

Khouri, Roger K., and Biggs, Thomas, et al. *Your Natural Breasts: A Better Way to Augment, Reconstruct, and Correct Using Your Own Fat*. San Pedro Publishing, 2012. Print.

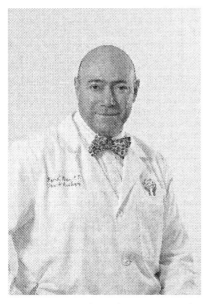

Roger K. Khouri M.D.

is a Plastic Surgeon with more than 20 years of experience with breast reconstruction. Fifteen years ago, while a Professor of Plastic Surgery at Washington University he published what was then the world's largest experience with microsurgical breast reconstruction. Over the past 8 years, he has perfected a much more patient friendly alternative method of breast reconstruction. He is invited with great acclaim all over the World to present and teach this minimally invasive new procedure. The procedure is minimally invasive, done as outpatient; it involves no incisions, no new scars, no implant, and gives the patient the bonus benefit of a few liposuctions body-contouring improvements.

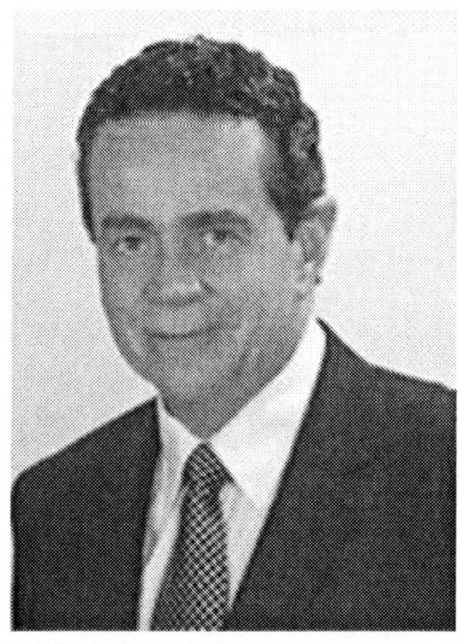

Richard D. Nadal, M.D., F.A.C.S., Board Certified in Plastic and reconstructive Surgery.

He earned his medical degree in 1979 and the University of Puerto Rico School of Medicine. He then continued his training in general surgery at the University of Florida and Washington D.C. in Georgetown University. In 1985 he received his certification from the American Board of Surgery.

Dr. Nadal continued his training in plastic surgery at the Indiana University which included six months of neck and head surgery. He then continued his training and finished a fellowship at the prominent Manhattan Eye, Ear and Throat Hospital. In 1989 he was certified by the American Board of Plastic Surgery after completing a total of 8 years in the surgical training alongside the best in his field.

Afterwards he established himself in Miami, Florida where he continued practicing surgery for 18 years.He is an active member of the following organizations: American Society for Aesthetic Plastic Surgery, American Society of Plastic Surgeons, Fellow of the American College of Surgeons and Colegio de Médicos-Cirujanos de Puerto Rico.

Learn more about Dr. Nadal at www.miamibreastcenter.com.

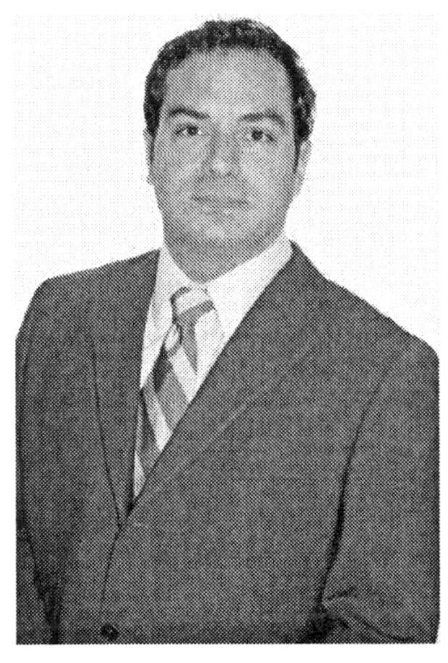

Daniel Calva, M.D.

Dr. Calva completed his training at the prestigious Johns Hopkins/University of Maryland Plastic & Reconstructive Surgery program. His main focus is on aesthetic/cosmetic and complex head-to-toe reconstruction. The Johns Hopkins Hospital has been ranked by *US News and World Reports* as the #1 hospital in the US for 23 years.

Dr. Calva obtained his Bachelor education at Georgetown University, where he graduated with honors. He then attended one of the top medical schools in the country, the esteemed Carver College of Medicine. After medical school he completed seven years of training in General Surgery (Board Certified) at the University of Iowa Hospitals and Clinics, one of the top residency programs in the US. During his General Surgery training, he did two years of molecular genetics, where he conducted award-winning research on cancer biology, and was awarded two grants by the NIH (National Institutes of Health) to performed cutting edge molecular research in cancer genetics.

Currently, Dr. Calva sees patients at the Miami Breast Center located in 580 Crandon Blvd. Suite 102, Key Biscayne, FL 33149. He can be reached by email at DrDanCalva@gmail.com or by phone at either (305) 365-5595 or (888) 488-5886.

Chapter 8

Chemotherapy Treatment

Elisa Krill-Jackson, M.D.

BREAST CANCER

Breast cancer is the leading cause of cancer in US women, but not the leading cause of cancer death. More than 80% of women diagnosed with breast cancer are cured, and that is because of the improved understanding and treatments we have for this disease, due to 40 years of research. In this chapter, I will explain what breast cancer is, what treatments are available, and genetic causes of breast cancer.

WHAT IS CANCER?

In its simplest terms, cancer is a group of cells with unregulated growth and the ability to invade normal tissue and spread. Cells in our body are constantly multiplying and dying, with the new cells replacing the old. Built into our cells' DNA are instructions for both dividing and dying. To divide, each cell will duplicate its DNA, and then split into two separate cells. However, sometimes cells make mistakes when they duplicate their DNA or when an agent damages the DNA. Although we have proteins that check for mistakes, sometimes errors get by. If the cell makes an error in an area of DNA that controls cell division, the cell may lose its controls over division and death; consequently, it will divide and multiply uncontrollably and lose its programming for dying at a certain time. The abnormal cells will accumulate and the mass will grow in size. This is what a cancerous tumor is.

Because these abnormal cancerous cells continue to divide, they can accumulate more mistakes in their DNA, which may allow them to spread throughout the lymphatics or blood stream and grow in different organs. These mutations can also make them resistant to therapies, just like bacteria become resistant to antibiotics. The ability of the cancer cells to mutate (change) allows them to escape many of our bodies' and science's efforts to control and kill them.

HEREDITARY BREAST CANCER

Some people are born with a predisposition to breast cancer, although only 5-10% of breast cancers are hereditary. There are genes in the cells of our body which are call tumor suppressor genes and oncogenes. Tumor suppressor genes are designed to control cancer by controlling cell division. When they are abnormal, or mutated, cells are more likely to make mistakes when dividing, and develop into cancers. Oncogenes are cells that are normally not active in the body, but when abnormal, can become active and predispose to cancer.

There are many genes which predispose to breast cancer. These include BRCA1, BRCA2, PALB2, CHEK2, RAD51, and P53, among others. Clearly the most common genes causing breast cancer are BRCA1 and 2.

BRCA1 and 2 mutations predispose to both breast and ovarian cancer. BRCA2 also predisposes to breast cancer in men, melanoma, pancreatic cancer, and prostate cancer. However, the risks for these latter cancers are not extremely high. The risk for ovarian cancer in women with BRCA1 mutations is up to 40% and BRCA2 up to 25% lifetime. For breast cancer, both of these genes increase the lifetime risk to nearly 85%.

Breast cancers associated with BRCA 1 and 2 generally are more aggressive cancers that occur at younger ages. It is not uncommon to see BRCA-associated cancers in women in their 20s. For women with BRCA mutations or family histories of BRCA gene mutations who have not yet been tested, breast screening with MRI's is recommended, beginning at age 25!

Although BRCA mutations can been seen in all ethnic groups, certain populations have a higher prevalence of them. These include Ashkenazi Jews and people of Dutch, Icelandic, or Norwegian ancestry. BRCA mutations are common as well in African Americans, and in fact are a leading cause of breast cancer in the Bahamas.

Diagnosing a cancer as hereditary is important for both management of a patient's cancer and for prevention of future cancers in both the patient and her family. Because of the risk of a second breast cancer in patients with a BRCA 1 or 2 mutation is up to 60%, many women will opt for bilateral mastectomies. Other mutations such as PALB2 and CHEK2, for example, do not confer such a high rate of cancer; therefore, increased screening with six monthly exams and yearly MRI's may be appropriate. BRCA 1 and 2 mutation carriers should also have their ovaries removed when they have finished childbearing. The newest recommendations advise oophorectomy at age 35 in BRCA1 carriers and 40 in BRCA2 carriers.

If a patient has a gene mutation, it means that one of the two copies (one each from their mother and father) is abnormal. Thus, the abnormal gene could come from either parent, and therefore a patient's father's family history is important in diagnosis. One in two sibling and children of an affected patient statistically will have also inherited the mutation, and therefore it is important to test all family members to prevent cancer in those unaffected.

GENES AND BREAST CANCER

Cancer cells behave differently based on the genes that are active inside them. All the cells in our body begin with the exact same DNA, but a colon cell is a colon cell based on what genes are turned on (or "expressed"). These genes are different from those present in a breast cell or a pancreas cell or a lung cell. So when a cell becomes cancerous, it starts out very much like the cell from which it came. Breast cancers, therefore, behave differently than lung cancers, even if the breast cell spreads to the lung or liver.

Cancer cells can be characterized by the genes that are "turned on" in the tumor and the proteins these genes produce. So a breast cancer cell that's "estrogen receptor positive" produces a protein that allows it to recognize and respond to estrogen. A cancer cell that's HER2 neu positive, makes excess of the HER2 neu protein. These characteristics are of the particular cancer cell and the changes it has developed as it has transitioned from a normal cell to a cancer cell. It does not refer to the genes or cells a person was born with – just to that particular cancer. With time, a cancer cell can develop more mutations and changes, just like in evolution. Therefore, when a cancer recurs or changes behavior, it is important to get another sample of the tumor to determine if its characteristics have changed.

PATHOLOGY

There are a number of important factors to know about a cancer that influences prognosis. Many of these can be found in the pathology report.

SITE OF ORIGIN

The breast is made up of milk glands, called lobules, and ducts, which connect these glands to the nipple. The cells lining the lobules or ducts can transform into cancer cells by genetic mutations, developing into lobular or ductal carcinoma.

IN-SITU VS INVASIVE BREAST CANCER

Ductal carcinoma in situ means that that tumor cells are inside the duct of the tumor, and this is therefore a "pre-cancer," as the abnormal cells trapped inside the duct walls do not have the ability to spread. Invasive (or infiltrating) cancer means that the cancer has broken through the wall of the duct or the lobule of the breast, infiltrated into the breast tissue, and has the ability to spread.

One term that has gone out of parlance is lobular carcinoma in situ. This is now known as lobular neoplasia, because it is not a cancer or pre-cancer in and of itself, but a lesion that signals that a woman has a higher risk of breast cancer in the future.

SIZE

The larger a cancer, the higher the risk of it spreading. A tumor smaller than one centimeter is considered very small and usually can only be found on an imaging study such as a mammogram or MRI.

LYMPH NODES

The number of lymph nodes involved also correlates with the risk of the cancer spreading.

STAGE

Stage is determined by the size of the tumor, the number of lymph nodes involved, and whether or not the cancer has spread outside of the breast and lymph node area. This is known as the TNM system: T, for tumor size; N for nodes; and M for metastases outside the breast and lymphatic area (or not). A Stage I tumor is under 2 centimeters in size with no involved lymph nodes, TINOMO.

A Stage II tumor is either over 2 centimeters in size or has 1-3 lymph nodes involved. Stage III tumors typically involve 4 or more lymph nodes or the skin of the breast.

While the stage is very important, we're learning that changes deeper inside the tumor, at the level of active genes, is really what determines the prognosis of the tumor. The simplest tests we have to evaluate these changes are:

- The tumor grade;
- The estrogen and progesterone receptors;
- The HER2 neu protein;
- The Grade; and
- The Ki67.

GRADE

The grade of the tumor refers to how much the breast tumor looks like normal breast tissue. A tumor with cells appearing similar to normal breast cells would be called a "grade 1" tumor. A tumor that is dividing rapidly, with cells appearing less regular would be called a "grade 3" tumor, which indicates a more aggressive, rapidly growing tumor more likely to metastasize.

Normal breast tissues respond to estrogen and progesterone via proteins on the cell surface called the estrogen and progesterone receptors. These are like locks that activate the cell when the key – the estrogen or progesterone hormone – is inserted. Most breast cancer cells retain the estrogen and progesterone receptors. These particular cancers are less likely to metastasize (spread outside the breast and lymphatic area) and can also be treated with hormonal therapy, conferring on them a better prognosis in general.

The Ki67 is a test that looks at what percentage of breast cancer cells are actively dividing into new cells: the higher the number, theoretically the more aggressive and risky a cancer. However, this test is often unreliable.

The HER2-neu protein is an important indicator of both prognosis and treatment. Tumors are classified as HER-2 0, 1+, 2+, or 3+. The 15-30% of tumors that are 3+ are considered HER2-neu positive, or HER2-neu amplified. Tumors that are 2+ are considered equivocal and a special test called a FISH (fluorescence in situ hybridization) is performed. The FISH test is considered positive if there are twice as many HER2-neu genes found as the number of a normal control gene. The HER2-neu test is vitally important to know. HER2 amplification makes a cancer extremely aggressive: even a 5 mm tumor has a significant chance of spreading!

However, since the introduction of the antibody Herceptin, an antibody that attacks cells with the HER2-neu protein, the prognosis of these tumors has become very favorable as long as appropriate treatment is administered.

Currently, our most difficult tumor to treat is known as a "triple negative" breast cancer. Triple negative refers to the fact that these tumors do not have estrogen or progesterone receptors or HER2-neu proteins on their surface. They tend to be aggressive, more likely to spread rapidly, and unresponsive to hormonal therapy or Herceptin. They do respond well to chemotherapy, however.

Although the pathology report offers much of what we need to know to treat a cancer appropriately, it is not complete. Estrogen and progesterone receptors and HER2 protein are only a small fraction of the characteristics of a tumor. Therefore, looking deeper into the genes that are turned on inside the tumor cell and the proteins contained within the tumor cell provides us with much more information. In the last 10 years, several tests have been devised to determine the "genomics" of the tumor – the genes turned on inside the tumor cells – to determine the prognosis of the cancer based on these changes. Some of these tests include Oncotype DX, Mammaprint, and Breast Cancer Index.

Genomic tests are currently most useful for the estrogen-sensitive cancers. Such tests allow us to determine if these cancers have a good or poor prognosis, and whether or not the patient would benefit from chemotherapy, or if hormonal therapy is sufficient. After surgery, a specimen of the tumor can be sent for the genomic test. It will be analyzed for the activity of genes related to hormonal sensitivity, proliferation, and invasion, and given a score which corresponds to the risk of the tumor eventually recurring or spreading. There are several of these tests including Oncotype DX, Mammoprint, and Breast Cancer Index.

The Oncotype DX test in particular has validated not only the relation of the score to the risk of metastasis over 10 years but also to the benefit of treatment with chemotherapy. Therefore, tumors with a "low recurrence score" have a good prognosis with hormonal therapy alone and do not benefit from chemotherapy. However, patients with a "high recurrence score" have a statistically large reduction in the risk of cancer recurrence and death with chemotherapy. These genomic tests have spared many women from the side effects of chemotherapy; those that are high risk receive it appropriately.

ADJUVANT TREATMENT

Radiation and surgery have been discussed in other chapters, so I will concentrate on "systemic therapy." Systemic therapy refers to the fact that this treatment – unlike surgery or radiation – is meant to kill cancer cells throughout the body.

WHY IS THIS A NECESSITY?

The same reason cancers can recur years later in other parts of the body: often, cancer cells have spread microscopically to other locations at the time of a patient's diagnosis. Although a PET scan, a CT scan, bone scan, and physical exam may not detect it, there may be microscopic cancer deposits at the time of the tumor's discovery in the breast.

The good news is that when a tumor is microscopic, the cells are much more vulnerable to therapies aimed at killing them. By the time it grows to a size that can be seen or felt outside of the breast region, it is not curable. That is why the treatment rendered after surgery, known as "adjuvant treatment," is so important. This is our one chance to kill any isolated tumor deposits and change the prognosis of the cancer. From years of studies we know that adjuvant therapy can improve the prognosis of some brea cancers by 50%!

Currently, there are three types of adjuvant systemic therapy in use: Hormonal therapy, chemotherapy, and antibody therapy.

HORMONAL THERAPY

Hormonal therapy is a "targeted therapy," the very first type of personalized medicine. Tumors with the estrogen and progesterone receptor proteins can be stimulated by estrogen and killed by limiting estrogen's ability to get to these receptors. The very first type of hormonal therapy used for breast cancer to eliminate estrogen was the removal of the ovaries in premenopausal women. We are still using this therapy successfully in many women, and recent studies have suggested improvement in the cure rate of cancer through the removal of the ovaries or the suppression of them chemically.

There are also medications that can be used as hormonal therapy. The first of these was Tamoxifen; which is still an excellent drug used for both premenopausal and postmenopausal women. Tamoxifen is an anti-estrogen, which means it attaches to the estrogen receptor and turns it off, thus blocking estrogen's ability to activate the cell. Tamoxifen has been shown to reduce the risk of breast cancer recurrence by more than 30%. It will also reduce new breast cancers by 50%.

As with all drugs, Tamoxifen does have side effects but is generally very safe. It can cause irregular menstrual periods, hot flashes, a vaginal discharge, or leg cramps. It can also cause two more serious side effects: blood clots, especially in the legs (known as DVT), and in postmenopausal women, can increase the risk of uterine cancer. However, the risks for both of these side effects is less than 1%, while the benefit in terms of breast cancer recurrence and death is usually much greater.

Tamoxifen is given for 5-10 years after a diagnosis of estrogen-sensitive breast cancer. Recent studies have shown that 10 years is somewhat more effective than five years, but treatments are usually individualized in terms of the risks of the cancer and the side effects of the drug.

A newer class of hormonal agents currently in use are the aromatase inhibitors such as anastrozole (also known by the brand name Arimidex), letrozole (Femara), and exemestane (Aromasin). Even in postmenopausal (whether due to natural age-related menopause, removal of the ovaries, or chemical suppression of the ovaries) women, estrogen is being manufactured in fatty tissue and the adrenal glands. Aromatase inhibitors turn off the enzyme that makes estrogen in these tissues, thereby decreasing the levels of estrogen that can stimulate a breast cancer cell and depriving the cells of estrogen. Because these drugs will not work on the ovarian production of estrogen, they cannot be used in women who are not in menopause.

These drugs have a different side-effect profile than Tamoxifen, often causing arthritis-like stiffness, especially in the hands and feet, and – rarely – severe muscle aches. They also cause vaginal dryness and can increase the risk of osteoporosis. Therefore, patients on aromatase inhibitors should have their bone density monitored.

Aromatase inhibitors have been compared to Tamoxifen as adjuvant therapy for breast cancer and are slightly more effective. They have been shown to be more effective than Tamoxifen alone when given for five years initially after diagnosis, for 2-3 years after 2-3 years of Tamoxifen, or for 5 years after 5 years of Tamoxifen. Again, they can only be administered to patients who are in menopause. Current studies are investigating whether 10 years of an aromatase inhibitor are better than 5 years.

Other agents are being investigated to see if they can improve the effects of hormonal therapy to cure breast cancer. Two exciting new agents in trials for higher risk breast cancer patients are everolimus and palbociclib.

CHEMOTHERAPY

Chemotherapy is routinely used in patients with more

aggressive estrogen receptor positive cancers (i.e. those with multiple nodes involved, or those with a genomic test showing the tumor to be aggressive), triple negative cancers, or HER2 positive cancers. Three classes of agents are typically used for chemotherapy:

- Anthracyclines (doxorubicin-Adriamycin or epirubicin)
- Cytoxan
- Taxanes (paclitaxel-Taxol or docetaxel-Taxotere)

These can be combined in multiple different combinations and administered before surgery (especially for large tumors), or after surgery, generally for 3-6 months. An older regimen still in use is Cytoxan, methotrexate, and 5-fluorouracil, which causes hair thinning but not total hair loss. However, it may not be as effective as the newer regimens. These combinations generally cause hair loss in addition to some unique side effects related to the specific drugs. The anthracyclines have a small risk – about 0.5% -- of causing heart damage, and about the same chance of predisposing to leukemia. Their use is declining and the Taxoter-Cytoxan regimen omits them. Studies are underway to determine if they are an essential part of breast cancer treatment. These taxanes can typically cause neuropathy, pain, and/or numbness in the hands and feet after multiple treatments.

Although chemotherapy can cause fatigue and hair loss, and lower blood counts, most women continue to work and generally feel well during much of their chemotherapy protocol. Only when the white blood count is very low is the immune system extremely compromised. Newer anti-nausea agents have virtually eliminated vomiting after chemotherapy, and nausea is for the most part, well controlled.

TARGETED THERAPY

The 15-30% of tumors that are HER2 positive have been shown to respond well to Herceptin, an antibody to the HER2 protein. The addition of Herceptin to chemotherapy has been shown to improve the prognosis of these risky tumors by more than 50%! The chemotherapy is generally a combination of Carboplatin and Taxotere with Herceptin; or an anthracycline and Cytoxan followed by a taxane and Herceptin for 3-6 months, with Herceptin continuing for the course of a full year, usually at three weekly intervals. Herceptin can cause a reversible decrease in heart function, so echocardiograms are used prior to treatment and every three months during the year of treatment to monitor heart function.

A newer agent, pertuzumab (Perjeta) has been approved for 3-4 months in combination with Herceptin when given before surgery, and has been shown to improve the chances of eradicating all traces of tumor in the breast. Ongoing studies are focusing on whether it increases the ultimate cure rate of breast cancer.

A WORD ON CLINICAL TRIALS

Although we have made major advances in the cure of breast cancer – the vast majority of women are cured – some cancers still do recur. The current knowledge we have is thanks to the thousands of women who have participated in clinical trials of breast cancer therapies. Over the last 30 years, women who have participated in clinical trials have in general had a better prognosis than women treated off trials. Since we still have work to do, participation in current clinical trials should be encouraged to further our understanding of breast cancer.

METASTATIC BREAST CANCER

When breast cancer recurs outside the breast and lymph node areas of the breast, it is called metastatic or stage 4 cancer. Breast cancer typically spreads to the bones, liver, and lungs, and sometimes to the brain. No matter what organ it inhabits, we still refer to it by the place it started: breast cancer. It still behaves like breast cancer and is treated as breast cancer. This is a good thing, because even though metastatic breast cancer is typically incurable, it is very successfully treated with a myriad of therapies. Metastatic breast cancer can be viewed as a chronic disease, often remaining under control with therapy for years at a time. Some women with HER2 positive stage 4 cancers have never had recurrence of their cancer with the advent of Herceptin antibody therapy!

With all of our new therapies, women with breast cancer are living longer and better quality lives. It is not uncommon to see women with HER2 positive or estrogen positive stage 4 cancers living 5 to 10 or even more years. I tell my patients that they must learn to live with cancer because they will be doing so for a long time.

Metastatic breast cancer that is estrogen sensitive is almost always initially treated with hormonal therapy. When the initial therapy stops working, there are many different types of hormonal therapy to try, and women can be on hormonal therapy without ever needing chemotherapy for years.

Multiple new chemotherapies are useful in treating metastatic breast cancer. In addition to the chemotherapies used for adjuvant treatment listed above, these new chemotherapies include:

- Capecitabine (Xeloda)
- Gemcitabine (Gemzar)
- Venorelbine (Navelbine)
- Liposomal doxorubicin (Doxil)
- Ixabepilone (Ixempra)
- Eribulin (Halaven)

HER2 positive cancers are initially treated with chemotherapy and Herceptin, but if a patient has a good response, they can be switched to the antibody alone and experience minimal or no side effects. Research has developed multiple new drugs for HER2 positive cancers, including pertuzumab (Perjeta), another anti-HER2 antibody that combines with Herceptin, and lapatinib (Tykerb), an oral agent that can be used alone, with chemotherapy, or with Herceptin.

Our newest approved agent is Kadcycla, which is a smart-bomb version of Herceptin. This drug is a combination of a small amount of chemotherapy attached to a Herceptin molecule, so that the Herceptin antibody can deliver chemotherapy directly to the breast cancer cell via its HER2-neu protein on the surface, thus bypassing normal tissues. This prevents the side effects of chemotherapy but not the effectiveness.

Although triple negative cancers have been notoriously difficult to treat, science is making some headway. The platinum chemotherapy agents, cisplatin and Carboplatin, have been found to be especially effective treatments for this type of cancer. Additionally, in triple negative cancers related to a BRCA mutation, new agents called PARP inhibitors are in clinical trials. These may increase the efficacy of chemotherapy.

With all of the new and exciting findings about the basic molecular mechanism of breast cancer cells, medical research is making great strides in the treatment of this disease. Most patients are cured and even those who cannot be cured are living longer with less toxic therapies, allowing for excellent quality of life. The future for breast cancer treatment is very bright, and hopefully this will one day give us the ability to cure or even prevent it.

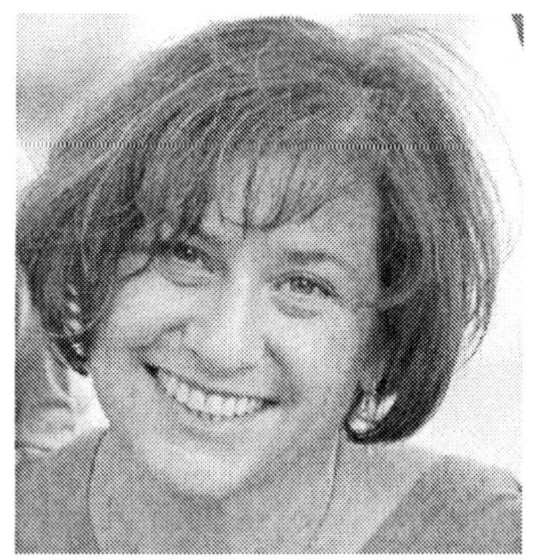

Elisa Krill-Jackson, M.D.

is a medical oncologist at Mount Sinai Medical Center in Miami Beach specializing in breast cancer and genetics. She attended medical school at the University of Michigan and did a residency in internal medicine at Brigham and Women's Hospital in Boston. She did her fellowship at New England Medical Center in Boston and at the University of Miami. Dr. Krill-Jackson is a Yale graduate and currently has a practice at Mount Sinai Medical Center in Miami, Florida.

Chapter 9

Radiation Oncology

Nicolas Kuritzky, M.D.

Why Radiation Therapy?

Typically, by the time they are ready to start radiation, most patients have had the cancer removed with negative margins. Inevitably, one of the first question asked by a patient at consultation is something along the lines of, "If my surgeon told me the cancer was taken out, why do I need it?" The simple answer is that while it is certainly a favorable sign that the margins are negative, this does not mean in reality there is no cancer left.

Let's briefly discuss what conceptually goes on during surgery and pathological analysis. When a surgeon removes a breast tumor, it is tempting to think of the tumor as a discrete, well defined mass; i.e. patients conceptualize the tumor as appearing like a bright red ball. As an analogy, when I remove a can from my refrigerator, there is no question whether part of the can is remaining in the fridge. It is clear whether it is entirely outside or inside.

This however is not the case with breast cancer. In reality the tumor often blends into the surrounding breast tissue and the borders are, to the surgeon's eye often indistinguishable from the surrounding breast tissue. Frequently the surgeon is only able to locate the tumor by cutting around a wire that had been preoperatively inserted under radiographic guidance. This clump of indistinguishable material is then sent (often during the middle of the operation) to pathology who then examine it under a microscope for the presence of tumor cells at the borders.

This is also true of lymph nodes. Patients also often imagine lymph nodes as well defined, "visible" nodules in the axilla. In fact, many times lymph nodes are not visible to the surgeon who is often removing an indistinct mass of fat located between vessels that he was guided to by the injection of dye or radioactive tracers.

During pathological analysis, the pathologist makes "cuts" or "slices" through the mass removed by the surgeon and reports on the presence of tumor cells at the margin. These "slices" are just a surrogate for the 'true margin." It is theoretically possible that between these cuts, "tentacles" or projections of a tumor are extending outside of the margin and disease is left in the patient. A tumor often is more similar to a dandelion than a ball. The name cancer actually refers to the Greek word for crab because tumors have projections or extensions into the surrounding tissue.

Based on thousands of patients who took part in multiple trials over many decades that randomized patients to receive radiation after mastectomy or lumpectomy, we know that post-surgical radiation reduces the chance of local recurrence by at least 60%.

For patients who have had a lumpectomy (breast conservation surgery), the rate of local recurrence may range from 10% to over 30% without radiation. A variety of indicators can be used to estimate the likelihood of local recurrence. Factors that affect the rate of local recurrence include size of tumor, lymph node status, tumor grade and receptor status, patient age, delivery of chemo or hormonal therapy, etc.

(http://www.ncbi.nlm.nih.gov/pmc/articles/PMC3254252/)

Historically radiation is typically recommended following breast conservation surgery for invasive breast cancer. In elderly women, there have been two studies that have shown for early stage tumors women who receive five years of hormonal therapy can consider omitting radiation. The rate of failure in the breast at ten years is around 10% without radiation and 1-2% with radiation. This improvement may not be enough for some patients to warrant radiation. My personal view however is that three weeks of radiation is much more tolerable and convenient than five years of hormonal therapy. If one of the therapies was going to be omitted, consideration should be given to doing without the hormones not the radiation.

TREATMENT PROCESS

Prior to the actual radiation treatment, a "simulation" is performed in which the patient is placed in the optimal treatment position and a CAT scan is given. This usually involves fabricating a custom mold or cushion to reproduce and maintain this position. In addition, tiny tattoos are placed that aid setting up that position on a daily basis for treatments.

Once the CAT scan is performed, the patient's body is digitally reconstructed on the computer in 3 Dimensions. The radiation oncologist and planner are then able to set beams that conform to the breast but minimize the amount of non-target tissue that is irradiated including heart and lungs. Sophisticated computer programs are used to calculate the dose distribution of radiation. These programs allow the planner to vary the intensity of different parts of the beam, effectively breaking the radiation beam into subfields. (Think of covering the head of flashlight with paper that is thicker in areas and thinner in others to create a non-uniform light beam.) This type of radiation is called IMRT (Intensity Modulated Radiation Therapy). When the computer work is complete, a physicist typically double checks the computer calculations.

Finally, prior to the first treatment, images are obtained to ensure that patient is in the appropriate position. Imaging is generally performed regularly throughout treatment to ensure that positioning is accurate.

RADIATION TREATMENT

No sensation is involved in the actual radiation treatment just like with any diagnostic radiological procedure. Major side effects that can occur during treatment are skin irritation and fatigue. Skin reactions typically occur after several weeks. (Skin changes in the first week of treatment are not due to radiation!) The skin may become darkened, red and itchy like a sunburn. Moisturizing lotions such as Aquafor may provide symptomatic relief. No moisturizing lotion has been proven to prevent or diminish the intensity of the skin reaction. A steroid cream, mometasone furoate has shown some benefit in several large studies in improving the severity of the skin reaction. Steroid creams such as mometasone or over the counter hydrocortisone do help reduce itch.

In addition to skin irritation, radiation may cause fatigue. Fatigue is most likely secondary to inflammation and is best addressed with regular exercise and increased physical activity. The fatigue is almost never severe enough that it would prevent a patient from working.

Long term side effects that can occur from radiation include effects on the heart, lungs and musculoskeletal tissue. For left sided breast cancers, radiation has been shown to slightly increase the risk of coronary artery damage and heart attacks. Therefore, modern treatment planning will attempt to minimize the dose to the heart. There are a number of techniques to minimize radiation dose to the heart. These include IMRT, delivering the radiation with respiratory inspiration to push the breast away from the heart or treating the prone position with the breast falling away from the heart.

Lung irritation (pneumonitis) from radiation is extremely rare but can occur several months following the treatment and generally resolves with high dose steroids. With regard to the breast itself, radiation can cause some increased thickening (fibrosis) of the breast or in extreme cases, shrinkage of the breast. Modern treatments have minimized the magnitude and risk of these side effects.

Can radiation cause cancer? While radiation is in fact a carcinogen, the absolute magnitude of the risk of therapeutic radiation for breast cancer resulting in a cancer is quite low; under 1%. In fact, most patients have a higher risk of dying in an automobile accident than from radiation induced cancer. Some studies have shown risks of well under 1% while other studies have not shown a measurable increased risk.

HOW MANY TREATMENTS?

Historically, a course of breast radiation therapy lasted approximately six weeks in America. Two large randomized trials from Canada and Britain showed that an equivalent dose of radiation could be delivered in approximately three weeks. Both of these trials have very long follow up and actually employed less sophisticated radiation than is in use today. Even though the shortened course involved higher doses of radiation per treatment, it was actually associated with *less* short and long term cosmetic side effects and was equally effective in terms of cancer control.

REFERENCES

Br J Cancer. 2004 Aug 31;91(5):868-72.

Radiation-induced malignancies following radiotherapy for breast cancer.

Roychoudhuri R[1], Evans H, Robinson D, Møller H.

J Clin Oncol. 2000 Jun;18(12):2406-12.

Second malignancies after treatment of early-stage breast cancer: lumpectomy and radiation therapy versus mastectomy.

Obedian E[1], Fischer DB, Haffty BG.

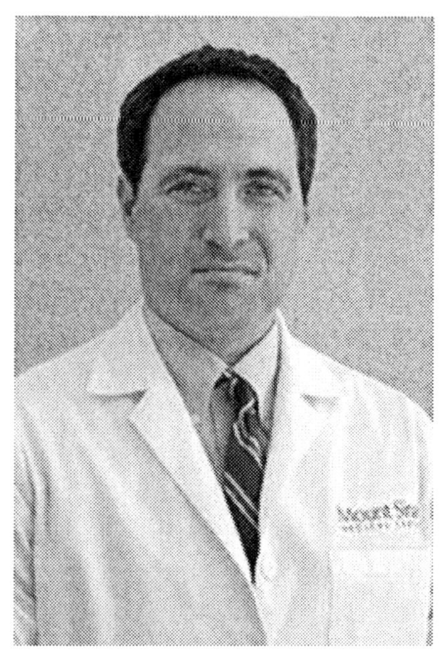

Nicolas Kuritzky, M.D.

is chairman of the Radiation Oncology Department at the Mount Sinai Medical Center Comprehensive Cancer Center in Miami, Florida. With 11 years of experience, he is an expert in the treatment of prostate and breast cancers, and innovative treatment techniques such as stereotactic radiosurgery, intensity-modulated radiation therapy, image guided radiation and brachytherapy.

Dr. Kuritzky completed his undergraduate studies at Stanford University and his medical degree at the University of Pennsylvania. He trained in radiation oncology at New York-Presbyterian Hospital-Weill Cornell Medical Center in New York City, where he was chief resident of radiation oncology.

Dr. Kuritzky is an active member of the American College of Radiology and the American Society of Therapeutic Radiation Oncology and is board-certified by the American Board of Radiology.

CHAPTER 10

NEW STRIDES IN BREAST CANCER TREATMENT

BEATRIZ AMENDOLA, M.D. F.A.C.R. FASTRO FACRO

There is no denying that more and more women are having double (bilateral) mastectomies these days. For some with more aggressive or advanced breast cancer it may be medically necessary; however, for most women it may be possible to conserve their breasts. It is true that for those women facing early-stage disease, deciding which type of surgery is best may not be easy. As a Radiation Oncologist for more than 30 years, I can confidently say that in women with early breast cancer the real choice is not between saving your breast and saving your life. This might be shocking news to some.

However, the truth is that women with early-stage breast cancer who have breast-conserving surgery such as lumpectomy live just as long as those who have a single or bilateral mastectomy. Survival is the same no matter which surgical approach is taken, as systemic management and local radiation improves the chances of keeping the breast. Even in women with advanced disease, using either chemotherapy or hormone therapy to reduce the tumor and then receive conservative radiation treatment might be an option.

Advanced or Aggressive Breast Cancer

Technology has made it possible to be able to treat the entire chest wall and regional lymph nodes after receiving chemotherapy and surgery with minimal side-effects. In many cases, patients will be treated in supine (lying on their backs) or prone (lying on their stomachs) positions. If a woman has more advanced or aggressive breast cancer, in many instances she might feel like giving up....don't. This is mostly because of lack of knowledge of what innovative Radiation Oncology can offer. If a woman has presented after many years of battling cancer with metastatic disease to the bones, brain, or liver there are techniques today that can focus and target only the tumor using image guidance while completely avoiding normal structures (healthy tissue). This technology is called Radiosurgery and it is usually delivered using a special piece of equipment specifically designed to destroy the tumor by using X-rays rather than surgery. The procedure is called radiosurgery, and is done as an outpatient procedure without anesthesia or hospitalization. It is bloodless and also painless and can be done in minutes, so women should not be afraid to ask for this technology.

Early Stage Breast Cancer

When breast cancer is diagnosed early and there are no genetic factors that can change the course of the disease, we can reach 95% cure rates with modern conservative treatment. Breast conservation treatment (BCT) is the preferred method of management in the overwhelming majority of women who present with early stage breast cancer. It consists of a minimal invasive surgery which provides a wide local excision of the primary tumor most often called a partial or segmental mastectomy (synonyms:

lumpectomy, tylectomy, tumorectomy, quadrantectomy) followed by adjuvant radiation therapy (RT) to the whole breast. The addition of RT to conserving surgery is necessary because it has been shown in multiple studies to result in an absolute risk reduction of 25-30% for local recurrence and an absolute improvement in overall survival of 5-7% at 15 years (1). So then why is it that we keep seeing so many women go for the extreme procedure, with chances of severe complications when we now have data supporting otherwise? Could it be vanity and the enticement of getting a tummy-tuck and a breast augmentation at the same time? Advances in plastic surgery promise more attractive artificial breasts than years ago. Unfortunately we do not think about the consequences of such a drastic approach.

Treating the Patient as a Whole

Breast cancer is not a local disease, it is systemic. In other words, it is a disease of the entire body. This is one of the reasons why we need to use some form of systemic hormones or chemotherapy to prevent the tumor from spreading to other areas of the body. For a small number of women, bilateral mastectomies are necessary because of multicentric disease (cancer in multiple breasts quadrants) or genetic mutations such as BRCA 1 or 2 most commonly seen in women of Ashkenazi Jewish heritage resulting in a lifetime risk of breast cancer in the 65-85% range. However, most double mastectomies are done on the breast with cancer, and a prophylactic mastectomy of the healthy breast in women without known genetic mutations. There are many scenarios in which the decision to proceed with bilateral mastectomies is based upon unfounded fear or an inaccurate assessment of the risks and benefits that a woman may face. Clearly a major factor is "the Angelina Jolie effect." She made her BRCA1 gene mutation public in 2013 when she detailed her path to a bilateral mastectomy after learning that this mutation carries an 85% risk for developing breast cancer. However, the BRAC1/2 genes linked to breast cancer are rare (0.25%). In the USA only one in 800 women in the general population are affected by this genetic mutation.

Present cancer guidelines discourage bilateral mastectomies for most women and recommend it only be considered on a case-by-case basis for women at high risk of bilateral breast cancer, such as those who carry a *BRCA1* or *BRCA2* mutation, or those who have a higher risk of contralateral breast cancer. It's important for women to always get a second opinion and discuss the options with specialists: breast cancer treatment calls for a multidisciplinary team approach involving the breast surgeon, the radiation oncologist and the medical oncologist. Then you can make an educated decision. It's interesting that when shopping, women actually shop around looking for choices – be it for a new car or clothing. Yet when dealing with breast cancer, most women see only one surgeon and perhaps a plastic surgeon without getting a second or even third opinion. Shop around! It also helps to talk to other women who have "been there" and can tell you of their own personal experiences.

For women with advanced tumors, it is crucial to be educated in all the new techniques and therapies available. Today, we are changing cancer from a fatal disease to a chronic disease that will require maintenance and follow-up, same as any other chronic illness. Breast cancer is particularly well-known for having a phase where disease is metastatic, but has only spread to a few body sites (5 or less). This phase of cancer is known as oligometastatic disease (2). It needs to be addressed properly, because if managed aggressively using modern technologies, patients may be cured. We have been very successful curing breast cancer with less aggressive treatments for many years. As noted above those treatments consist mostly of lumpectomy followed by radiation. There have been many advances in the field of radiation oncology for breast cancer patients. Below are two of the most advanced forms of radiation treatment available, although they may not yet be available at all medical centers.

Radiation Treatment Advances

Accelerated Partial Breast Irradiation (APBI) Brachytherapy: Only for Early Disease

Brachytherapy, derived from the Greek term for close, indicates placing a radioactive treatment source close near or inside the tumor. The advantage is the quick dose fall-off sparing adjacent tissues from radiation while providing high focal doses (3). High dose rate brachytherapy (HDR) refers to the delivery of a high dose of radiation in a relative short time. The pathways to the insertion of the radioactive source are usually created using catheters inserted into the tumor bed. The radioactive source is inserted at any time post-surgery and hence it is called an "afterloader" technique. Due to the high activity the source is inserted remotely into the patient using a remote afterloading unit. (Fig 1) After the treatment is completed the source is removed from the patient.

Accelerated Partial Breast Irradiation (APBI) using HDR is a high-dose, remotely controlled radiation that treats only the part of the breast which needs it. It is a shorter course (usually 5 to 7 days), as opposed to conventional external radiation treatment which usually requires 5 to 6 weeks of daily radiation treatments. This treatment delivers radiation to the area where it is needed most with minimal radiation exposure to the adjacent normal tissues reducing the potential for side effects (4-6). It represents an alternative to conventional external irradiation for early breast cancer.

FIGURE 1

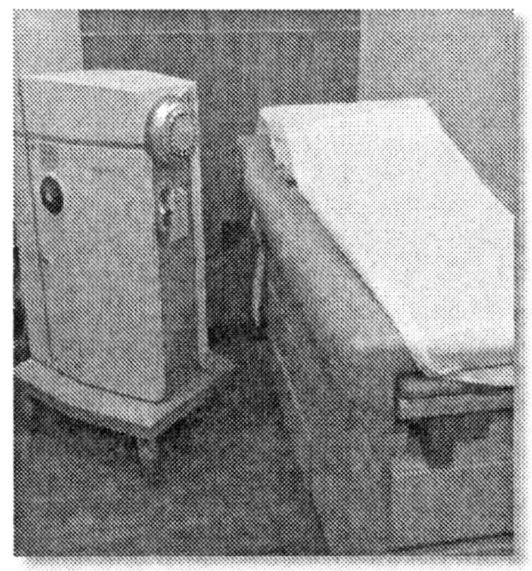

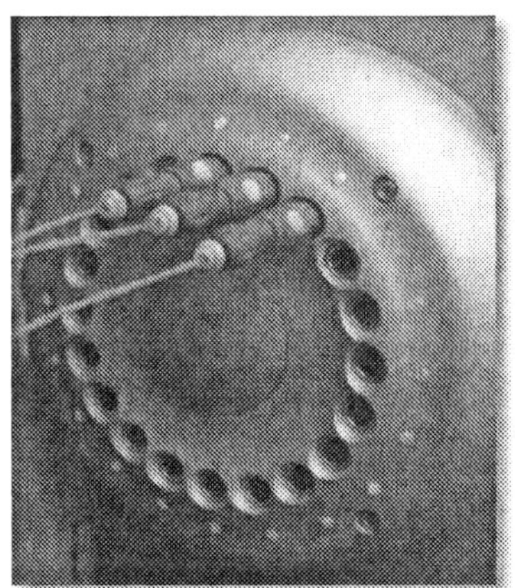

FIGURE 1A -1B Remote afterloader unit for High Dose Rate (HDR) Brachytherapy using catheters

FIGURE 2

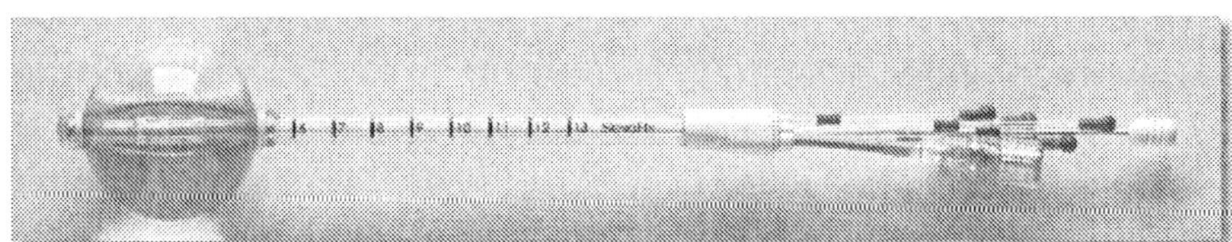

FIGURE 2 A

Balloon-based multicatheter device for delivery of ABPI to treat breast cancer using HDR

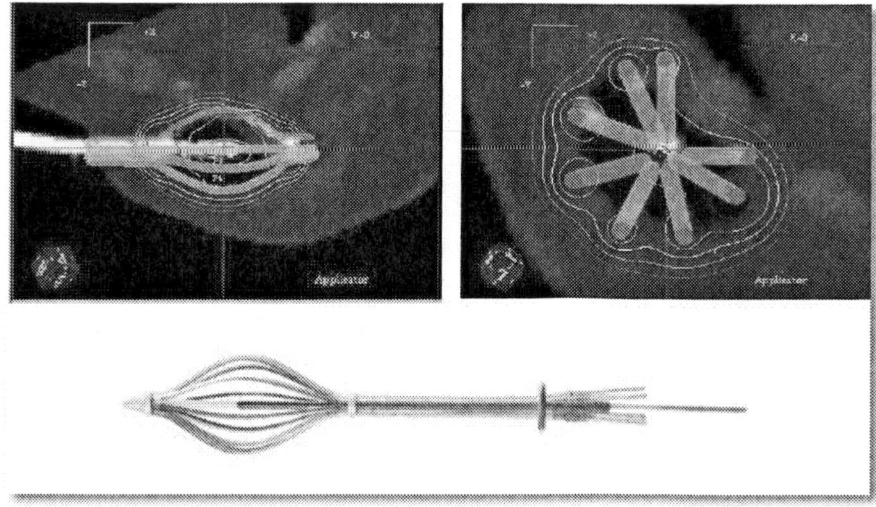

FIGURE 2 B Another type of catheter device for delivery of ABPI to treat breast cancer using HDR with dosimetric schema

Advantages of APBI Brachytherapy

Brachytherapy treatment offers several advantages compared to the traditional external-beam radiation therapy:

- Radiation only targets the area surrounding the tumor bed (after removal of the tumor- by surgical lumpectomy) rather than the whole breast.
- Radiation is delivered in fewer treatments at larger doses, so the total number of treatments is usually completed in only 5-7 days.
- The fewer number of days required for treatment is especially helpful for patients who live far away from the radiation center or have a busy schedule.
- Elderly women are excellent candidates, because all patients are treated with a shorter course of radiation on an outpatient basis.
- The cosmetic results are excellent.
- Most women feel little or no discomfort during the treatment.

PRONE BREAST RADIATION THERAPY

Prone Breast Radiation Therapy: designed for treatments of the left or right breast, including whole breast, partial breast, and accelerated partial breast treatments.

Prone breast radiation therapy is a concept that has been recently perfected to treat all stages of breast cancer. Several new studies have shown that receiving radiation to the breast while lying in the prone, or face down position has many benefits for women who are candidates for this type of treatment (7). This approach, while obtaining the same quality results as treatments in the traditional supine position, where women lay flat on their back for the radiation treatment, significantly avoids the radiation exposure to adjacent internal organs like the heart and lungs. The heart is especially vulnerable to damage when the left breast is treated because of the location of the heart on the left side of the chest just beneath the breast. Furthermore, respiratory motion may be reduced in the prone position, helping to improve treatment accuracy. Consequently, the prone breast position is most often used when radiating left breast cancer, although it can be used for treatment in both left and right breast cancer patients.

Figure 3

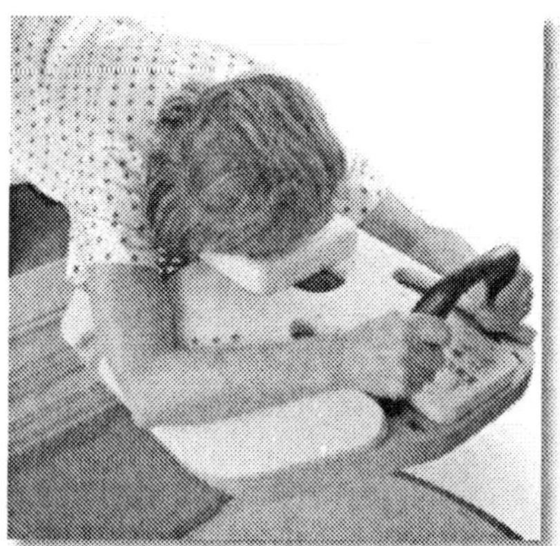

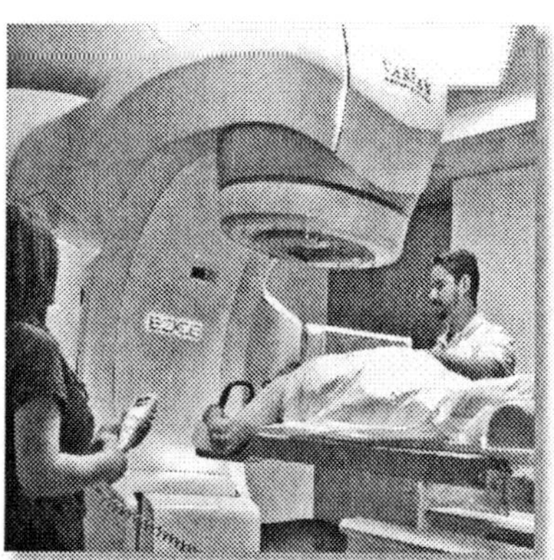

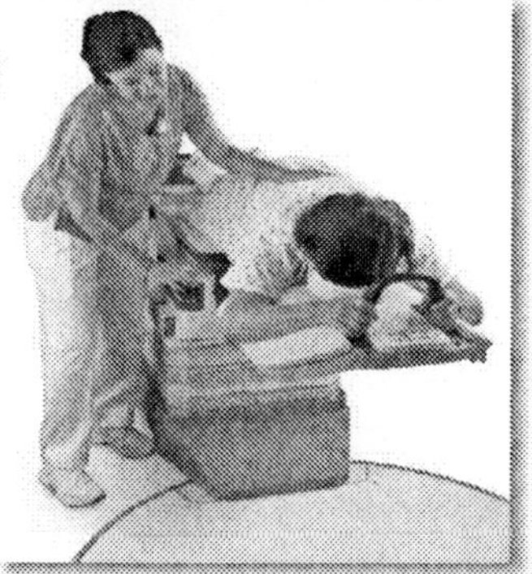

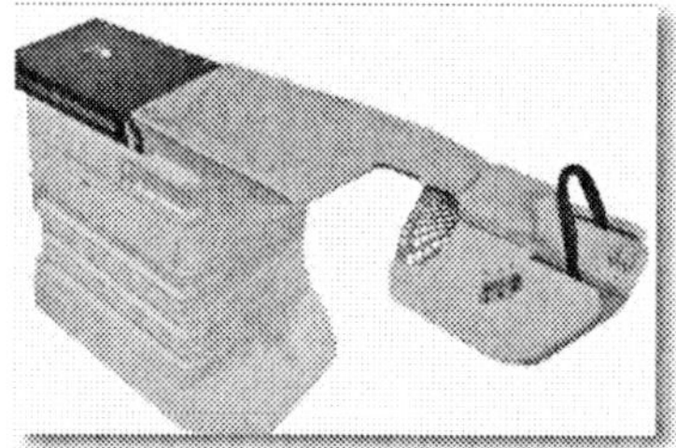

FIGURE 3 A-B-C-D Examples of patients undergoing external beam radiation therapy in a modern linear accelerator unit (upper left corner) using a dedicated prone breast treatment table device (pink device in right lower corner of the illustration).Please note how the breast cut-out in the board where the patient rests facilitates full access to the targeted area of the breast without any obstruction beneath the breast.

Prone breast radiation therapy is effective in delivering a consistent and precise dose of radiation throughout the course of treatment. Before the development of the prone breast technique, women with larger breasts were placed on their backs in the traditional position to receive radiation. Gravity pulls the breasts close to the body, causing exposure to internal organs and also making treatment less consistent because larger breasts may lay flat differently with each radiation session. With the prone position, we can ensure radiation is distributed evenly, consistently and accurately during each treatment.

Advantages of Prone Breast Radiation Therapy:

- Radiation dose is evenly distributed in the breast
- Protecting the heart and lungs from unwanted radiation
- Minimized skin irritation
- Optimal cosmetic results

Summary

The decision to have bilateral mastectomies should not be made without considerable thought and research. In my view, women should proceed cautiously and think carefully about the advantages and disadvantages of all the medical choices involved so they can lead a happy and healthy life post cancer.

References

Di Lascio S, Pagani O. Oligometastatic Breast Cancer: A Shift From Palliative to Potentially Curative Treatment? Breast Care. 2014;9:7-14

Clarke M, Collins R, Darby S et al. Effects of radiotherapy and of differences in the extent of surgery for early breast cancer on local recurrence and 15-year survival: an overview of the randomized trials. Lancet 2005;366:2087-2106

Saw CB. Brachytherapy: High Dose Rate (HDR) implants. In Encyclopedia of Radiation Oncology, Brady LW and Yaeger TE ,Eds. Springer Verlag, Berlin Heidelberg 2013

Amendola B.E, Amendola M.A, Perez N, et al. Five-year follow-up for MammoSite APBI – from a single community practice. Am J Clin Oncol. 2008, 143

Wobb JL, Shah C, Chen PY, et al. Brachytherapy-based Accelerated Partial Breast Irradiation Provides Equivalent 10-Year outcomes to Whole Breast Irradiation: A Matched-Pair Analysis. Am J Clin Oncol. 2015;

Husain ZA, Lloyd S, Shah C, et al. Changes in brachytherapy-based APBI patient selection immediately before and after publication of the ASTRO consensus statement. Brachytherapy. 2015;15:490-495

Huppert N, Jozsef G, DeWingaert K, Formenti SR. The role of a prone setup in breast radiation therapy. Frontiers in Oncology 2011,1:1-8

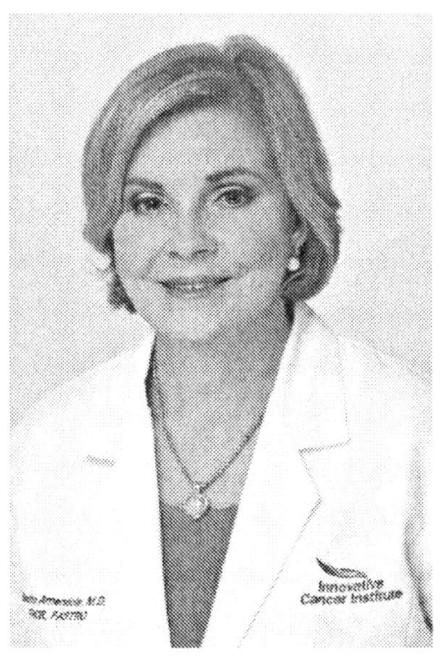

Beatriz Amendola, M.D.

is a highly respected radiation oncologist and an honored member of the leading medical societies of the specialty in the United States, Latin America and Europe. She has been a highly successful practicing physician of radiation oncology in the U.S. for more than 35 years.

She has been awarded Fellowship from the American Society of Radiation Oncology (ASTRO), from the American College of Radiation Oncology (ACRO) and from The American College of Radiology (ACR). Her main areas of interest include breast, lung, head/neck and prostate cancer as well as brain tumors. Dr Beatriz Amendola has extensive knowledge in the field of radiation therapy, with expertise in Brachytherapy, as well as in radiosurgery using Gamma Knife, CyberKnife, and LINAC based radiosurgery.

Dr. Beatriz Amendola completed her residency in Radiation Oncology at the Medical College of Virginia in Richmond, Va., with Board Certification in Therapeutic Radiology by the American Board of Radiology in 1980. She has held several academic positions, including Acting Chairman of the Department of Radiation Oncology at the University of Michigan and Associate Professor and Director of Residency Training at the University of Miami, Department of Radiation Oncology. She has edited a textbook on Radiation Oncology and she has published more than 60 scientific articles in peer-reviewed medical journals of the specialty.

Dr. Beatriz Amendola has delivered more than 500 scientific presentations, scientific exhibits, and lectures nationally and internationally. She has received multiple honors and awards including the Gold Medal from CRILA (Circulo de Radioterapeutas Ibero Latino Americano). Dr. Beatriz Amendola was recently awarded Honorary Membership in the Spanish Society of Radiation Oncology (SEOR) at the Biannual Congress of SEOR in Valencia, Spain, June 1-3, 2015 because of her multiple contributions to the specialty of Radiation Oncology in Spain.

Chapter 11

"THE RED BALLOON" – LYMPHEDEMA

Elizabeth Anne Ouellette, M.D.

Lymphedema is a swelling in the arm caused by lymph fluid accumulating in the tissues. The lymph fluid is made up of proteins, cellular materials and bacteria that return from the tissues in an effort to maintain tissue fluid balance. This fluid and cellular debris return centrally in the body through lymph channels that have valves similar to the venous system to prevent backflow of the fluid. The channels move the fluid by using muscle within the walls of the vessel and are controlled by the sympathetic nervous system. The fluid builds up in an arm or a leg when the lymph vessels or the nerve supply to those nerve vessels are injured.

This buildup of fluid can occur after surgery, trauma to the tissues, radiation or injury. The lymph system is our defense mechanism that helps to keep us healthy, and when cancer, bacteria, or disease appear, our lymph nodes overwhelm it and can become tender and painful. Since breast cancer can spread through the lymph nodes, surgeons must remove some of them to see if the cancer has spread which is known as axillary node dissection. Sometimes after surgery, radiation is needed to make sure there are no remaining cancer cells.

Surgery and radiation can put a woman at risk for developing lymphedema because the pathways that normally drain the fluid from the tissues back to through the lymphatic system have been impaired. Lymph fluid is rich in proteins which rebuild our tissues, but these proteins can also accumulate in the tissue spaces causing the limb to enlarge and the skin to stretch. After time the tissue become hard or fibrotic. It does not necessarily affect the entire arm, but does affect the forearm where you might lean against a table or rest on the arm of a chair.

One of the predictors of lymphedema can be a patient who has high lymph flow pre-surgery which may indicate a lymphatic overload and failure. This then creates a situation where the person with breast cancer may be more likely to develop lymphedema. (SK Bains, 2014; "The Breast") By increasing surgery and increasing reconstruction rates there are some interesting facts coming to light regarding reconstruction. Women who have undergone immediate breast reconstruction with an implant appear to have less lymphedema, but the reasons for this are unknown. Lymphedema did not appear if there was any difference in the severity of the cancer staging nor with the extent of the surgical procedure, radiation or neoadjuvant chemotherapy. Another option in an attempt to reduce the formation of lymphedema is to try to reduce the amount of axillary node dissection with the surgery. Performing a sentinel node dissection instead of an axillary lymph node dissection has a significant decrease in the frequency of lymphedema postoperatively although it does not eliminate lymphedema from occurring entirely. (McLaughlin, et al. "Journal of Clinical Oncology" 26 (22) 5213-5219).

This condition affects between 35-89 percent of the two million breast cancer survivors in the United States. (Brorson H, et al., "Lymphology" 41(2): 52-63) (Kissin MW, et al., Br J Surg 72(7): 580-4) (Segerstrom K, et al., Scand J Plast Reconstr Surg Hand Surg 26 (2): 223-7) Doctors are still not sure exactly what triggers the lymphedema to occur, however there are some predictors: infection of the surgical site, radiation to the axillary (armpit) area and obesity (Bergan, A., et al., "Progress in Lymphology" XX 40 (Suppl), International Society of Lymphology, pp. 96-106). In an article on lymphedema in breast cancer survivors twenty years after diagnosis, Dr. Jeanne A. Petrek and her colleagues found that lymphedema occurred in 13 percent of patients, 77 percent of whom noticed the onset within three years after surgery.

It is important to guard against even minor mishaps and maintain a healthy weight. Sometimes it is the chicken-and-the-egg question; did the infection from the scratch in the garden or an overly playful cat cause the lymphedema to occur, or did lymphedema make the skin more vulnerable to infection that requires medical attention? Was it the change in barometric pressure from the plane trip recently taken? Other simple precautions include:

- Using sun block to protect the skin from sunburn;
- Applying mosquito repellent when outside to protect against insect bites;
- Wearing gloves when gardening;
- Care when cutting or filing your nails;
- Keeping skin moisturized;
- Eating a healthy diet low in salt and fat;
- Wearing a compression garment when flying or in situations with barometric pressure shifts.

Lymphedema can occur right after surgery (though many times this can be temporary) or up to thirty years later. This type of lymphedema is termed secondary lymphedema because the lymphatic system is intact in other parts of the body but damaged in the area where the cancer, surgery or radiation has occurred.

The other type of lymphedema is primary where the lymph vessel themselves are not functioning properly in that there may be too many or too few vessels. This type of lymphedema is seen mainly in women and primarily in the leg. Sometimes it can run in families.

Early signs of lymphedema include mild swelling under the armpit or around the shoulder blade and heaviness in the arm though the hand and forearm may not show signs of swelling. Sometimes women report that their bra is uncomfortable or too tight. It may be helpful to elevate the arm at night and do simple arm exercises and deep breathing to stimulate the lymphatic system. You can also measure the circumference on one arm and compare with the other to see if there are any changes in the size. It is still difficult to make a clear diagnosis as there are no widely accepted criteria of lymphedema at this time. One tool that may be helpful in making a diagnosis is bio-impedance measurements that measure the amount of fluid in a limb. As this becomes a more established tool, it may be easier to detect and quantify lymphedema.

Other times the hand or arm begins to swell and it may be uncomfortable to wear your rings or a watch. You should see your physician to make sure there are no other medical problems occurring. As there is no specific test to diagnosis lymphedema, your physician usually has to rule out other medical conditions that can cause swelling. Lymphedema is usually not painful. However sometimes radiation can affect the nerves leading from the shoulder or neck region. There may be some tingling sensations or mild pain. Light exercise or stretching can assist in relieving some of this discomfort. As the limb increases in size, the fluid can put pressure on surrounding nerves and joints also leading to pain or discomfort. Unfortunately at this time there is no cure for lymphedema but the condition can be managed and you can still lead a very healthy and productive life. Therapy today for lymphedema includes complex decongestive physiotherapy which is manual lymph drainage, compression bandaging to reduce the swelling in the arm, exercises and education so you know how to manage this condition. An option that has now become available is low-level laser treatments (LLLT), but exactly how this effective in some women is not known. Please check in your community for certified experienced therapists that know how to do the manual lymph drainage and bandaging. You can learn how to keep your arm healthy and a near-normal size.

Once you realize that you have lymphedema, other options include wearing a compression sleeve and glove. These garments support the limb and do not let the fluid refill. A certified fitter should fit arm sleeves and gloves so you get the most comfortable fit. It does no good to purchase a sleeve and keep it on the shelf it needs to be on you.

Some other therapies include a compression pump that inflates and deflates the cuff in a cycle. Some have tried hyperbaric oxygen as a lymphedema treatment. A small pilot study at the University of South Carolina found a 38 percent reduction of lymphedema in the hand which persisted for 14.2 months. Exercise is important to keep the muscles toned and flexible. There are specific exercises that are recommended if you have lymphedema, however it is safe to do your exercises in the pool. Water acts as resistance to the working muscle moving the fluids from the arms to the trunk of the body and back into the circulatory system. One of the best exercises is to swim as it gets the arm elevated to the level of the heart and the motions required of swimming help to reduce the arm swelling.

Sometimes even with the best of care an infection or cellulitis can occur in the arm at risk. The signs are redness, swelling, pain, fever and chills. You must see your physician immediately to get antibiotics. Many times after an infection the arm can increase in size or lymphedema can start. That is why skin care is so important. It is also important to be aware that the little injuries in life can trigger the otherwise quiet lymphedema to flare. A fracture to a finger which in the average person causes the hand to swell, in the breast cancer patient will cause the whole arm to swell. In this setting, start treating the lymphedema with exercises and therapies along with the care required for the injury.

A surgical procedure for issues other than breast cancer can trigger the lymphedema, but patients undergoing hand surgery have been found to tolerate the procedures well with and without tourniquet application during the surgery. Patients with breast cancer should not be afraid of having surgery on the affected limb if it is necessary to regain function of the hand. Examples of this would be carpal tunnel release, a fracture that requires fixation, etc. It is important to be aware of the prior breast surgery and begin additional exercises that will decrease swelling in the arm at the time of the surgery and for some time after the surgery.

Patients that have a flair up of their lymphedema after a surgery or trauma to the arm generally take about three months of additional therapy to return back to their baseline swelling. As long as you are diligent in the exercises and don't allow yourself to get frustrated, things will improve!

If the lymphedema becomes severe, there is a staging system. Other options can be considered that are surgical, but usually these would be addressed at the time of the breast reconstruction.

Untreated and treated lymphedema can progress, however with diet, exercise, good skin care and a compression garment, life can be enjoyed and lived to the fullest.

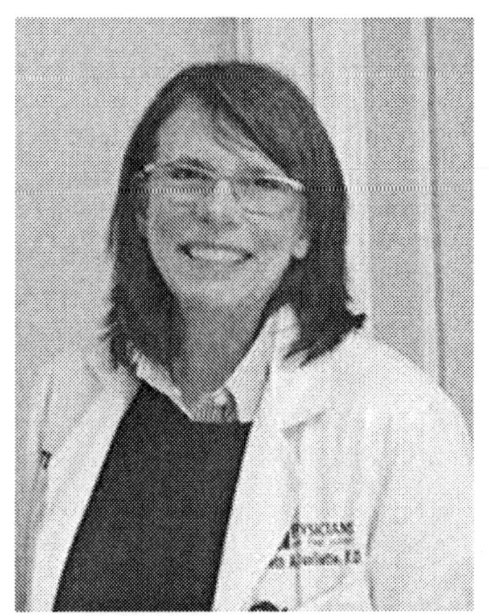

Elizabeth Anne Ouellette, M.D.

obtained her medical degree at the University of Texas Medical School in San Antonio, Texas in 1978. She attended the University of Washington School of Medicine for her Orthopaedic Residency training which was completed in 1983. She came to Miami in 1984 for her Hand Fellowship at the University of Miami.

Following her fellowship she remained at the University of Miami for twenty three years where she became the Chief of Hand Surgery in the Department of Orthopedics and achieved rank of Professor Emeritus. In addition, Dr. Ouellette became the Chief of Hand Surgery at Jackson Memorial Hospital and the Director of their Hand Fellowship program. Among Doctor Ouellette's many talents, she is a gifted violinist.

Visit the Oulette group at http://www.theouellettegroup.com

Chapter 12

What You Need To Know About Lymphatic Drainage Therapy

Samara Christy, LDT, CLT

BREAST CARE THROUGH LYMPHATIC DRAINAGE THERAPY

WHAT YOU NEED TO KNOW ABOUT LYMPHATIC DRAINAGE THERAPY

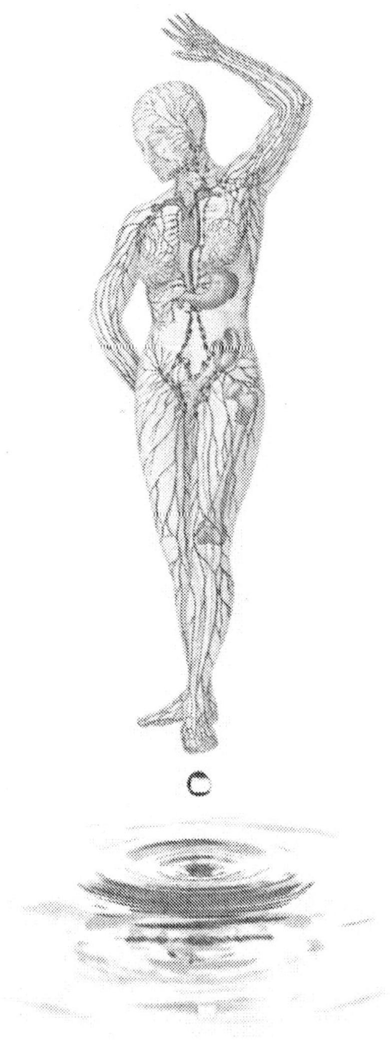

Here we are again. The year is 2014, and it is October: Breast Cancer Awareness Month. Unfortunately, it is Breast Cancer Awareness every day for millions of breast cancer survivors. I, like many of you, have read reams of material on Breast Cancer Awareness. Every year thousands answer the call to attend marches for breast cancer awareness and to raise millions of dollars for research—yet breast cancer statistics remain dismal at best. At present, one out of every eight women will develop breast cancer in her lifetime; one in every ten men will also. And although we have managed to save more lives through breast cancer awareness, early detection and treatments, millions of women continue to be diagnosed with breast cancer every year. It's clear that more needs to be done in the area of *prevention*.

Yes, diet and exercise, a healthy diet and a more balanced and less stressful lifestyle are major preventative steps. But in one of those "Aha!" moments I realized I had vital information, information that most people have never even heard about, information that needs, in my opinion, to be shouted from the mountaintops. So here goes:

Most people are unaware that <u>we all have cancer cells</u>, and the only way cancer cells leave the body is through the lymphatic system. By decongesting your lymphatic system, it will assist your body in doing what it was designed to do—keep you cancer free.

You are probably asking, "How would I go about decongesting my lymphatic system?"

Most people are unaware that there is a medically recognized therapy designed to do just that. It's called Lymphatic Drainage Therapy .

First, I would like to share with you how important your lymphatic system is to your well-being. You may not know that your body has three times more lymph fluid than it has blood, and that all that lymph fluid circulates through your body every 24 hours. In a congested lymphatic system, lymph is thick, sticky, stagnant, laden with toxins and unable to circulate and eliminate waste. Most importantly, your lymphocytes (white blood cells, which fight infection in your body), reside in your lymph nodes—of which you have between 600 and 1,000. Your lymphatic system is responsible for supplying plasma-rich protein to your blood as well as carrying away toxins and other debris. Further, your lymphatic system is your primary defense against bacteria, viruses and fungi. Most women—and men too—are unaware of how important a role their lymphatic system plays in having healthy breasts. Our breasts have hundreds of lymphatic lines that carry toxins and precancerous cells out of the breast tissue through the lymph nodes located in the armpit—meaning that a healthy lymphatic system is essential.

Since the fluid in the lymph system must be pumped by the movement of our muscles, the less we move, the more stagnant our lymph system becomes. With today's sedentary lifestyles, pollution, diets low in nutrients and high in fats, sugars, additives, and preservatives—and also because most of us fail to drink enough pure water to assist our body in eliminating toxins—our lymphatic systems can easily become overloaded, congested and clogged. In other words, if your lymphatic system is congested, your whole immune system will be compromised.

Here are a few easy steps you can take that will make a tremendous difference in your lymphatic health:

1. Drink plenty of pure water (rule of thumb: take your weight and divide it by two; that is the amount of ounces of water you should be consuming every day). Remember, your lymphatic system needs lots of water to flush out toxins.
2. Unlike your heart, since your lymphatic system has no pump, it needs exercise or other physical, manual or electro-sonic stimulation to help it move. To get you started, let me suggest

   this very simple exercise. Sit on a large, high quality exercise ball and bounce gently for twenty minutes every day, while watching your favorite television program, listening to music, or working on your computer. This exercise is something that most everyone can do, and it's very effective in moving the lymph system as it was designed to operate.

3. For women: stop wearing underwire bras. Underwire bras go over lymph nodes on both sides of each breast, causing stagnation.
4. It is my sincerest hope that you will make a pledge to yourself this month to find out all you can about your lymphatic system and make an appointment with a Lymphatic Therapist (see www.Rightwayhealthandwellness.com for names and contact information of certified electro-sonic lymphatic practitioners in your area).

HOW IT ALL BEGAN

In 2010, a breast cancer survivor came to my office for lymphatic drainage therapy treatments clutching one of my brochures. Sandy (not her real name) had read how lymphatic treatments could boost her compromised immune system, the aftereffects of a mastectomy followed by chemo and radiation. As a result of having fourteen of her lymph nodes removed, Sandy's right upper arm was four inches bigger than her left, a condition called lymphedema. During her treatment Sandy asked me, "Is it really true that you can take down the swelling in my right arm?" I assured her that I could. Sandy was to be married in six months, and it was her dream to wear a sleeveless dress for her summer wedding, which was to be held in Florida.

Like many women who have undergone a mastectomy, Sandy had to have all her lymph nodes in her armpit removed, causing her to have to wear a compression garment 24/7 to keep the lymphatic fluid from pooling in her arm and keeping her arm from getting any bigger than it already was. Sandy confided to me that she hated the fact that the sleeve was a constant announcement to the world that she had gone through cancer. I treated her twice a week for the first two weeks, and then once a week for four months, using a protocol called rerouting .

After four months of weekly lymphatic treatments, her right arm was almost the same size as her left, and she no longer had to wear a compression sleeve (except when she had to travel by plane). I can't adequately convey how much my heart was touched when Sandy showed me a picture of herself on her wedding day, without her compression sleeve, and wearing a beautiful sleeveless dress. She continues having follow-up treatments every six to eight weeks. Shortly after treating Sandy, I decided to become certified as an XP2 Lymphatic Trainer. I wanted the credentials not only to be able to train other lymphatic practitioners, but to train more people in rerouting – this this life-changing technique – as well.

To locate a lymphatic practitioner trained in rerouting in your area, go to www.rightwayhealtandwellness.com.

*We are able to reroute other conditions such as lymphedema of the legs, or removal of lymph nodes in the groin.

MOST AILMENTS CAN BE LINKED TO THE LYMPHATIC SYSTEM AND A COMPROMISED IMMUNE SYSTEM

The lymphatic system plays a vital role in the body's immunity to disease. Its complex network of fluid-filled vessels continuously bathes cells and carries away the body's "sewage" – toxins, metabolic waste products, globules of fat, excess liquid – to the lymph nodes. The lymph nodes are the body's filters, trapping and neutralizing these harmful substances.

The body contains three times more lymph fluid than blood. While the circulatory system has a pump—the heart—to keep the blood moving, lymph fluid must be pumped by the movement of muscles. The less we move our bodies, the more stagnant the lymph system becomes. So how does lymph fluid move? Without a heart-like pump, the lymphatic system depends on motion – exercise, massage, or other physical stimulation – to propel lymph fluid through its vessels. Here are some methods that are currently in use:

Manual Lymphatic Drainage (MLD)

A therapist massages and virtually (though gently) squeezes the lymph fluid along the lymphatic pathways.

Electro-Sound Lymphatic (ESLD)

The Lymph Drainage XP2 technology uses specific high frequencies of electricity and sound to break down congested lymph fluid. As mentioned before, your body has 600 to 1,000 lymph nodes scattered throughout the body. 30 percent of these lymph nodes are in the stomach, and they are about six inches deep. Manual Lymphatic Drainage cannot reach those deeper lymph nodes, while the XP2 can easily and painlessly can penetrate them. Because body fluids are a conductor of electricity, the lymph fluid is effortlessly moved through the lymphatic pathways.

What is Electro-Sound Lymphatic Drainage?

Electro-sound lymphatic drainage is an accelerated one-hour method of detoxifying the lymphatic system. If the lymphatic system is congested, the lymph fluid is thick, sticky, stagnant and laden with toxins, rendering it unable to circulate and eliminate wastes. Lymphatic congestion and toxicity reduces the electrostatic fluid of the proteins in the interstitial fluids, and contributes to thickening and clumping of the lymph. Breaking down congested lymph fluid is painlessly achieved using the Lymph Drainage XP2.

Electro-Sound Lymphatic Drainage (ESLD) is used as a complementary modality by a wide range of practitioners, including physicians, naturopathic doctors, plastic surgeons, general practitioners, oncologists, osteopathic doctors, chiropractors, dentists, nurses, massage and physical therapists and colon therapists.

How Does Electro-Sound Lymphatic Therapy Work?

This therapy is a two-step process. As the client reclines on a massage table, the therapist increases electro-static tension and stimulates lymph flow with the Lymph Drainage XP2 Machine. This state-of-the-art device uses two hand-blown glass tube transmission heads containing rare noble gases—argon, xenon and krypton—that devitalize bacteria and viruses while causing no harm to healthy body tissue.

Moving the XP2's two transmission heads over the skin, the therapist manually directs the lymph along the client's limbs and torso in the direction of the lymphatic pathways. The glass tubes deliver a high-frequency signal that stimulates the lymphatic system, increasing circulation and proper elimination and detoxification while enhancing cell nourishment and immunity.

The Miracle of Rerouting

Clients who have had all their axillary nodes removed as a result of a mastectomy can develop lymphedema in that arm.

After-care for those individuals in the past has been as follows: manual lymphatic drainage, compression wrapping and the wearing of a compression sleeve 24/7 to keep the lymphatic fluid from pooling in the affected arm.

With Electro-Sound Lymphatic Drainage Therapy, the practitioner is able to reroute the lymph fluid in the affected arm by placing one of the probes on the anastomosis about 2" below the clavicle on the sagittal watershed in the center of the chest. This causes a draw of the lymphatic fluid to that area. Simultaneously, the other probe is set at a high intensity setting and is used to treat at two to three inch intervals, starting three inches down from the top of the arm, and slowly moving up the arm in a circular motion. This process is followed by doing five to seven sweeps up the arm with the probe towards the anastomosis. We repeat this process by slowly moving down the arm two to three inches at a time. When we reach the finger tips, we do full arm sweeps from the finger tips to the probe at the anastomosis for fifteen to twenty minutes.

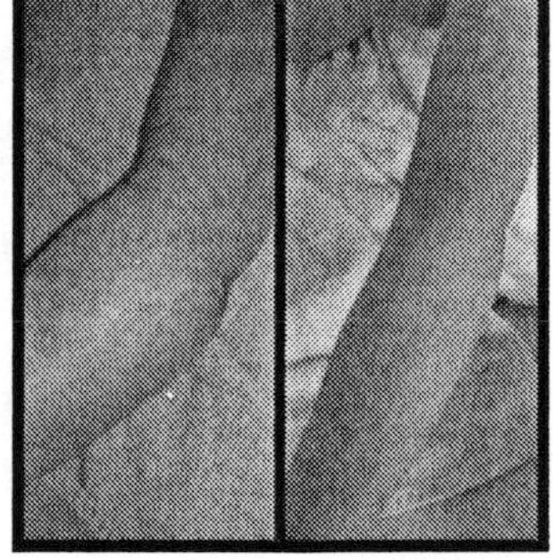

After treatment, the patient will see immediate reduction of the swelling, and over a course of 10 to 12 sessions given once or twice a week, the lymphatic collectors of the patient with Stage One Lymphedema will reroute a new pathway and the patient's arm will no longer swell. This rerouting precludes the wearing of a compression sleeve (except when traveling on an airplane) to keep the swelling down.

Rerouting patients with Stage Two to Four Lymphedema can take up to a year. Recommended follow-up maintenance after a patient's arm has been rerouted would be one LDT treatment every four to six weeks.

Samara Programs, Inc. | 305.323.1994 | www.samaraprograms.com | samaraprograms@hotmail.com

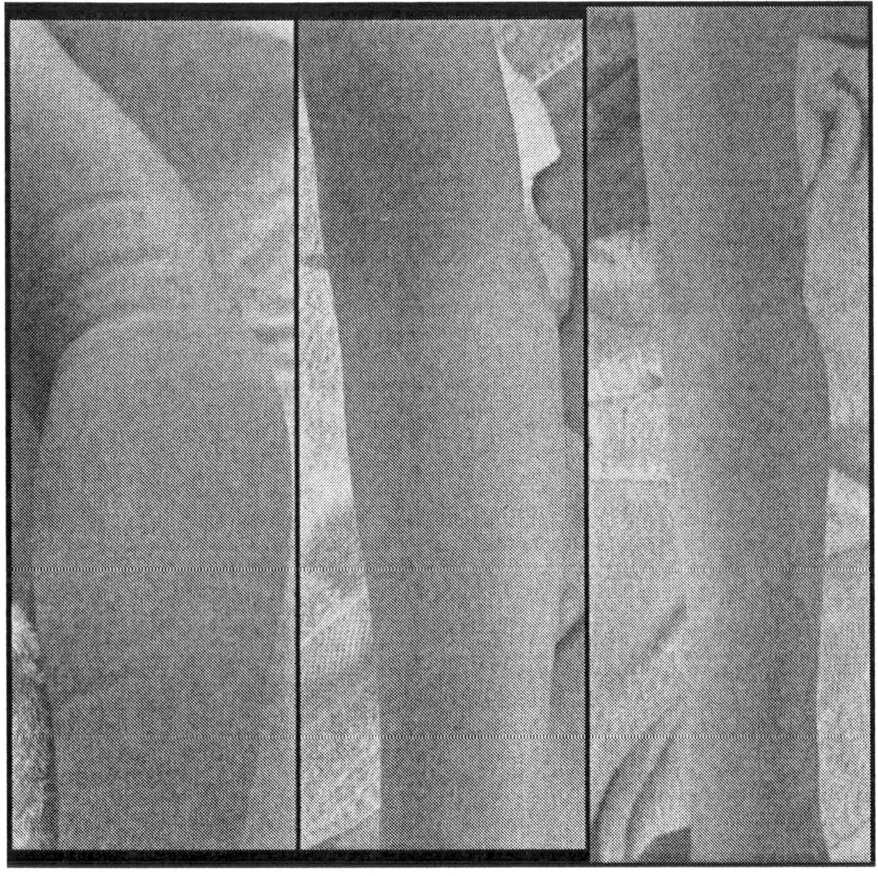

CASE STUDY - Stage Four Lymphedema of Arm

This client (name withheld at client's request) came to us with severe Stage Four Lymphedema due to a mastectomy of her right breast and all of her axillary nodes having been removed from under her right arm.

We were able to give her relief by getting her arm swelling down (see before and after pictures below) by seeing her once a week for ten months (44 weeks).

It is worthwhile to note that if this client had come to us sooner, the time for her to receive relief could have been dramatically shortened.

BEFORE rerouting

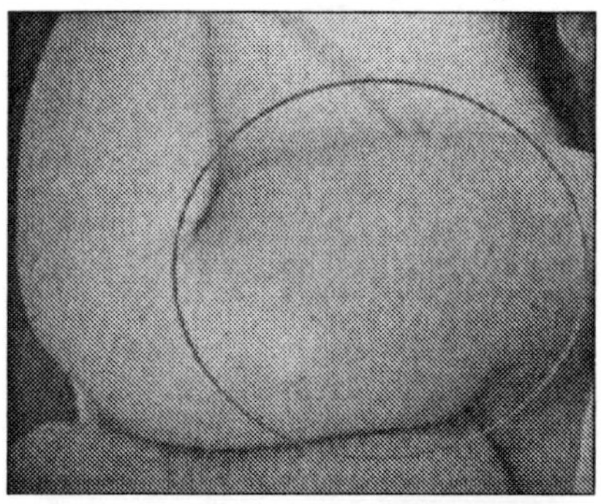

AFTER rerouting

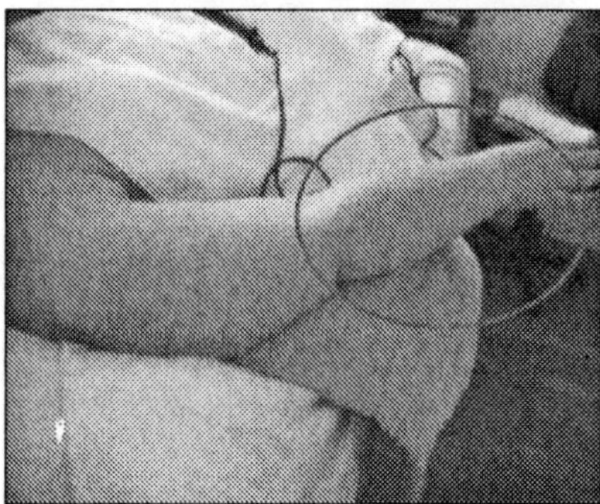

Samara Programs, Inc. | 305.323.1994 | www.samaraprograms.com | samaraprograms@hotmail.com

Adrenal Failure in Patient (Year 2006)

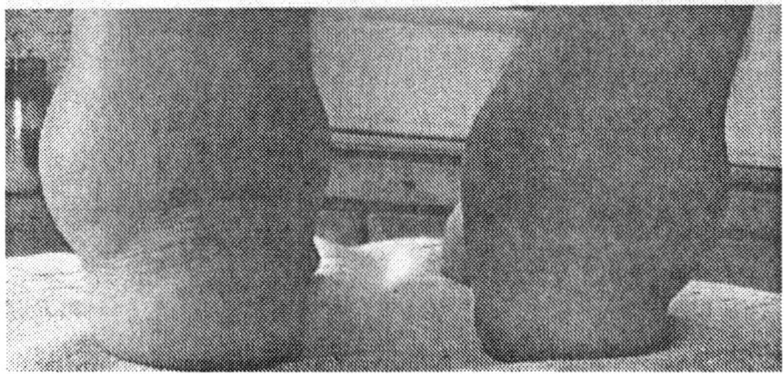

Results after 2 ½ months treatment twice monthly

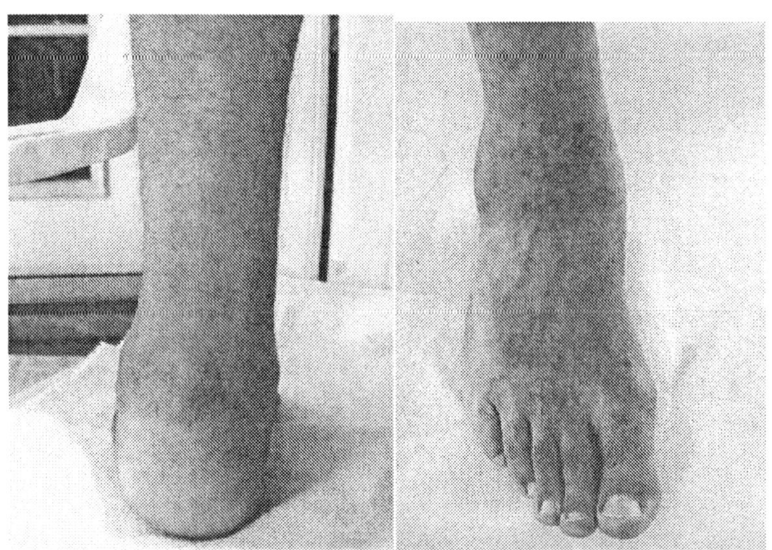

THE SCIENCE BEHIND IT
How Inert Gas Ionization Instruments Work On the Body

Inert elements have the same amount of protons and electrons, so they cannot interact molecularly with any other element. Thus they remain in their elemental state and do not form molecules. This is what gives them their unique properties (inert). The Inert Gas Ionization Instrument's (IGII) high voltage discharge excites the electrons, causing them to jump to an outer orbit. When this occurs, the atom has to go back to stability or back to its natural state. The return to stability is given off as radiant energy through the transmission head, which would technically be called a transducer (transducers change or transform energy). This radiant energy is given off through a combination of light, sound vibrations and through the flow of electrons (also known as ionization), which is discharged into the nearest ground (living body tissue). This effect is far more biologically compatible through the transduction of the Inert Gas Ionization process than, say, broadcasting at low voltages into metal plates, such as with an ultrasound. The reason for this is that inert elements create a buffering effect in the exchange of energy in the ionization of the inert gases, rather than the direct RF transmission created by the actual circuitry of the instrument. The effect created by the light and sound vibration, and by the flow of electrons as they are ionized through the transmission head, causes a disassociation of the trapped proteins within the interstitium. Trapped proteins in the interstitium hold water and cause swelling and blockage as the threadlike vessels swell beyond their capacity, and can no longer effectively pass along the lymph through its normal means of transport in the lymphatic system. Trapped proteins (not to be confused with nutrient proteins) are highly electrical in nature, and when they are exposed to the discharging ions in the transmission head, they become disassociated and release their bond among themselves and release the stagnant lymph. This allows the lymph vessels to release the excess blocked, stagnant or retained fluid, and to flow out into its normal filtration and reabsorption channels.

But what if those normal filtration and reabsorption channels have been compromised? What if, as in the case study presented here, those channels were destroyed by breast cancer treatment?

The use of an Inert Gas Ionization Instrument in conjunction with the proper therapeutic techniques can provide results beyond that of manual lymph manipulation alone and/or the use of tight-fitting garments. Just look at the case studies that preceded this. Why not address the trapped and sticky proteins directly? Why not provide substitute nodes to replace those that were destroyed?

New pathways can be created by rerouting (described above) in combination with the use of alternative anastomoses, which moves lymph fluid from one quadrant to another.

What Are Some Of The Benefits of Lymphatic Drainage Therapy?

Some of the many benefits of ESLD:

- Supports post-mastectomy health
- Reduces edema (swelling and lymphedema of many origins
- Relieves discomfort from fibrocystic breast
- Regenerates tissue, such as pre-and post-surgical scars, stretch marks and wrinkles – especially on the face
- Supports preventative health maintenance
- Detoxifies body tissue
- Assists with weigh loss
- Reduces cellulite tissue
- Helps relieve chronic joint and muscle pain
- Promotes T-cell development

Reduces symptoms of chronic fatigue and fibromyalgia

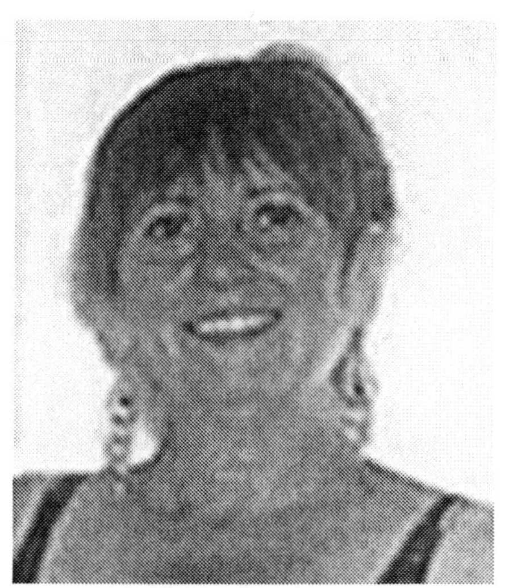

Samara Christy LDT, CLT

has more than twelve years' experience as an XP2 Electro-Sound Lymphatic Drainage therapist, trained by Doctor Jennifer Johnson Gramith in Alpharetta, GA. In 2006, she went on to become certified as a XP2 Lymphatic Drainage trainer, qualifying her to teach and certify others to be practitioners. Her passion is working with breast cancer survivors who have been left with lymphedema in their arm(s) as a result of their lymph nodes being removed at the same time they had a mastectomy. As part of their recovery, these clients are instructed to wear a compression sleeve for the rest of their lives, to help prevent swelling from the lymphatic fluid pooling in the affected arm(s) as a result of the lymph nodes being removed at the site where the lymph fluid drains. Samara is able, with the XP2 Lymphatic Drainage Machine, to reroute the lymph flow to other area of the body, thus reducing the swelling and eliminating the need to wear a compression garment. Currently Samara practices in the Miami, FL area, where she works with clients and trains new lymphatic drainage therapists. She has assisted hundreds of clients with their lymphatic health, enabling them to embrace a healthier lifestyle. Visit Samara's website at www.samaraprograms.com. You can reach her at samaraprograms@hotmail.com.

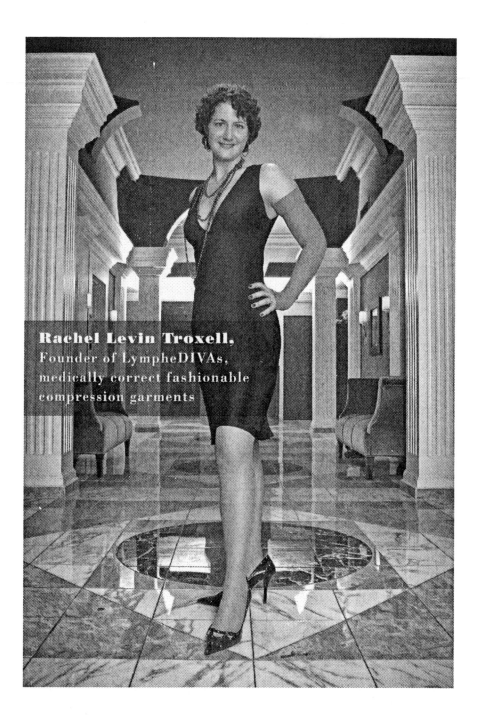
Rachel Levin Troxell,
Founder of LympheDIVAs,
medically correct fashionable
compression garments

Lymphedivas: Medically Correct Fashion for Lymphedema

The story of LympheDIVAs began in Philadelphia when two young breast cancer survivors Rachel Troxell and Robin Mille developed lymphedema, a side effect of breast cancer treatment that can cause permanent swelling in the arms. Their physicians and lymphedema therapists recommended a compression sleeve as the most effective way of controlling the swelling. When they researched their sleeve options, they found that the only ones available were rough textured, heavy, hot, beige, and bandage-like. Frustrated and dismayed, Robin and Rachel met with fashion designer Kristin Dudley to discuss their idea of creating a more elegant and comfortable compression sleeve.

In late 2007, Robin left the company. Soon after, Rachel discovered her breast cancer had returned. While she was being treated, she continued building LympheDIVAs, which brought her much joy during this difficult time in her life. Although Rachel's body succumbed to breast cancer on January 22, 2008 at the age of 37, she continued to be a vital presence at LympheDIVAs until the end. Her determination and compassion to improve the lives of breast cancer survivors is very much ingrained in the spirit of LympheDIVAs.

Today, LympheDIVAs' products can be found in retail locations nationwide and internationally. At Rachel's request, her father Dr. Howard Levin and her mother, Judy Levin took over the responsibility of running the company which their daughter helped found. In August of 2010, Rachel's little brother Josh Levin joined . They all hope that LympheDIVAs' compression apparel will continue to inspire breast cancer survivors everywhere to feel as beautiful, strong and confident as Rachel. For more on Rachel's story and Lymphedivas, visit www.lymphedivas.com.

Chapter 13

Pain Management

Dennis Patin, M.D.

It is hard to believe that more than seven years have passed since the initial publication of *The Empty Cup Runneth Over*. It is an honor for me to have been asked to write a follow up chapter on anesthesia and pain management. The name of the original chapter was *Reaching Nirvana – Pain, Pain, Go Away – Anesthesia Saves the Day*. While that title remains appropriate, in this updated chapter I will seek to incorporate additional information on advances made in the field and how those advances have led to a safer and more pleasant experience for a woman undergoing any type of diagnostic or surgical procedure related to a potential or actual cancer diagnosis. Also, we will discuss contemporary pain management in the acute and chronic setting.

Anesthesia literally means "without sensation," and is generally referred to as a service or treatment a patient may receive to allow a diagnostic or surgical procedure to take place without discomfort. Discomfort can be emotional or physical. Emotional discomfort can be alleviated by reducing anxiety, and by providing amnesia for the procedure. This is the building block or base of anesthetic care, and it starts with the anesthesia care provider-patient relationship.

Before any procedure, you will have a meeting with that provider, where you'll have an opportunity to ask questions about your anesthetic and the choices you may have. This anesthesia care provider could be your doctor, administering local anesthetic and/or sedative medications, or it could be a physician anesthesia specialist known as an anesthesiologist, working alone or with the help of an anesthetist known as a CRNA (Certified Registered Nurse Anesthetist) or AA (Anesthesiologist Assistant) a type of PA (Physician Assistant). Such a care team is quite common, and is believed to be associated with superior outcomes, especially in more complicated cases. A good discussion of anesthesia options goes a long way toward building trust and minimizing anxiety.

Very minor procedures may require only local anesthesia, which is typically injected into the site where a needle biopsy on incisional biopsy is to take place. The local anesthesia literally "numbs" the area for hours, wearing off gradually. Depending on physician, institution, and patient preference, the local anesthesia may be supplemented by oral or intravenous sedative medications designed to relieve anxiety and provide amnesia. These can be administered by or under the supervision of the physician performing the procedure, where it is known as Sedation/Analgesia, or by the anesthesia care team specialists, where it is known as MAC or (Monitored Anesthesia Care). MAC is typically used for more invasive or painful procedures, in patients who have more complex medical conditions, and in those where simple local anesthesia is insufficient.

General anesthesia is administered for more complex and painful procedures, and only by the anesthesia care team. In addition to the reduction of anxiety and procedural amnesia, a benefit of general anesthesia is absence of sensation, absence of pain, absence of movement, and reduction in abnormal reflexes during the procedure. The anesthesia care team will monitor and support your vital signs continuously, often with the aid of a breathing tube inserted after you are asleep and taken out just before you return to full consciousness.

A common fear is awareness under anesthesia, that the patient will remember parts of their procedure and be unable to signal or notify their anesthesia care provider. Fortunately, the incidence of this is extremely low. If you are particularly concerned, mention it to your provider and special steps will be taken to further minimize the risk.

Modern-day anesthesia is very safe, so safe that malpractice premiums for anesthesiologists are similar to that of general medical doctors such as internists and family physicians. Contributing to that safety is a preoperative evaluation, where your medical history, surgical history, medications, and allergies are reviewed, indicated laboratory and diagnostic tests such as an EKG are performed, and conditions are optimized. No patient is too sick to receive anesthesia, and no patient is too healthy not to benefit from the proper anesthetic care for their procedure or condition. During this preoperative evaluation, you will receive instructions regarding which medications to take or stop taking, and how long to fast before the procedure. It helps to have a friend or family member with you, as it can be confusing. For outpatient procedures, you will be asked to have a caregiver take you home.

In the recovery room, you may be given additional pain relievers known as opioid analgesics orally or intravenously, and this treatment may be continued in the inpatient setting with what is known as PCA (Patient Controlled Analgesia). For home use, you may receive a prescription for common oral pain relievers such as morphine, oxycodone (Percocet), hydrocodone (Vicodin), hydromorphone (Dilaudid), and others.

Post-operative or post-procedure discomfort is normal, and will rapidly improve in several days. Any significant pain lasting more than a week or two should be brought to the attention of your surgeon. He or she may then wish to refer you to a pain specialist, a medical doctor with unique knowledge and skills to help you further. After a consultation, the pain specialist may recommend a number of options ranging from acupuncture and physical therapy, to additional medications or procedures such as nerve blocks and injections. Fortunately, the number or percentage of patients undergoing procedures and surgery and later developing pain requiring a pain specialist is very small.

Should you be diagnosed with cancer, there may be associated pain from the tumor itself, or from surgery, chemotherapy, or radiation treatments. The most important thing you can do in this regard is to inform your health care team about your symptoms. They will ask questions to assess your pain in more detail. In fact, pain is considered the "fifth vital sign" after blood pressure, heart rate, respiratory rate, and temperature. Assessing pain is done at all healthcare visits, inpatient and outpatient.

After assessment, several decisions can be made, ranging from no action needed because of minimal pain or patient request to urgent consultation with a pain specialist. A pain specialist is a physician with additional training and experience in the medical specialty of pain management. These physicians are usually also anesthesiologists, neurologists, physical medicine and rehabilitation specialists, or psychiatrists. They can be found in solo practice, group practice settings, or university based academic centers.

A pain specialist will take a more in-depth history, perform a focused pain exam, review medical records, and come up with several treatment plans, ranging from the simplest, to the most involved. Keeping a pain diary may be useful, in addition to involving and bringing a friend or family member to the consultation and follow-up appointments.

Treatments are either considered noninvasive or invasive. All things on the outside of the body are noninvasive; this includes physical therapy, acupuncture, exercise, improving sleep, and psychologic and spiritual support.

Invasive includes anything that goes into the body, and the most common treatment here is medication. Three broad categories of medications are:

1. Nonsteroidal anti-inflammatory medications such as ibuprofen and acetaminophen. They are general

purpose pain relievers and several are available over the counter.

2. Opioids such as morphine, oxycodone (Percocet and Oxycontin), hydromorphone (Dilaudid), oxymorphone (Opana), transdermal fentanyl (Duragesic), buprenorphine (Butrans), tramadol (Ultram), tapentadol (Nucynta), and methadone.
3. Adjuvants. The most common are the anticonvulsants and antidepressants, topical medications, and everything else that doesn't fit the above categories.

Your primary care physician or cancer specialist may start you on some of these medications while reserving others for the pain specialist.

In up to 20% of patients, medical management will be insufficient, either failing to satisfactorily relieve pain or secondary to unacceptable side effects such as sedation. In these cases, selected nerve blocks can be performed or the delivery route of medication changed. A very effective route is intrathecal, also known as intraspinal or neuraxial. Here a small catheter is implanted into the fluid surrounding the spinal cord and the catheter is connected to a delivery system, usually an implanted drug reservoir known as a pump. Pain relief can be substantially better than systemic administration, with a marked reduction in side effects as well.

This is a natural time to discuss the concepts of palliative care and hospice. Palliative care is simply attempting to relieve various symptoms of a disease process that has no cure. Hospice is palliative care at the end of life. Palliative care is a medical specialty like pain management, with various physician specialists receiving additional training. Many, if not most, also work in the hospice field. They are excellent pain management specialists as well, with a slightly different focus and perspective.

In summary, a woman facing a potential cancer diagnosis or actual diagnosis will come to interact with the medical specialties of anesthesiology and pain management. We are all committed to allaying your physical and emotional pain and suffering, no matter where you are on the cancer treatment continuum.

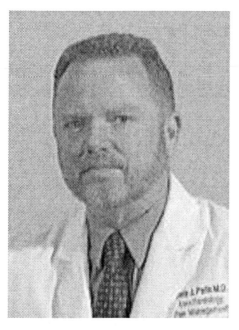

Dennis Patin, M.D.

is a specialist in anesthesiology and interventional pain medicine. He earned his M.D. from the University of Miami School of Medicine/Jackson Memorial Hospital in 1985 before completing an internship at Oakland Naval Hospital in 1986, followed by a residency at Jackson Memorial Hospital in 1992. He is an Associate Professor of Clinical Anesthesiology at University of Miami, Miller School of Medicine and is certified by the American Board of Anesthesiology – Pain Medicine. Licensed to treat patients in California and Florida, Dr. Patin currently practices in Miami, Florida and Plantation, Florida.

Chapter 14

Through the Eyes of an Oncology Nurse

Janet Villalobos, ARNP

My name is Janet Villalobos. I was the first person in my family to attend college. Today I am a Board Certified Acute Care Nurse Practitioner, working in Pain Management at the University of Miami, Sylvester Comprehensive Cancer Center. There, our practice focuses mainly on cancer pain, which provides for a very rewarding career. There is no limit to the satisfaction I feel from seeing these patients obtain the pain relief they so desperately desire. I consider myself very lucky to have the opportunity to be part of that team.

I began my career in healthcare at Baptist Hospital, where I volunteered my time during my college years and later worked as an emergency room technician. Since then, I've worked as a registered nurse with over 15 years of healthcare experience in different specialty areas including pediatric oncology and ICU nursing, medical/surgical telemetry, home health, case management and adult oncology.

In addition to my extensive clinical background, my academic achievements include two bachelor degrees, one in biology and one in nursing, graduating Magna Cum Laude from Barry University School of Nursing. Throughout my nursing career, I have forged a path which has led me toward helping patients deal with disease. For this reason I felt that a Master's degree in nursing would give me the tools to better serve my patients by integrating the medical model and nursing model.

I am also the mother of a very beautiful 12 year-old daughter who is the light of my life and my reason for living. She has been with me through all the tough times, even when she didn't know it. She is an exceptional human being and a loving child with everyone she interacts. She always displays good manners around others and has a very unique quality which I wholeheartedly admire; she is very polite and discreet with others. She makes her mother proud every day.

Nursing was not my first choice. In fact, it wasn't even my second choice, but it was the best one I could have ever made. It has definitely changed my life. As a young girl, I wanted to be a teacher. I knew I wanted to do something that involved children. Don't all kids think alike? My daughter now says the same thing... she would like to be a teacher or a neonatal nurse. It almost always involves working with young ones. Whenever I would tell my mother about my dreams of becoming a teacher, she would reply that it wasn't a good idea because it paid too little; that I wouldn't be able to make a good living as a teacher. The best thing for me to study, she would say, was medicine. After all how many physicians in the United States do you see driving around a beat up car and living in the projects?

Encouragement without guidance led me to enroll as a premed major in college to earn a Bachelor's in Biology. Eventually I wound up in medical school, but because I wasn't part of the elite and just an average student, I ended up attending a foreign medical school. Needless to say, this would not be my calling; in the end the hurdles became too overwhelming so I left medical school to start nursing school. Since I had already been accepted to Barry University School of Nursing, I decided to give that career a shot. Never in my life did I imagine the personal satisfaction I would gain from entering into a field with such immense responsibility and such little appreciation for what one does. You may ask: *How can she obtain gratification from doing something that very few appreciate?*

Trust me, I ask myself the same question at times. Especially on the nights I'd come home after a long shift and felt as if I had left my heart and soul on that unit; I had nothing left inside when I returned to my home. Sometimes I was an empty shell. But then there were those "other" days. I call them "The Glory Days."

Don't get me wrong, I loved medical school and I didn't leave because of academic reasons. I would've finished had circumstances been different.

Nursing school was a breeze compared to medical school, I must admit. I graduated Magna Cum Laude without any effort outside of the classroom; I couldn't wait to finish and get on with my life. When I first graduated from nursing school, I attended an open house at Jackson Memorial Hospital with the hopes of going into ICU nursing, but it didn't go beyond the initial interview. I was discouraged because there was too much red tape.

Then I heard about Miami Children's Hospital hiring graduate nurses. There I interviewed and got hired on the spot as a pediatric oncology nurse. That is how my relationship with oncology started. I was very excited to be able to work with children. I wasn't a teacher, but I was looking forward to interacting with kids and making an impact in their lives. Working with kids in the medical field is quite different from adult nursing. Much of this divergence is due to the parents – to whom I never gave a thought.

When you take care of children, you take care of the entire family. It's like dealing with a gangster who is surrounded by all his body guards or a politician by his advisors! I didn't know what I was getting myself into at the time. I definitely met some beautiful souls there, no doubt. Others were not so beautiful and in fact very difficult to deal with. Throw in the parents and you have a recipe for disaster. I remember one in particular whose port I was trying to access. Both parents and family members were present throughout the entire process. Imagine the pressure to not lose my sterile field, especially having other more experienced nurses critiquing my technique in front of everyone and the child screaming and thrashing about while he was held down.

How do you gain that child's trust after sticking him with a needle? If I missed and had to try again, how would I deal with the vocal disapproval of his angry parents? So here I was, a new nurse, fresh out of school who hadn't yet passed my Boards and already inflicting pain on those little souls I wanted to help. In particular, I remember one incident where a boy spat on my face because I had to re-access his port. While I didn't like what he did, I disliked his punishment even more. With one swift movement his mother slapped him so hard his face swung to the side and back causing him to hit his head against the side rail. It was not a pretty experience, but unfortunately one that I will never forget.

He and I never connected, but I loved that child and he will remain a part of me as long as I live. Not because of that incident – although it has marked me forever – but because he was "special" as his parents would call him. He wasn't a typical nine year-old boy who reasoned and cooperated. He had the mind of a four year-old. Yes, he was mentally challenged but what was sadder than his disability was the fact that his parents had not come to terms with it. They loved their boy but didn't know how to deal with him. Hell, I gotta give it to them, it was hard for *anyone* to deal with him.

But he won my heart because he was sweet when he wasn't fearful due to being poked. During these times, he'd be very affectionate and play endlessly. Sometimes he would sit in his room and sing while he played. That always touched my heart so I would finish my hourly rounding and to-do's before taking off to his room to spend time with him – even if just to watch over him and pray we would be able to cure him. He was one of the lucky ones; he survived cancer and was discharged after just two treatments.

Others didn't fare so well. Death is one aspect of oncology

nursing I have never come to terms with. I remember a nine month-old boy with blond hair and blue eyes. He looked like cherub angel. Both his parents were young and he was an only child. It was approximately six months from the time of diagnosis to death. I recall that moment vividly. His father held him in his arms while he fought for breath. He'd lovingly rock him and say "it's okay buddy, it's alright sweetheart." Heart-wrenching.

Writing about it now brings tears to my eyes. More than 50 percent of those children died from cancer during those years. I would meet a new child and his family and fall in love with them only to have the child ripped away from us by this devastating disease. At that time, I couldn't identify what was going on in my head. I dreaded going to work and I would torture myself thinking about those kids and their parents when I wasn't there. I never identified what was happening to me. Although I was an effective nurse who never made mistakes, I demonstrated somewhat aberrant behavior with my colleagues and I didn't get along too well with some parents.

Of course, I never thought about talking about my feelings and worries with anyone; I simply went on day-to-day trying to cope with becoming too attached to the children and then having to say goodbye. I felt that oncology treatments were a failure. *What was the point of putting all these children through hell if they were only going to die in the end?* I remember one mother took me aside and asked me what I would do if I had to make a choice of putting my child through a bone marrow transplant. At first, I tried the usual response. I remained professional, noting that giving her my personal opinion would not be the right thing to do. In response, she broke down and started crying. Since we'd become quite close during the treatments, I had no choice but to be a friend.

After warning her that she had asked me for my sincere advice and that I was going to offer it, she said she would consider whatever I told her. My answer was a resounding NO. I would never put my child through a bone marrow transplant. I had seen what that treatment did to the children and I had not seen one survive in the year I had been a nurse. I said, "If he were my son, I would get him out of here and spend the time he has left doing things he wants to do."

Please understand I was not a parent at the time; I had no idea how protective one becomes with their own child. Back then it was easy for me to decide. After all he was not my son. I regret to say that I'm not so sure anymore what my answer would be to that question. In the end, she put him through the transplant and he did not survive. But had she not attempted to save her child, could she have lived with herself? I look at it as a no-win situation; any decision she took would have been mired in regret.

Although it is doesn't make up for her loss, she had three other children; I was comforted by that to some extent because she'd still have a reason to live. Her other small children still needed her and their father. I also took note of family dynamics. While many families are supportive, others are remarkably dysfunctional. Whenever I encountered these kinds of families I'd wonder, *why in the world did God allow these children to get sick?*

There was a little girl with whom I became especially close. She had leukemia and I remember the first time she came in for her first round of treatment. At the time of diagnosis, she was just nine years-old and led into the unit by her mother and three other siblings. Her mother was a young woman wearing high heels, tight jeans and top and hair extensions, with a face covered in make-up. She was overly bejeweled with thick gold hoop earrings and several gold teeth. Each of her children – including the newly diagnosed angel – was poorly groomed, dressed in clothes about several sizes too small, with wet noses and disheveled hair.

To my dismay, this tiny patient was dropped off and left alone with no spare clothing or shoes. I remember she was too big for the smaller hospital gowns, forcing us to give her adult gowns. She would walk around the unit dragging the gown behind her and bunching it up in her hands in front of her. I made it a point of sharing good times with her and requesting her as my patient whenever she was there. I dreaded going home and leaving her all alone overnight; a helpless, innocent child with no one to dry her tears or hold her through the night to soothe away her fears. She didn't ask for this. She hadn't done anything to deserve her misfortune. Didn't other people see this?

I would observe the other nurses around me and found them so distant from the patients. Some would tell me that I would get used to it eventually. They seemed like business as usual at all times. I wonder if some of them had undergone counseling where they'd learned to deal with the stress and profound sadness that comes from losing a patient. After some more lives loved and lost, I decided I couldn't deal with it anymore and resigned.

Have you ever heard the expression "whoever does not like soup gets two servings?" Well that saying definitely applies to me. I went back into oncology nursing at the University of Miami about five years ago, but this time with adults. As I mentioned earlier, working with adults is definitely different than working with children. Although my heart still goes out to them due to their devastating diagnosis, I have comfort in the knowledge that they have lived already and are, for the most part, fully capable of taking care of themselves and understanding their diagnosis – sometimes even capable of embracing it, accepting it, and fighting it consciously. With the advancement of science in the field of oncology, many patients who once got a death sentence with this diagnosis are now surviving to live another day. With this said, my outlook on the treatments and the diagnosis itself has molded into one of hope for the future; perhaps I can shed some light on this for you if you are battling this tough disease and need some tips.

Getting a cancer diagnosis can be overwhelming. The worst emotion that will probably keep anyone up all night is fear of the unknown. For this reason alone, many patients will not seek medical attention, even when they are aware that their bodies have undergone some kind of change. The best advice I can offer as a nursing professional is for patients to become informed about their diagnosis and treatment options. It is okay to get a second opinion. Often this involves seeking another healthcare provider who can review your records and test results, and confirm the initial diagnosis and treatment or suggest a different approach.

New innovative treatments are discovered continuously and a second opinion may also lead to a change in the diagnosis and treatment approach. It may even save your life. Once a cancer diagnosis is received, it is important to make a list identifying important questions like the type of cancer, the specialists able to treat the type of cancer, and the treatment choices available. Another important question to ask involves the effectiveness of one treatment modality over another.

Take for example, breast cancer. Breast cancer types can vary quite extensively. There are many treatments which could be effective in eradicating this disease. In addition to the most common treatments such as surgery, chemotherapy, and radiation, there are more innovative interventions such as targeted therapy and hormone therapy which provide personalized treatment. Breast cancer, like any other type of cancer, has the best chance of being cured if caught in the earliest stages. Knowing the stage of the cancer can shed light on how extensively the cancer has expanded throughout the body, whether to nearby lymph nodes of other organs. This will usually dictate how it is treated.

Knowing the grade of the tumor is also important. The higher the grade, the more likely it is to grow more quickly. The use of hormone therapy will be determined by whether or not the tumor is receptive to estrogen or progesterone. Some breast cancers overproduce a substance called HER2. In these cases, they can be treated with targeted therapy. Once the type of breast cancer is determined, then a treatment plan will be recommended.

So now that you have a cancer diagnosis and a treatment plan, what's next? Once you and your healthcare provider decide which treatment is best for you, getting prepared for what lies ahead is key. Most importantly, you'll need a positive attitude. I have seen patients on both side of this psychological spectrum, and guess who did better? Next, know what to expect after surgery. For women who choose to undergo a mastectomy to avoid the risk of recurrence, there are usually two different approaches to reconstruction.

One approach involves the use of a flap, which is tissue

obtained from another part of your body. Another is the use of a tissue expander which slowly expands your breast tissue in order to accommodate an implant which is done with a second surgery. Surgeries times can vary depending on the extent of intervention needed. It can be either an outpatient or inpatient procedure and it may even require you to stay several days in the hospital. You can definitely expect swelling, scarring, and possibly a change in breast sensitivity. Overall recovery can take up to six weeks.

Expect to take pain medication and be sure to ask your surgeon if performing surgery on the natural breast simultaneously with your reconstruction would be a good idea so that both look more symmetrical. Many women fail to think about this and often undergo unnecessary surgeries to get their breasts to look the same. Remember nipple reconstruction too! Working in a cancer inpatient unit, in addition to administering the treatments ordered by providers to our patients, I also dealt with the side effects that often plague these patients, mostly nausea and vomiting, fatigue, neutropenia, and hair loss.

Most breast cancer patients are given chemotherapy and radiation on an outpatient basis, but I can still offer some savvy advice for these patients as they will experience these at home. Prevent nausea and vomiting by eating small, frequent meals consisting of foods you like. Most chemo regimens will change your palate; therefore, the the foods you ate previously might now be unpleasant for you. Drink plenty of fluids in small sips throughout the day instead of trying to chug down a whole glass. For combating fatigue, take advantage of frequent rest periods during the day. Don't do too much at one time.

Maintain regularly scheduled time for physical activity whether walking, light jogging, or even bike riding. Make sure you stay tuned to your inner self with relaxation techniques, yoga, or meditation. For times when you are neutropenic (low white blood cell count/low immune system activity) from the chemotherapy, make sure you practice a good hand-washing technique since this has been known to be the best prevention of infection. If you develop a fever, contact your oncologist right away. You will need immediate hospitalization and antibiotic therapy. Stay away from crowded places, children, and pets while you are neutropenic. Children can carry lots of bugs around from picking toys up off the floor or playing outside and I don't have to explain about dogs who roam around outside in the yard and come into the house without cleaning their feet or washing their hands!

For many women, losing their hair in addition to losing a breast can mean losing their feminine identity. While undergoing treatment, do not use abrasive shampoos or heat styling devices such as blow dryers or flat irons. Also if you know your treatment is going to cause you complete hair loss, give yourself a shorter cut or shave your head completely. If you decide to shave, you can choose different hair coverings from hats and scarves to wigs. You can even buy these before you need them so you are prepared when the time comes. Hair and make up are integral to feeling feminine. You can optimize your look by applying make up to help you feel more like yourself and you can even use a self tanner to combat the pallor that more often than not accompanies cancer treatments. Remember to trim, file and color your nails to cover any discolorations which may result from some chemo treatments. Be sure to do this yourself or have a friend do it with your own tools to avoid getting an infection from shared tools.

Unlike children who are automatically cared for by their parents, grandparents and other family members willingly and without asking for help, many adults isolate themselves from family and friends when faced with a cancer diagnosis. They don't want to overburden their loved ones. But to you I say this: enlist the help of family and friends. Everyone pitching in equally means there is less to do for any one caregiver, providing for adequate time off and a more effective support system. Caregivers should take turns staying with you overnight in the hospital and at home. Take inventory of what each person is good at doing and don't be afraid of asking them for help – from cooking to cleaning, laundering, medication administration, errand running and child c, are.

No one person should be left to care for someone with cancer by themselves. It can cause something called caregiver burnout and it's not fair to the caregiver – especially if there are others willing to help. I took care of a patient whose daughter stayed with him during the day and whose wife would come in and keep him company overnight. During the weekends, his son-in-law would stay with him while his sister would cook his favorite homemade meals. They worked in sync, each knowing what needed to be done. One day I asked them how they did it. They told me that they'd gotten together when he was first diagnosed, made a list of responsibilities, and divided them up. It worked like a charm! It's important for caregivers to accept help from others and continuously communicate with one another.

At the beginning of this chapter I related that nursing had been the best career choice I ever made. Well if you read this chapter in full, now hopefully you understand why. Oncology nursing is a tough field because it showcases our mortality as human beings and involves giving of oneself as a person as well as a professional, and those lines can be blurred at times. As a nurse I have been able to make a difference in my patient's lives by preparing them to face their cancer treatment, accommodating them while hospitalized, educating them on a daily basis and comforting them through their most critical time. Dealing with a cancer diagnosis, its treatment and its aftermath can be daunting for even the most well-adjusted individual with the best support system. I have been blessed to be a part of many patient journeys and I wouldn't trade this for anything else.

Janet Villalobos, ARNP

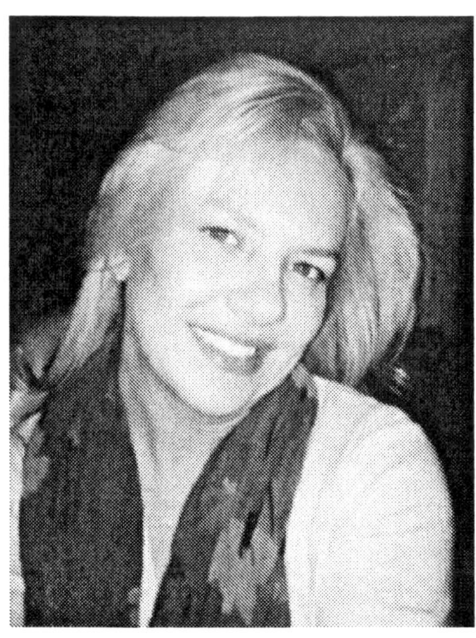

is a Board Certified Acute Care Nurse Practitioner working in Pain Management at the University of Miami, Sylvester Comprehensive Cancer Center, where she focuses mainly on cancer pain. She has worked as a registered nurse with over 15 years of healthcare experience in different specialty areas including pediatric oncology and ICU nursing, medical/surgical telemetry, home health, case management and adult oncology.

Chapter 15

Nutrition

A Higher Level of Wellbeing

Sabrina Hernandez-Cano, RDN, NC, CDE

Any one of us who may not have obvious risk factors can still be diagnosed with breast cancer. A female's lifetime risk is one in eight. From friends, cousins, aunts, colleagues, clients – even my own mother – I've known many who were shocked when test results revealed there was a lump in their breast. Given that most of them felt as if they'd been eating well and following a healthy lifestyle, news of such a health crisis took them by surprise. That is why I believe there is so much frustration with a diagnosis of breast cancer. We do the best we can with our food, exercise and our environment; however, health is a journey, not a destination. We need to become aware and vigilant of risk factors and aim to lower them.

My goal in the following nutrition chapter is to review my years of experience and knowledge and offer what I have gathered from nature, science, and survivors so that we may rise to higher level of wellness. That way, if must face a breast cancer diagnosis, we may have a stronger mind and body to heal and recover with optimum cellular strength.

I strongly believe in nourishing thyself first. It starts when we choose natural foods, activate our bodies, and positively feed our mind and spirit to the best of our ability. Wellness is an interior mirror looking from the outside in and reflecting from the inside out. Poor nutrition, stress, a sedentary lifestyle, and a toxic environment are a pretty good recipe for most types of cancers.

We need to ask some basic but important questions. Are we choosing chemical-laden, artificial junk food? Do we neglect our basic need for the proper amount of water? Do we lack movement and become so rigid and tight that our bodies just don't flow? Do we know the distribution of our weight so we know how much fat mass or muscle mass we carry? Do we give into excess sugar and alcohol because we buy into sweet and sexy marketing?

It is time to become aware and to question why, in our nation, losing weight has become a 50 billion dollar industry. If we continue to buy junk food, manufacturers will continue to package it nicely for us. Our future generations may find themselves eating from boxes and wrappers filled with processed and non-nutritious strange things that may not even classify as food. I invite you to a higher level of wellbeing. A switch to natural foods and nourishment of our physical, emotional, intellectual, social and spiritual being. Wellness will have you humming like a hummingbird and reflecting strength, flexibility and endurance. Mental focus clarity and longevity will be yours.

My own nutrition has improved ever since my life experience as an overweight kid inspired me to change. The struggle to fit in and not get called names was so strong that I found myself making better food choices, eating smaller portions, and dancing my way into a career that I would choose again if I had another life to live. My greatest joy and gratification comes from seeing the transformation in my clients when they eat right and find daily enjoyable movement. When good nutrition and wellness transcend through the life cycle of human beings, it leaves behind a better planet for those to come.

Prevention is Paramount

Keeping abreast of the latest research is key in prevention and care. Thanks to the impact of research, scientists, and the latest technology, lives are being saved and the quality of life improved. There are habits and practices that we know for sure can lower risk factors and then there are things that are still not so clear. However, one thing is absolutely indisputable: weight matters. Scientists are telling us that gaining weight as we age increases the risk of post-menopausal breast cancer. A combination of excess weight and higher levels of estrogen and insulin may also be a detrimental triangle.

Avoiding obesity, which is correlated with high circulating insulin levels, is crucial in preventing breast and other cancers. Post-menopausal women do not produce estrogen. Their fat cells become responsible for making estrogen; therefore, the more fat cells in the body, the higher the amount of estrogen as estradiol in their blood, which increases risk.

Overwhelming evidence supported by in-vitro, animal, and epidemiologic studies suggests that lifestyle and diet influence cancer initiation, promotion, and progression. Currently, according to the American Cancer Society (ACS), 60-70 percent of all cancer cases are directly related to the foods we eat and the way we live. The ACS also estimates that almost half of all cancer deaths could be prevented by simply choosing a better lifestyle and getting screened by your physician. This suggests we have control over our health.

It is never too early or too late to be mindful of healthful eating and take charge of our very own well-being. Dietary guidelines for cancer prevention are very much like those for avoiding the risk of other health problems including heart disease, diabetes, Alzheimer's, and high blood pressure. Although approximately 17,500 diets exist and there is an industry worth over fifty billion dollars in health –promoting ideas and products that may (or may not) work, the bottom line relies on the most scientifically convincing evidence for cancer-fighting potential.

Maintaining or achieving a healthy weight, becoming physically active, exploring the power of nutritious foods, and staying nutritionally strong during the fight are our ammunition; they define what a promising lifestyle is all about. In this chapter you will also find super nutritious, delicious recipes and meal plans that promote optimal health.

Weight Matters

Healthy weight is not determined by charts or scales alone. Your own healthy weight is unique to you; just as you are special in many ways, so is your height, size, and shape. This is why your genetic makeup plays a strong role. A genetic link may also exist to body fat. However, we cannot blame genes alone.

Metabolism (the rate at which your body burns energy) differs from woman to woman. Patients love it when they finally understand body composition. A machine called the Tanita Body Composition Analyzer runs a small current up one leg and down the other. There is no pain during this procedure. The patients get a readout that shows not only their weight but their muscle and fat mass. Because muscle burns more calories than fat, it is advisable to become physically active and increase muscle mass. Healthy weight is also determined by your body mass index (BMI). This is simply your weight in relation to your height (see Chart) for an easy way to figure your BMI.

Simply plot your height in inches: for example, if you are five feet tall, that's sixty inches; if you are five feet, two inches tall, that's sixty–two inches. Now find your weight across and your BMI above. This tool also helps determine your risk for weight-related health problems. BMI is usually higher in women with more percentage of fat than those with higher percentage of muscle.

Women with excess body fat are at greater risk for health problems including cancer. The higher the BMI the greater the risk. A BMI of 18.5 to 24.9 indicates a healthy weight; 25 to 30, overweight; and 30 and higher, obesity.

Body Mass Index (BMI)

Weight in Pounds (lbs) and Kilograms (kg)

Height in Feet and Inches and in Meters (m)	100 lbs 45 kg	110 lbs 50 kg	120 lbs 54 kg	130 lbs 59 kg	140 lbs 63 kg	150 lbs 68 kg	160 lbs 73 kg	170 lbs 77 kg	180 lbs 82 kg	190 lbs 86 kg	200 lbs 91 kg	210 lbs 95 kg	220 lbs 100 kg	230 lbs 104 kg	240 lbs 109 kg	250 lbs 113 kg
4'8" 1.46 m	22	25	26	29	31	34	36	38	40	43	45	47	49	52	54	56
4'9" 1.47 m	22	24	26	28	30	33	35	37	39	41	43	45	48	50	52	54
4'10" 1.48 m	21	23	25	27	29	31	34	36	38	40	42	44	46	48	50	52
4'11" 1.50 m	20	22	24	26	28	30	32	34	36	38	40	42	44	46	48	51
5'0" 1.52 m	20	22	23	25	27	29	31	33	35	37	39	41	43	45	47	49
5'1" 1.55 m	19	21	23	25	26	28	30	32	34	36	38	40	42	44	45	47
5'2" 1.57 m	18	20	22	24	26	27	29	31	33	35	37	38	40	42	44	46
5'3" 1.60 m	18	20	21	23	25	27	28	30	32	34	35	37	39	41	43	44
5'4" 1.63 m		19	21	22	24	26	28	29	31	33	34	36	38	40	41	43
5'5" 1.65 m		18	20	22	23	25	27	28	30	32	33	35	37	38	40	42
5'6" 1.67 m		18	19	21	23	24	26	27	29	31	32	34	36	37	39	40
5'7" 1.70 m			19	20	22	24	25	27	28	30	31	33	35	36	38	39
5'8" 1.73 m			18	20	21	23	24	26	27	29	30	32	34	35	37	38
5'9" 1.75 m			18	19	21	22	24	25	27	28	30	31	33	34	35	37
5'10" 1.78 m				18	20	22	23	24	26	27	29	30	32	33	35	36
5'11" 1.80 m				18	20	21	22	24	25	27	28	29	31	32	34	35
6'0" 1.83 m			16	18	19	20	22	23	24	26	27	28	30	31	33	34
6'1" 1.85 m			16		19	20	21	22	24	25	26	28	29	30	32	33

Healthy Weight   Overweight   Obese

Aim for BMI of 18.5 to 24 and you will be in a healthy weight range. But don't forget that a healthy you comes in many different sizes and shapes. This makes you a special individual and a beautiful woman.

The most important thing about your weight is to keep it within a healthy range so you can enjoy a fuller, more productive life and reduce your risk of diseases. If your BMI is above 25 or 30, there is some work to be done. Clearly, there is a link between obesity and breast cancer. *Why do I know?* Because at this moment at least 107 articles from research on my desk tell me so.

Experts and researchers on diet and cancer prevention note that obesity (BMI 30 or above) affects hormones and hormone-related cancers. Cancer is on the rise every year and, unfortunately, so is our weight as a nation. We are facing an epidemic of obesity and we must stop it or we will continue to see more health problems in the future. Just as we fight to find a cure for breast cancer, we must use our ammunition to fight obesity.

The National Cancer Institute says obesity and inactivity may account for up to 20-30 percent of breast, colon, uterine, kidney, and esophageal cancers. It seems that obesity is a major risk factor for breast cancer in post-menopausal women, but not for premenopausal women. Studies are also suggesting that excessive body fat also decreases chances of recovery from cancer. The reason is that excess fatty tissue is a main source of circulating a hormone called estrogen in your body. And breast cancer risk is linked to how much estrogen you are exposed to during your lifetime.

A research study found that women who gained weight after their breast cancer diagnosis increased their risk of recurrence. Excess weight also increases levels of another hormone called insulin, which in turn fuels estrogen. Estrogen is linked to breast and endometrial cancers.

By now, you have seen that although research always has something new to say, many sources from all over the world say the same thing when it comes to weight. Research in achieving or maintaining a healthy weight and lowering the risk of first–time breast cancer also suggest that overweight women have an increased risk of breast cancer – especially after menopause – as compared to women at a healthy weight during this time in their lives.

In a 2005 analysis, Harvard Medical School indicated that losing five to twenty pounds may reduce your cancer risk by 10 percent. Losing more may provide more protection. No matter how much weight you need to lose, even a small loss will offer benefits. So then, how do you lose weight?

This is the fifty-billion-dollar question. First, beware: Almost all of us have contributed to this amount by buying headlines that are just too good to let pass by, even if they don't make sense at all. You know, the ones that read, "Lose 10 pounds in three days."

Yeah, right, sure – only in my dreams.

It just doesn't make any scientific or mathematical sense at all. Before I even attempt to explain how to lose weight, let me remind you that I was an overweight child. Eating on smaller plates, commitment, determination, and a bit of physical activity helped me achieve a healthy weight. You can do the same.

A healthful diet requires that you eat not only the right kind of food, but also the right amount. Excess food that is more than the amount your body requires turns into excess energy or calories that get stored as fat. Since proper nutrition is one of the cornerstones for cancer prevention, let's figure out how many calories promote a healthy weight.

Even though you may need to reach weight goals, it is not advisable to lose weight during cancer treatment. During cancer therapies such as chemotherapy and radiation therapy, you need to eat to your full potential to maximize the amount of nutrients so that your body can be strong to fight along with the medical treatments.

The American Cancer Society has reported that one third of cancer deaths were related to nutrition, physical inactivity, and obesity. Let's do the math. If we are going to lose or gain weight, we need to know that there are 3,500 calories in one pound of fat. The cause of overweight is an energy imbalance: more calories consumed than used. To figure out how many calories you need, simply take your healthy weight in pounds from the BMI chart and multiply by 10 for women and 11 for men. Calories for basic needs, depending on how active you are, would be added 20 percent for light activity, 30 percent for moderate activity, and 50 percent for high activity.

Required Daily Calorie Intake for a 140-Pound Woman

140x10=1,400. Add 20 percent or 280 for light activity.

1,400 +280 =1,680 calories and activity= total calories need

If your BMI is 25 or above and you need to lose weight, take your present weight and divide it by 2.2. Then multiply by 25 and subtract 500 calories to reveal the number of calories you need to eat on a daily basis to promote one pound of fat loss per week: 1,700 calories for a 200–pound woman will promote 1 pound per week weight loss, which is safe.

Although this should give you an idea of how important it is to consider calories in weight management, it is not a substitute for a consultation with a registered dietitian who can provide an individualized program.

Using medical nutrition therapy, a registered dietitian will tailor strategies to your budget, schedule, special needs, and the needs of your family. To find a registered dietitian in your area you can go to the Academy of Nutrition and Dietetics and web site at www.eatright.org.

Always consult with your physician before starting any weight–loss or physical activity program. In order to be successful in any weight–loss endeavor, you must have internal motivators – things like your good health, increased energy and stamina, self-esteem, and a commitment to yourself and your health goals. Your commitment should be for a lifetime – not just for the summer to fit into that cute bathing suit.

Ten Strategies and Ammunition for Successful Weight Loss

1. **Commit** as if you were getting married.
2. **Forget** your total weight. Know your Fat Mass in pounds. Don't weigh yourself daily.
3. **Tweak** all your meals. That means cut the portions of the foods you choose in half.

4. **Whatever** you do, don't start_a diet. It only a few days away from ending and making you feel like a failure. Just know your calorie intake.
5. **Make** a wish list of all the foods you wish you were eating. Buy at least three every time you grocery-shop.
6. **Don't** buy anything in large quantities. Even children should get used to smaller containers and bags.
7. **Eat** several times throughout the day.
8. **Read** labels and know what they mean.
9. **Leave** emotions out.
10. **Get** physical.

The Best Diet is knowledge

- **Calories** come from carbohydrates, proteins, fats, and alcohol. Calories that come from fat and alcohol supply more calories than carbohydrates and proteins, per gram.
- **Carbohydrates** and proteins have fewer calories per gram, while fats supply nine calories, and alcohol seven calories Carbohydrates are the main energy source for the body. They are the body's basic fuel. We need them in the right quantity and of the right quality. This means choosing whole grains such as whole grains, bulgur, quinoa, high–fiber cereals, and brown and wild rice. These are more nutritious because they have the bran and germ, which are rich in vitamins, minerals, fiber and phytochemicals. Go easy on refined white grains such as pasta, rice, and white bread and rolls. Avoiding them in excess is best. They do not contribute as much nutrition and increase the need for more insulin. I find this makes one hungrier and therefore more prone to overeating.

  Research is now suggesting that these carbohydrates, which are low in fiber, may cause spikes in blood sugar because they are quickly converted into glucose. Whole grains are digested slowly and have a lower impact on blood sugar.

A study co-sponsored by the American Institute for Cancer Research reported that women who ate the most carbohydrates were more than twice as likely to have breast cancer as those who ate less. The lowest rates of breast cancer were in women who ate higher amounts of insoluble fiber found in whole–grain carbohydrates such as bran cereals, whole wheat bread, and vegetables. Fiber is a variety of compounds which have different effects on the body. There are two categories of fiber, soluble and insoluble. Soluble fiber is the one that evidence suggest helps to lower cholesterol and may reduce the risk of heart disease. Soluble fiber sources include oats, oat bran, barley, beans or legumes, fruits, vegetables, and brown rice. Insoluble fiber is the one that aids in constipation when consumed with plenty of water. In one reported study in the Journal of the American Medical Association a diet high in fiber helped in controlling weight gain and insulin levels. I encourage my patients to consume 20-30 grams of fiber daily, and to look for good sources of fiber on the labels: 3 grams or more per serving. The research on fiber is ongoing and not yet conclusive, but researchers agree there is plenty of evidence that a diet rich in fiber based on whole grains, fruits, and vegetables may protect against many chronic diseases. This may be because fiber curbs insulin secretion and fiber-rich carbohydrates often contain anticancer substances.

- **Proteins:** This macro nutrient earns the superlative for most popular; everyone wants to eat it for power and strength. It's true our bodies use protein to build and repair; however, it is important to understand that there are the same calories – 4 to be exact – per gram in both carbohydrates and proteins. Extra protein also gets stored as fat. It is important to be mindful of portions. Choose lean meats such as chicken, fish, shellfish and more vegetables proteins. Good source of vegan protein include garbanzo beans, lentils, soybeans and edamame. Vegetables such as peas, spinach, broccoli and Brussel sprouts also contribute protein.

➢ **Fats:** Research is still not yet conclusive on the association of eating a low-fat diet and the prevention of breast cancer. Some scientists are suggesting that there might be a link between estrogen and fat intake: When dietary fat increases, estrogen levels in breast tissue also go up, which may provoke cancer growth. What we are sure of is that overall food choices that are lower in fat such as fruits, vegetables, and whole grains do offer protection not just for your breasts but for your heart as well. A high–fat diet, especially from animal fat such as saturated fat and Trans fatty acids, has been linked to some types of cancers including breast, colon, rectum, and lung. In addition to aiming for a low-fat diet, it is also important to consume the right kind of fat. But let's first define fat and the role it plays in our system.

Fat, according to Webster's dictionary, is fleshy, plump, oily, rich, and resinous. Fat means so many different things to so many different people. Most women have something to say about "fat" in their lives. I remember Oprah Winfrey talking about it when I was a kid. It was a great, informative show.

"Too much on the thighs, hips, and booty" or "too little on the breast, legs, and ankles." Whether women struggle with obesity or battle anorexia, fat in the last decade has become a hot topic. And with the latest research on the overall health benefits of oils, it seems the whole country is turning toward a positive attitude about fats. Fats are essential to good health; they perform crucial bodily functions. No human being can live without them. Fats are like a fancy jet plane. They transport special vitamins such as A, D, E and K, as well as carotenoids into the bloodstream. That is why these important vitamins are called the fat-soluble vitamins. Fat also aids in the maintenance of cell membrane, structure, and function. And most importantly, it preserves one's immune system.

The kind of fat that we choose to eat can actually benefit or harm us. There are healthy and harmful fats. So let's set the record straight. You can start choosing the best oils for overall health, including breast cancer prevention.

Monounsaturated

Monounsaturated fat is called mono because there is actually one (mono) hydrogen on the carbon chain. The body can process one hydrogen more easily than a chain that is fully saturated with hydrogens. Okay, enough organic chemistry. Monounsaturated fats are liquid at room temperature and begin to solidify in the refrigerator. Monounsaturated fats such as olive, peanut, and canola (avocados and most nuts also have high amounts of monounsaturated fat) are excellent quality of oils.

Too much fat, even the good kind, can add excess calories. The U.S. Department of Agriculture (USDA) and the Department of Health and Human Services (HHS) recommend that fat make up no more than 20-35 percent of your daily calories. For example, 20 percent of 1,400 calories equals 280 calories; divided by 9 (the number of calories per gram of fat) is 30 grams of fat.

Polyunsaturated Fats

Poly (or "some", as the name implies) tells us that there will be more than one hydrogen on the carbon chain. Polyunsaturated fats are also liquid at room temperature. Foods high in polyunsaturated fats include vegetable oils such safflower, corn, sunflower, soy and cottonseed oils. Although these oils are not completely saturated, many times they are partially hydrogenated soybean oil or corn oil. Laboratory tests have shown that breast tumors appeared more often in animals fed diets high in safflower and corn oil than those fed olive oil. Researchers have also noted higher levels of toxic chemicals such as dichlorodphenyltrichloroethane (DDT), and polychlorinated biphyenyls (PCB) in women with breast cancer. Toxic environmental waste have been also found in fatty tissue.

Since the breast is comprised primarily of fatty tissue there is a higher chance of waste being stored there. This means it's not simply the amount or the amount or the kind of fat, but what is in it that really counts. That is why fresh or even organic foods may be the best choice.

Omega-3 Fatty Acids

These are a type of polyunsaturated fat that is essential for good health. They are called essential because the body cannot make these fatty acids on its own. Omega-3 must be included in the diet from fatty fish such as salmon, albacore tuna, and mackerel. Another source of omega-3 fatty acid comes from alpha-linolenic acid (ALA), which the body converts into DHA and EPA (docosahexgenoic acid and eicosapentgenoic acid). Alpha – linolenic acid can be found in certain nuts such as walnuts and vegetable oils like canola, soybean, flaxseed, and olive oil.

Include omega-3 in your diet by eating fish at least twice per week and including ground flaxseed in your cereal or salads. You can get flaxseed oil or seeds that have been ground. The seeds must be ground to get the benefit. Whole seeds aid in constipation.

Saturated Fat

Saturated fat is solid at room temperature and mainly in animal products, such as bacon, butter, sour cream, cream cheese, lard, red meat, poultry, and whole cream products. Other main sources contributing to saturated fats that are not from animals include coconut, palm, and other tropical oils.

Trans Fats

Avoid them at all cost. These fats start out as good old unsaturated oils and then are blasted with hydrogen gas to solidify them, creating an acid that raises bad cholesterol and your risk of heart disease. Aim for zero grams on the labels of foods you bring home. Fortunately and finally, the U.S. Food and Drug Administration (FDA) found partially hydrogenated oils (PHO's) – the primary dietary source of trans-fat – unsafe. Manufactures will have to eliminate trans-fats from their foods. They have three years from today.

Moving Our Bodies

Exercise: A commitment to a healthful lifestyle also means getting physically active. Studies have found that people who exercise have a lower risk of developing cancers of the breast and other cancers. Regular activity can help you achieve and maintain a healthy weight, which has also been found to reduce risk of chronic diseases. In preventing cancer initially, the American Institute for Cancer Research reports that women who are physically active have 30 to 40 percent less risk of breast, endometrial, and lung cancers. Regular exercise after breast cancer diagnosis may reduce the risk of death, especially in women with hormone-sensitive tumors, according to the Harvard Nurses' Health Study.

Health Study: Three thousand women with cancer were studied. Those who were physically active by walking three-to-five hours per week at an average pace had the greatest benefit.

The American Cancer Society recommends that we exercise thirty minutes and preferably forty-five to sixty minutes five or more days a week, at a moderate to vigorous pace. Always consult your physician before engaging in any physical activity. Remember to have fun and incorporate a variety of activities like dancing, yoga, playing a sport, Pilates, marathons, or even boot-camp fitness routines. Make it a habit by scheduling it in as a priority. After all, not only does exercise prolong your life, but it reduces daily stress and makes you feel a live and full of stamina.

Moving our bodies and taking the time to do it is an expression of self-love. The new smoking is inactivity. We need to be in harmony and balance with our physical being. Twenty to thirty minutes of exercise should be part of the work day. If it were mandatory we would not have a choice. We would have to do it in order to get our paycheck. Our companies would have a stronger, energetic, and healthful employee. We would spend less on medical bills and have fewer sick days. It should be part of our work and healthcare system. Incentives should be given to the "worked out" employee. A fit staff member is a more productive employee, manager, and teacher. A more effective executive and professional.

Any form of moving our bodies' counts: Yoga, Tai chi, Pilates and gentle stretching are beneficial for preventing injuries and for overall health and well-being. Studies on breast cancer have shown that walking as much as five hours a week helps prevent recurring cancer. The most important thing about exercise is that it's an opportunity to have fun and enjoy ourselves with friends and family. So walk, dance, or toss that ball. But do move now. Because while we wait our bodies are slowly but surely breaking down. I ask myself every day, "What kind of 90 year old body do I want to have"? My answer: just like my dad. At age 90, he has never sat for very long and is always walking, biking, stretching, and deep breathing. He's my champion. One of the greatest ways to get up and get moving is the buddy system. In my case, I call it the Kathleen project. Kathleen, my dear, strong, and muscular friend, picks me up at 4:55 a.m. so we can spin, "No Excuse" at 5:15 a.m. I owe her my "work in progress body mode." Her famous words are "give me a month" – somehow this has turned into years. Thanks Kathleen, your body rocks! And so does your inspiration and motivation. Please pick me up for spinning even when we're 90 years old!

A Diet Rich in Wellness

Although there exist well documentation of over 17,500 diets the best diet is one that is rich in phytochemicals and antioxidants – in other words, lots of color. These foods are nature's medicine. Our bodies form free radicals when oxygen is metabolized by the body. This is a necessary process to ward off viruses and bacteria. A toxic environment can also promote free radicals. Too many free radicals, and not enough antioxidants can lead to aging and cancer. A combination of phytochemicals or plant chemicals with antioxidants such as (ACE) Vitamin A, vitamin C, and vitamin E should be the fabric of protective and great diet. Phytochemicals can be found in whole grain, beans, fruits, vegetables, nuts, seeds, wine, coffee, tea and dark chocolate.

We are pretty convinced that inflammation is the fire that fuels may diseases including cancer. Inflammation occurs when the immune system is triggered to release chemicals that are damaging, especially when the inflammation occurs for long term. Good nutrition and certain foods can help balance the immune system and insulin levels.

A Mediterranean, Asian, and Indian diet is recommended. All are rich in vegetables, fruits, and vegetable proteins including lentils, peas, beans, and tofu. They also incorporate the use of herbs and spices such as turmeric, mint, thyme, rosemary, and garlic and multi and whole grains like quinoa, bulger, brown rice, and sweet potato.

Choose healthy fats such as olive, canola, flaxseed and Omega–3 oils and butters and eating less animal protein and dairy while opting for more fish and organic meat and eggs. My sister Sandy and I spent some time in Bali and discovered that eating this way gave us enough energy and courage to practice yoga twice a day, meet with the guru and visit three more islands all on the same day. The funny thing is that upon arrival of such a life changing experience she met a French fellow and became his fiancé. They both relocated their lives from Los Angeles to our hometown of Hialeah to open the first French Café, “La Fresa Francesa,” in the history of *The City of Progress*, something the Mayor is overjoyed about. This eatery provides an amazing fusion of worldly flavors; when I visit them I am reminded that balance and moderation is the core of wellness.

We can enjoy our favorite foods as long as we incorporate wellness guidelines for our everyday intake. Therefore limiting alcohol, sweetened drinks, fruit juices, sodas, refined sugars processed, bleached flours, breads, pastries, muffins, cookies and cakes is a good idea. Something I repeatedly hear in food and nutrition conferences is that "Sugar kills, but sugar and fat kill faster." A helpful reminder to make better food choices.

A diet rich in wellness and prevention is a diet that is naturally detoxifying and rids the body of carcinogenic substances. It supports the immune system, preventing malnutrition. A powerful diet is one that reduces oxidation, and inflammation to prevent tumor growth and spread. When I am asked about a detox diet my response is always the same. I detox 24/7. Our liver especially is working hard; why not eat a detox diet filled with natural, organic foods that will go to work all day? Eating right is an opportunity to detox 3-5 times a day.

Nutrients that can aid in the body's natural detox process include whole, organic foods, green cruciferous vegetables, probiotics, and adequate filter from beans, whole grains, fruits and nuts. Adding herbs and spices, garlic and anions. Drink green tea and plenty of water.

Whole organic foods – choose foods labeled USDA certified organic. The USDA, Environmental working group (EWG), shoppers guide to pesticides TM in produce is an excellent tool to help you choose the foods we should buy organic. They call them the "Dirty Dozen Plus" TM and the "Clean Fifteen" TM. Organically grown and raised foods have a positive impact on our health and our environment. Fresh produce can be cleaned by mixing a solution of 16 oz. water and 2 table spoons of vinegar for 2-3 minutes and then rinse and brush.

Functional Food

It is a very exciting time for the science of nutrition. For years we have focused on what foods we should avoid. But today, research is revealing a lot more about the benefits of certain foods that have a potentially positive effect on health beyond basic nutrition. These are call functional foods. These foods contain phytochemicals – and "phyto" means plant. These plant substances fight for our health. Therefore, we also call them super foods.

Just as the public developed an interest a hundred years ago about the discovery of vitamins, today we are seeing great enthusiasm as scientist explore their "functional" benefits. Phytonutrients provoke health by slowing the aging process and reducing the risk for chronic diseases. They are bioactive substances that plants produce naturally to protect themselves against viruses and bacteria. There are thousands of phytonutrients, providing aroma and flavor to our foods. At least two thousand are responsible for plant pigments that make our plates a carnival of colors ad.

One orange may have more than 150 different phytonutrients. Carotenoids give oranges their bright color. Flavonoids give blueberries their blue tint. Both act as antioxidants and may neutralize free radicals. Quercetin, found in tea, onions, and other vegetables may reduce the growth and spread of cancer cells. Plant-based foods contains a variety of these protective substances, especially fruits and vegetables. Phytonutrients are grouped according to their characteristics and possible protective function (see List 1, Examples of Functional Components for functional nutrition phytonutrient list), Other foods that may lower cancer risk include catechins in white, oolong, green , or black tea, which on the oxygen-radical absorbency capacity (ORAC) score ranked as high or higher in antioxidant potential than many fruits and vegetables.

Researchers at the University of Rochester, New York Medical Center, have found that EGCG, another antioxidant component in green tea, has an affinity for a common protein in cancer cell, which may prevent the cascade of events that triggers cancer. The way EGCG may stop the cancer process before it starts is by binding to the most enjoyable when shared with a friend. My coauthor Cindy and I have tea together all the time. These foods mentioned along with many other ones in research today are most likely to have cancer-fighting potential.

It is important not to obsess about any one specific food. There is no single food that can prevent cancer. There are dietary strategies, however that can help make a difference.

Consuming a broad range of healthful foods and living a new, improved lifestyle is smart. A smart lifestyle includes not smoking. Talking to trained professionals about the best option to quit is crucial. Also avoid exposure to sun on your skin, but do get enough vitamin D, "the sunshine vitamin", Research tell us to avoid sun exposure between 10:00 A.M. and 2:00 P.M., Researchers also recommend protecting your skin with clothing or sunscreen.

Vitamin D is absorbed within just a few minutes of sun, several days, or a week. Consume fortified milk or fatty fish. If you do not get some sun or consume milk or fatty fish then consider taking a multivitamin with vitamin D or any other vitamin D supplement. There is mounting evidence that vitamin D may protect against several types of cancers including breast cancer.

Super Survivor Food

Broccoli: My favorite! I chop it up and put it in everything including beans, quinoa, and even hummus spread. Along with kale, Brussel sprouts, cauliflower and cabbage, broccoli has been extensively studied by scientists. The general consensus is that the chemicals in the cruciferous family can ward off and protect against cancer. Broccoli contains a much researched chemical called glucosinolates which breaks into indoles and isothiocyanates. It appears to be protecting against hormone–related cancers like breast cancer. The chemical indoles interrupts the replication of cancer cells. That is why broccoli has become one of my favorite medicinal foods. I call it my daily dose.

Paul Talalay, M.D., Professor of Pharmacology and Molecular Science at Johns Hopkins University in Baltimore was one of the scientists who discovered the potent cancer-fighting isothiocyanate sulforaphane in broccoli (try saying that five times fast!). He also found that tender broccoli sprouts are a superrich source of sulforaphane. According to Dr. Talalay, broccoli and other cruciferous vegetables such as cabbage, kale, cauliflower, and Brussel sprouts have anticancer substances: When plant cells are broken down during chewing, glucosinolates are released and converted to another protective substance called isothiocyantes. These chemicals induce enzymes that help detoxification and boost antioxidants, says Dr. Talalay. Other colorful vegetables with protective properties include tomatoes, squash, carrots, and dark leafy greens.

Probiotics - Friendly Bacteria: The health of our gut is crucial in the healing and prevention of diseases; the colon holds unfriendly bacteria and free radicals. Therefore, we must create a good environment in the gut for good health. Eating more fiber, drinking plenty of water and getting a probiotic supplement will make for a happy gastrointestinal tract. Always consult with your physician or dietician before staring any supplement.

Berries: I am wild about berries! I promote them daily for their wide range of phytochemicals, high fiber, and vitamin C. They are sweet, juicy, and a bit tart at times which makes them perfect to pair with a variety of foods such as vanilla yogurt, salads and as relish on chicken and fish dishes. The variety is abundant. From wild blueberries which have about 26 antioxidants to salmonberries which are part of the rose family. They are pink, salmon colored, but turned as red as they ripen. They are not easy to find but exquisite. I had these in Oregon when I stayed there for a while in my quest to the best ingredients for the Hummingwell wellness bar. The darker berries like blackberries and blue berries are literally under the microscope. Scientist are telling us that the phytochemicals and antioxidants may be potential cancer fighters. I buy a variety of fresh berries and freeze them so I can enjoy them all year round. I make warm berry desserts natural jams, relish, and even salad dressings with berries.

Seeds are the future. They take our food supply to the next generation and contain a concentration of nutrients and oils that are full of flavor, texture and nutritional benefits. I sprinkle, stir, grind, and crunch on seeds like chia, flax, hemp, pumpkin, sesame, sunflower, and watermelon.

Seeds are rich with minerals and healthful fats such as poly unsaturated fatty acids. I grew up watering my chia pet and now I eat them because they are packed with protein, omega–3 fatty acids, fiber, and minerals such as iron calcium, magnesium, and manganese. Chia makes an excellent nonfat thickener for soups and sauces. The gelatinous paste is a type of soluble fiber that is important in heart health.

Flax seeds are bursting with powerful antioxidants, omega-3 fatty acids, protein and vitamin B, zinc, magnesium and manganese. It's important to grind the flaxseed; otherwise it passes through the digestive tract intact. I sprinkle ground golden flaxseed on my oatmeal, berry smoothies, salads, soups, beans, and quinoa berry muffins.

Hemp seeds are getting lots of attention for their high protein and excellent omega-3 fatty acid and mineral content I sprinkle them over yogurt, cereal and savory dishes like stir–fry and soups. Toasting them a bit before you eat or cook with them makes them tastier.

Herbs and the Spice of Life

Spices are the easiest way to become creative in the kitchen; they help me cut back on fat for taste. The ancient healers have used them all across the world. They have exchanged them as medicines in the form of tinctures, teas, syrups, oils and extracts. Scientist today have found they may have phytochemicals that are antioxidant, anti-inflammatory and protect against bacteria's and viruses.

Buy them fresh and cook rosemary, thyme, oregano, basil, mint and ginger which are super fragrant and aromatic. Turmeric and curry, native to the orient, cultivated for least 5,000 years in India, and now found in the Caribbean, are the most powerful natural anti-inflammatories identified by scientists at the moment. Studies are emerging with news about turmeric's main compound, curcumin. This compound has been found to be helpful in playing a role against many diseases including Alzheimer's. It has been shown that curcumin may inhibit the growth of certain cancers. It's the anti-inflammatory and antioxidant spice. It's warm, golden color livens every stew, soup, chili, casserole and salad in my kitchen. On top of the list for inhibition of most cancers including breast cancer are garlic, leeks, scallions, and ginger root – all powerful anti-inflammatories and antioxidants.

Ginger tea eases nausea from chemotherapy and radiation side effects. I get creative and combine olive oil, turmeric, black pepper, garlic, leeks, wild blue berries, scallions, ginger, and balsamic vinegar for a cancer-fighting dressing I use on my salads and vegetable dishes. It was a favorite among my awesome colleagues when I worked at Cardiac Rehabilitation at Baptist Hospital. When I add plain yogurt it becomes the super dip. Even my football passionate son welcomes this dip during football season at game time with his friends. It's teen-approved. I call it the Miami Super Dolphin Dip in hopes this will be the year the Miami Dolphins will take us to the Super bowl. Go Miami!

Dark Chocolate, Red Wine, Coffee, and Self Love

Dark Chocolate

I've always had a passion for dark chocolate; however my true love affair began in a small island called Sao Tome and Principe, Africa's second-smallest country. I was there on a health mission with my husband Alex who is a passionate surgeon and wrote the chapter on Biopsies in this book. There I gained a deep appreciation for cocoa beans. I learned that chocolate means bitter water and that the Aztecs made a bitter drink from cocoa beans and spices. The Mayans believed the bitter drink would heal their hearts, minds and bodies. Now scientific research has revealed a type of anti-oxidant, phytochemical called catechins and flavonoids. These compounds are getting kudos for heart health. The Mayans may have been on to something sweet, while sipping their bitter cocoa drink. I've noticed that a piece of dark chocolate a day makes me happy, wholesome, and very satisfied.

Red Wine

For many of us wine lovers, there is not much convincing to be done here. Wine is a decadent and honorable socialite. It's also noteworthy for the great scientific evidence linking the phytochemical, resveratrol to a multitude of health benefits especially for decreasing risk of coronary disease and stroke. The powerful resveratrol has demonstrate to have antioxidant, anti-clotting, anti-inflammatory, and anti-cancer properties.

Alcohol

This is another subject that needs to be addressed because research is now saying that women who consume even a few drinks per week have an increased risk for breast cancer. The reason is that alcohol may raise estrogen levels, which increases the risk of breast cancer. According to the Nurses' Health Study, the increased risk for breast cancer link with alcohol occurs mostly in women who don't get adequate amounts of the B vitamin and folic acid. Limit alcohol drinks to one per day. However, women who have had breast cancer are at high risk should avoid alcohol altogether. Because there is evidence that alcohol may protect against heart disease, ask your physician if drinking in moderation may benefit or increase risk, based on your genetic predisposition.

Coffee

The aroma is captivating, alluring and as many of us know, addicting. With good varieties of coffee beans it's easy to fall and stay in love. Coffee beans have over 1,000 active compounds, phyto chemicals and a high anti-oxidant profile. The health benefits range from improved mental, and physical performance to cancer fighting properties. In one analysis of eighth studies on endometrial cancer risk and coffee. Involving 300,000 women, found a decrease of seven percent risk in developing endometrial cancer. As reported by the American Institute of Cancer Research. Another good reason to enjoy a cup of Jo.

H2O

Humans are made up of mostly water. The average person carries 10 to 12 gallons of it. It is essential in digestion and excretion. It lubricates our joints and is a major component of body fluids. It is our natural, calorie free, cleansing and purifying drink. The most beautiful skin and balanced body's carry it in abundance. Dehydration causes headaches, increased appetite, constipation, irritability, and lethargy. We cannot live without and would die inits absence in a few days. With the incredible burden we put on our kidneys, from toxins and pollutants from our environment it is a shame that for most people it's a struggle to get the recommended 8-8oz glasses per day. I have found that recommending drinking a couple of glasses of water in the afternoon helps as a pick-me up, much like when you water a dying plant and it quickly comes back to life.

Although calorie-free, somehow it energizes me. It also helps to curb my appetite during those hungry hours from 3 p.m. to 6 p.m. until dinner is ready. I call these the witches hours because if were not careful we can eat right through the pantry. A combination of accumulated stress from the day, appetite, and running around to wrap up our daily routine can create cause for over eating, even though we have probably consumed a pristine diet all day. I found eating a substantial, nutrient-dense snack and hydrating with water was the answer. These hours were the reason I created Hummingwell Wellness bar. Dark chocolate, vanilla, quinoa, oats, and 22 vitamins and minerals in 150 controlled calories solves this problem. I pair it up with a nice tall glass of infused H20. I love natural infusions of lemon or berries in my water but there is nothing like pure, crystal-clear, cleansing H20. If you need an extra boost, dipping Hummingwell Wellness bars into your coffee melts the dark chocolate for a delectable and mouthwatering experience.

Hummingwell Wellness Meal Plan

Designed using a variety of foods rich in phytochemical, anti-oxidants, omega 3 fatty acids and rich in vitamins and minerals. Hummingwell promotes a variety of super and functional foods to promote clean eating. Choose farm fresh, organic, non GMO and minimally or non-processed foods. Always check the first ingredient in your foods, that's what you are eating most of.

Use often: Garlic, leeks, onions, shallots, herbs, turmeric, curry, omega rich oils, and low-fat dairy products, and do wash all fruits, vegetables, and salads, Remove outer leaves to reduce exposure to pesticides.

Be mindful of your meal time. It is a sacred time of nourishing. Over eating happens when we are not connected to our core. Take a deep breath and be thank full before your meals. Eating is a ritual, a pleasure that if respected will in turn provide our bodies with all the nourishment we need. Including our soul and spirit.

DAY 1

Breakfast

1 cup oatmeal
¾ cup wild blueberries
12 almonds, slivered
8 oz. 0-1% fat milk, Almond or cashew milk
1 cup green tea

Lunch

2 slices light rye bread
2 oz. turkey breast nitrite free
1 oz. low-fat Swiss cheese
1 teaspoon olive oil mayo sprinkle turmeric makes
1 teaspoon mustard
½ cup baby carrots
2 tablespoons nonfat Greek yogurt dressing for carrots
2 kiwis

Snack

1 cup nonfat light fruit yogurt
12 cherries, sweet or fresh
1 tablespoons flaxseed

Dinner
1 cup brown wild rice
1 cup zucchini plus 5 tablespoons chopped /cooked onions
1 cup summer squash
4-6 oz. wild Alaskan salmon grilled, baked, broiled, or pan –fried
1 teaspoon coconut oil for cooking salmon

DAY 2

Breakfast
1 Hummingwell, wellness bar
½ cup pomegranate juice
1 cup low-fat light vanilla yogurt

Lunch
2 eight –inch whole corn tortillas
7 oz. grilled chicken cut into strips
½ cup fresh or already prepared salsa (chopped tomato, scallions, cilantro in a tomato sauce, sprinkle turmeric) over grilled chicken.
1 cup shredded kale or spinach in tortillas
1 cup mixed fresh berries-strawberries, blackberries, or raspberries add balsamic vinegar a dash of agave and freeze.

Snack
7 walnuts
1 cup white tea with fresh ginger

Dinner
8 oz. sautéed shrimp in marinara sauce
Marinara sauce, use lots of chopped up heirloom tomatoes
Leeks /shallots
3 cloves garlic
2 teaspoons olive oil
1 cup fresh tomatoes
1 cup ready-made tomato pasta sauce, low- fat
2 cups linguini or gluten free pasta
2 tablespoons grated parmesan cheese
1 cup broccoli, steamed

DAY 3

Breakfast
Almond smoothie
1 cup milk, vanilla almond milk
1 ¼ cup strawberries to mix in blender. May use variation of frozen or

fresh fruit. Peaches are an excellent stone fruit.

Lunch

1 serving of seed crackers

3 oz. canned tuna

1 tablespoon reduced-fat mayonnaise to mix with tuna, sprinkle turmeric

Chop scallions, leeks and black pepper

2 sliced plum tomatoes, baby spinach leaves, chopped onions

½ cup frozen yogurt

Snack

1 green apple cut into slices, powdered with cinnamon

1 tsp of almond butter

Dinner

5 oz. veggie burger

¼ cup mushrooms, ¼ cup onions, ¼ cup red bell peppers, sautéed with 1 teaspoon of olive oil and dried spices of choice.

1 cup brown rice with veggies

½ cup black beans

7 spears fresh asparagus

½ cup frozen mango

DAY 4

Breakfast

1 cup high –fiber cereal

1 small banana

8 oz. of 1% milk almond, cashew milk.

Lunch

Mini pizza

1 whole grain pita bread

½ cup tomato sauce

½ cup chopped tomatoes

3 oz. light mozzarella cheese

½ cup mixed veggies on top lots of chopped broccoli

1 slice apricot sprinkled with low-fat granola and a tablespoon of vanilla yogurt

Snack

Fresh large pear and a piece of dark chocolate

Dinner

8 oz. flounder, baked

1 teaspoon olive oil

Minced fresh garlic, scallions, leeks
1 large sweet potato
1 cup green beans
1 baked apple with low-fat vanilla frozen yogurt
Sautéed the olive oil with the fresh garlic and pour over the fish.

DAY 5

Breakfast

3 egg whites (cooked to your choice)
¼ cup fresh mushrooms, sliced
¼ cup chopped onions
¼ cup diced tomato
¼ cup diced red, green, or yellow bell peppers
1 tablespoon olive oil to sautéed the vegetables to mix with the egg whites
1 oz. low-fat cheese
4 oz. orange juice
2 slices whole –grain toast

Lunch

1 sweet potato with chives
4 oz. organic chicken strips
1 spinach salad
½ cup grape tomatoes
1 cup watermelon

Snack

1 cup low-fat blueberry yogurt or ½ cup fresh blueberries

Dinner

5 oz. eggplant parmesan cheese with cooked garlic spinach
7 asparagus spears
½ cup banana
¼ cup frozen grapes
¼ cup strawberries
½ cup low-fat vanilla yogurt

DAY 6

Breakfast

Pumpernickel bagel
½ teaspoon cashew butter
4 oz. blueberry juice
8 oz. low –fat milk or yogurt

Lunch

4 oz. roasted chicken

1 cup of quinoa
Add all ingredients below to quinoa
2 teaspoon of slithered almonds
2 teaspoon of golden raising
1 cup of mixed veggies
1 teaspoon of turmeric with ½ teaspoon black pepper
Garlic, pearl, onions, shallots, leeks.

Snack

¼ cup high –fiber cereal
½ cup low-fat vanilla yogurt
1 teaspoon honey, drizzled over cereal and yogurt

Dinner

6 oz. baked grouper
1 cup steamed broccoli with garlic and herbs
1 sweet potato
Romaine lettuce, green /red/yellow bell peppers chopped, cucumbers, tomatoes, onions, light vinaigrette dressing
1 cup of ginger tea

DAY 7

Breakfast

1 cup oatmeal
1 cup chopped fresh blackberries
1 teaspoon cinnamon
4 oz. pomegranate juice

Lunch

Bean vegetable soup buy a combination of beans and mix
Add onions, garlic, fresh herbs and seasonings to beans
Whole grain /pumpkin seed crackers
1 cup cherries

Snacks

1 Hummingwell bar
1 cup of jasmine green tea

Dinner

2 cups quinoa pasta
1 tablespoon olive oil.
4 oz. shrimp lightly pan fried with black pepper and salt.
2 tablespoon parmesan cheese
1 cup spinach leaves with ½ cup strawberries in a raspberry vinaigrette sauce, sprinkle walnuts

DAY 8

Breakfast
1 flat whole grain bread
1 tablespoon almond butter
1 egg. Sunny side up
2 strips turkey, thin sliced and pan fried with olive oil spray
4 oz. blueberry juice

Lunch
4 oz. smoked salmon with tomato and onion on a bagel
1 teaspoon low-fat cream cheese
2 cups green lettuce mixed with grated carrots, beets, cucumbers

Snacks
1 Hummingwell bar/ dipped in 1 tablespoon of honey peanut butter
1 cup of tea

Dinner
1 cup vegetable or bean soup with a variety of mixed veggies chopped in.
1 whole –wheat –grain roll or seed crackers
3oz. grilled chicken with diced mango and onions on top, on a ved of thinly sliced avocado
1 piece of dark chocolate

DAY 9

Breakfast
1 cup veggie omelet, spinach, broccoli, onions, shallots, leeks
1 cup almond cashew milk
½ cup raspberries

Lunch
1 cup tuna salad
2 slices whole grain /whole oat bread
1 teaspoon reduced-fat mayonnaise add turmeric
2 cups leafy greens like kale or broccoli
1 tablespoon olive oil with balsamic vinegar
1 cup green tea

Snack
1 Hummingwell bar
1cup of mango or papaya green tea

Dinner
1 cup lean beef or turkey chili, beans in a bowl with lettuce, tomato, onions, shredded low fat, cheddar cheese
1 cup steamed mixed vegetables

DAY 10

Breakfast
6 oz. grape juice
1 cup fresh strawberries
8 oz. low-fat almond cashew milk
1 tsp. vanilla
Oat muffins mix 1 cup oats and ¾ coconut floor, 1 ½ baking soda, ½ cup chopped walnuts
Bake 350º - 20-0 min, or until firm.

Lunch
8 oz. grilled Mahi Mahi
2 slices of whole –grain bread or roll
1 teaspoon tartar sauce
2 stalks of bok choy
1 cup tomato wedges and sliced onions
1 tablespoon salad dressing made with olive oil and balsamic vinegar

Snack
3 cups air-popped popcorn sprinkled with garlic powder and herbs.

Dinner
3 oz. broiled pork tenderloin
1 cup wild rice with mixed veggies
1 cup steamed broccoli
½ cup frozen fruit dessert
1 cup green tea

DAY 11
Breakfast
8 oz. green drink, kale spinach, green apple, ginger
1 cup cooked oatmeal with 2 tablespoons raisins
1 cup fresh blueberries

1 cup soy or low –fat milk

Lunch

8 oz. Baked halibut

1 cup wild rice with crushed walnuts, spice it up with tarragon and turmeric

1 cup mixed vegetables.

Snack

1 Hummingwell bar

Dinner

Broccoli, hemp soup, blenderiw, 1 large carrot, onion,

1 cup ginger or chicken,

1 tablespoon leeks, broth,

3 tablespoon times seeds, sheeed

1 piece dark chocolate

DAY 12

Breakfast

3 low-fat pancakes, whole –wheat preferred, with 1 large sliced baked apple with cinnamon

¼ cup real fruit compote

6 oz. fruit smoothie , made in blender with ½ cup blueberries , 6 oz. vanilla soy milk , and ice

Lunch

1 chicken sandwich with 2 whole grain wrap, lettuce, tomato, onions, 1 tablespoon low-fat mayonnaise add turmeric

1 piece dark chocolate

Snack

1 Hummingwell bar

Dinner

1 cup quinoa pasta primavera

½ cup marinara sauce with chopped spinach and 3 oz. shrimp or scallops

1 cup mixed veggies in sauce

1 whole –grain roll

1 cup diced strawberries, orange, kiwi or mangoes

Hummingwell Recipes

MEDITERRANEAN LEAFY SALMON

(2 Servings)

Ingredients

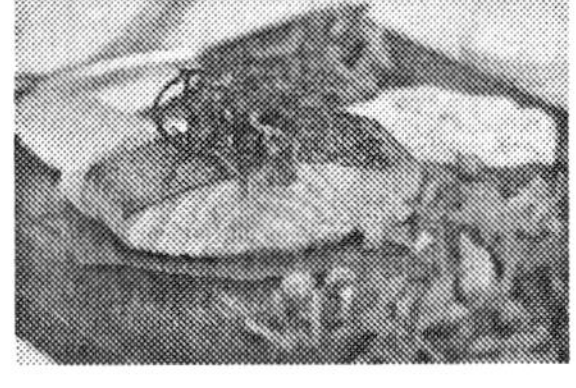

10 cups mixed organic leafy greens
8 oz. salmon
¾ cup crumbled feta cheese (if desired)
1 small sliced and cooked red bell pepper
4 sliced black olives
Salt and pepper to taste
2 tablespoons raspberry vinaigrette –sprinkle with 2 tablespoons of sliced almonds, if desired
Preparation:
Grill or bake salmon
Toss all ingredients and enjoy in a chilled bowl. Garnish with parsley leaf

Mediterranean leafy salmon is not only exquisite in taste, it also looks beautiful. It's like having a fruit festival on a plate. The combination of salmon and red bell peppers with black olives is very special. Salmon is rich in Omega -3 fatty acids, making it a heart healthy choice. The leafy greens and crumbled feta cheese makes this recipe appropriate for mid –day or evening. Enjoy especially under candlelight.

PUMPKIN SOUP

(Servings, 1 Cup each)

Ingredients

1 large Vidalia onion
2 garlic cloves
2 cup pumpkin, canned or fresh
6 cups chicken broth and a pinch of cumin powder and curry
½ teaspoon of allspice
Pinch of salt
1 cup skim or low-fat plain yogurt
Chopped leeks

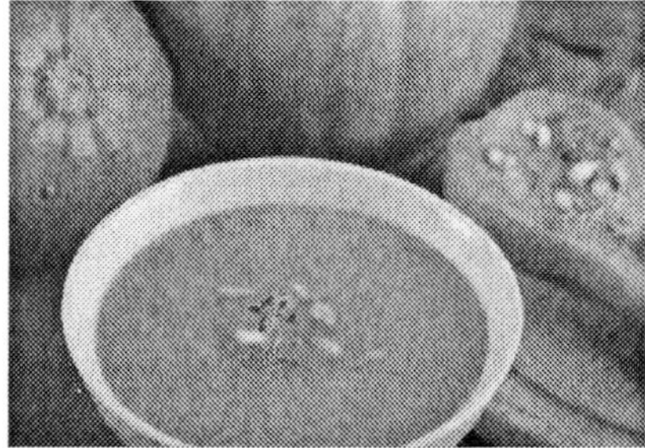

Preparation

Boil all ingredients except milk in a pot.
Simmer for 20 minutes and let cool.
Puree soup in a blender and return to pot.
Add skim or low-fat milk and stir.
Place low-fat plain yogurt in the middle of the soup, in each bowl, if desired.
Garnish with leeks.

Nutrition Analysis

Per Serving: 145 calories, 2 gm fat, 6 gm protein, 2 gm carbohydrates, 3 mg cholesterol

Pumpkin soup is rich in beta carotene.
Research suggests that its antioxidant properties may protect against some cancers. Beta carotene functions in immunity, vision, taste/smell, wound healing, and skin integrity. It is also found in carrots, sweet potatoes, apricots, cantaloupe, pink grapefruit, and other orange winter squash. This delicious soup also contains calcium, which is needed for bone and tooth structure, bone absorption, and blood clotting. This soup is easy to prepare, looks great, and tastes amazing. Enjoy!

BROCCOLINI A LA HOUDINI

(2 Servings, 1 cup each)

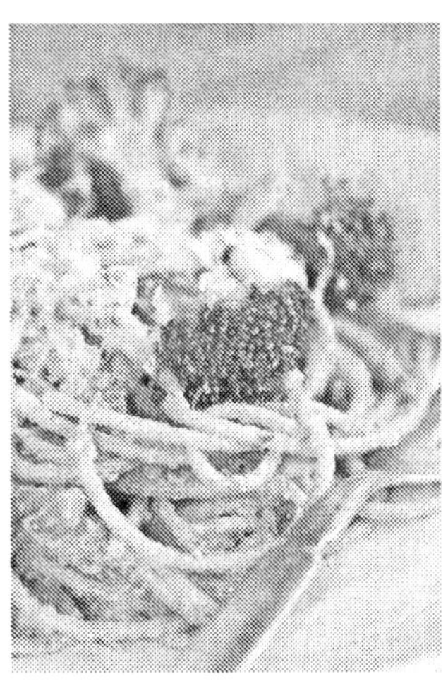

Ingredients

4 oz. multigrain or quinoa pasta
2 cups fresh broccoli
4 medium carrots
2 cups vegetable broth
4 garlic cloves
1 small onion
1 tablespoon of olive oil
2 tablespoons grated Parmesan cheese

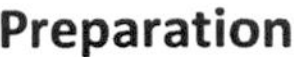

Preparation

Boil pasta as directed on package.
Put broccoli, carrots, vegetable broth, garlic, onion, and olive oil in blender; chop and mix all together. Heat in saucepan and pour over pasta. Sprinkle with parmesan cheese. Garnish with basil leaf.

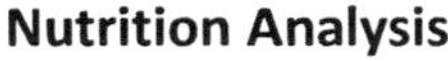

Nutrition Analysis

Per Serving: 350 calories, 7 gm fat, 12 gm protein, 38 gm carbohydrates, 2 mg cholesterol

Broccoli a la Houdini is an amazing recipe for those who do not put broccoli at the top of their favorite food list. The vegetable disappears when you blend it. However, the benefits remain.

Broccoli is known as one of the healthiest foods used by mankind. Experts agree that cruciferous vegetables contain cancer-fighting components. Cruciferous vegetables also include bok choy, brussel sprouts, cabbage, cauliflower, and more. Enjoy this recipe as you benefit from the increase of veggies in your diet.

TANGY THREE –BEAN SALAD

(2-3 Servings)

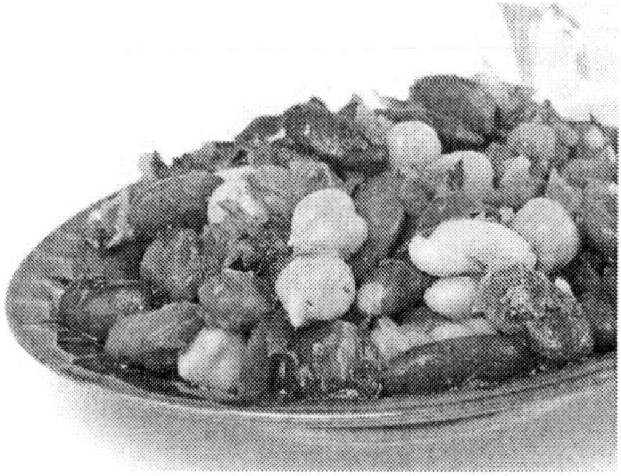

Ingredients

½ cup small white beans
½ cup red Kidney beans
½ cup garbanzo beans
¾ cup sliced green onions
¾ cup sliced black olives
3 garlic cloves, chopped
3 tablespoons of feta cheese, sprinkled
3 tablespoons olive oil
3 tablespoons cilantro chopped
½ teaspoon of hot sauce if desired, with ½ teaspoon of salt
1 ½ cups Romaine lettuce

Preparation

Cook beans (can also use canned). Sauté green onions, garlic, olive oil, and salt. Mix the beans into the pan with the sauté and add cilantro and hot sauce to taste. Garnish with lemon slices and parsley leaf.

Nutrition Analysis

Per Serving: 240 calories, 3 gm fat, 21 g, protein, 30 gm carbohydrates, 3mg cholesterol

Dried beans or legumes are the best plant source of protein that nature provides. Beans are also an excellent source of soluble fiber, which has been shown to aid in lowering cholesterol and controlling blood sugar. Insoluble fiber is also present, which increases bulk and alleviates some digestive problems. Beans are also known for being a good source of iron. This recipe is an ideal alternative to meat. Serve with a little rice to make it a complete protein and enjoy.

CANNON BALL SMOOTHIE

(2-3 8-oz SERVINGS)

Ingredients

½ cup frozen or fresh blueberries
(wild blueberries have 26 anti-oxidants)
½ cup frozen or fresh strawberries
1/2 cup vanilla yogurt
1/2 cup pomegranate juice
1 tablespoon flaxseed or chia seeds
1 scoop protein powder, if desired

Preparation

Mix all ingredients in a blender and serve chilled.

Nutrition Analysis

Per Serving: 220 calories, 1 gm fat, 7 gm protein (24 gm with protein powder), 45 gm carbohydrates,
0 mg cholesterol

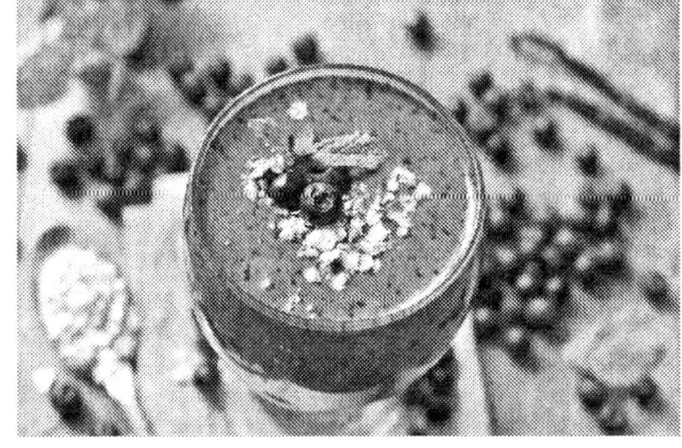

The Cannon Ball Smoothie can be made with just about any berry you like. Berries are full of vitamin C, potassium, fiber, and flavonoids, which according to research may bolster cellular antioxidant defenses. This recipe also contains calcium for strong bones and teeth, and flaxseed, a source of omega 3 fatty acids, which, according to research, may contribute to maintenance of heart health.
An excellent way to start your day or even enjoy as a midday snack.

HUMMING WICKED

The wicked, keep way low or way-out

The foods below should not be part of our regular everyday diet. Excess of these foods may cause inflammation which science tells us plays a key role in the development of diseases. There are creative ways of making many of these foods using fresh fruit and alternative natural sweeteners. Always avoid the following:

GMO
Processed
Artificial
Trans Fats
Hydrogenated oils
Fried
Chargrilled
Hormones
Refined Sugar
Excess animal protein

Excess white flour, Rice, Pasta, Potato
Candy
Cookies, Cupcakes
Cakes
Pies
Pastries
Jelly, Jams Syrup

Sodas
Juices
Sugar drinks
Excess Alcohol
Vegetable oils, corn soybean, sunflower
Eggs from poor caged chickens

Remember, excess sugar kills; excess sugar and fat kill faster. Excess calories, no matter where they come from, get stored as fat and cause excess weight.

Be mindful of the way foods make you feel. Go for Super Foods and leave the wicked out. Use aromatic oils as scents to soothe emotions instead of going for the sugar.

The Hummingwell Pantry

Here is a quick grocery list, to ensure you always have plenty of healthy options

STARCHES
Quinoa
Sweet Potato
Whole grain, wild rice
Pomegranate juice
Seed crackers
Oats
Bulgur
Multi-grain bread,
flat bread and pita

FRUITS
Wild blueberries
Raspberries
Strawberries
Any stone fruit like apricots
Cherries
Blackberries
Organic Apples

VEGGIES
Broccoli
Kale
Spinach
Cauliflower
Squash
Pumpkin
Peppers (all colors)
Cucumbers
Tomatoes
Eggplant

PROTEIN
Fish
Shellfish
Hemp
Tuna
Chia
Sardines
Flax
Cage Free eggs
Pumpkin,
Almonds
Walnuts
Lentil and colors beans
Cashews
Tofu and tempeh
Greek Yogurt

SPICES
Basil
Chives
Cilantro
Garlic
Ginger
Mint
Pepper
Rosemary
Thyme
Turmeric

Vanilla

FATS
Fish Oils/Omega 3
Flaxseed oil
Linseed oil
Olive oil
Fatty acid
Coconut Oil Virgin

DAIRY
Omega 3 grass fed
NonGMO Organic dairy eggs

EXTRA PLEASURE
Green Tea
Dark Chocolate
Humingwell bars

SUGARS
Agave Nectar
Stevia
Acacia Honey

Going through a Cancer Diagnosis

When I found out about my mother's breast cancer, it not only turned my world upside down, but I also lost my appetite for a few days, even months. A cancer diagnosis can do this not only to the people going through it, but to those who love and care for them. Do make an effort to make good nutrition a priority at this time. It is essential to helping you feel stronger and better.

I learned from my mother that proper nutrition helps you handle the side effects of cancer treatment. Eating right also reduces your chances of infection and assists with your recovery from treatment or surgery. Keeping foods fresh and safe food handling is also important because immune response may not be as optimal. When white blood cells are low the body has a harder time fighting infection or harmful bacteria.

During treatment with chemotherapy and radiation therapy, you may have friends and family who offer all kinds of advice on complementary or alternative therapies, vitamins, minerals, herbal products, and have miracle potions. They have good intentions and it is reassuring to know that your circle of loved ones are proactive in your care. However beware and have caution, because while some of these products may be safe and harmless and other not. They may interfere with the effects of radiation of chemotherapy. Some may even interfere with recovery from surgery and others may have harmful side effect. Be sure to consult your physician and or dietitian about any alternative or complementary therapies.

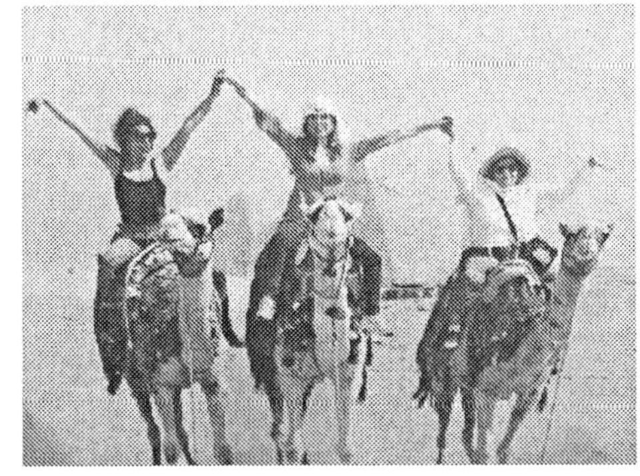

I am grateful to share that my dear mom, Maribella is doing awesome. We celebrate her life by taking her on fun adventures that include riding camels.

REFERENCES

Psychology Today - "6 Lessons We Can Learn From Eastern Chinese Medicine." https://www.psychologytoday.com/blog/the-doctor-is-listening/201301/6-lessons-we-can-learn-eastern-chinese-medicine

Academy of Nutrition and Dietetics - Eat Right: http://www.eatright.org/

American Cancer Society: http://www.cancer.org/

American Diabetes Association®: http://www.diabetes.org/

American Heart Association: http://www.heart.org/HEARTORG/

American Institute for Cancer Research (AICR) – "Protein vs Carbohydrates: A Weight Loss Choice?" http://preventcancer.aicr.org/site/News2?page=NewsArticle&id=7462&news_iv_ctrl=0&abbr=pub

Hopkins Medicine.org: "Cancer Protection Compound Abundant in Broccoli Sprouts." http://www.hopkinsmedicine.org/press/1997/SEPT/970903.HTM

Web MD.com: "Cancer-Fighting Foods: Diet to Help Prevent Cancer." http://www.webmd.com/diet/eating-good-health

Cancer.gov: "Eating Hints: Before, During, and After Cancer Treatment." http://www.cancer.gov/publications/patient-education/eatinghints.pdf

Chicago Tribune: "Environmental Nutrition: Celebrate Cruciferous Vegetables." http://www.chicagotribune.com/lifestyles/food/sns-201508311800--tms--foodstylts--v-f20150831-20150831-story.html

USDA.gov: "Food and Nutrition." http://www.usda.gov/wps/portal/usda/usdahome?navid=food-nutrition

"Food Circles: Envisioning How Eating a Variety of Foods Over Time Will Benefit Health." *The Journal of Integrative Medicine & Therapy* 1.1 (2014). Print

Hummingwell.com: "Tips."
http://www.hummingwell.com/tips/

Hummingwell.com

Food Insight.org: "IFIC Foundation - Your Nutrition and Food Safety Resource."
http://www.foodinsight.org/

India Diets.com: "Health, Nutrition, Fitness, Weight Loss."
http://www.indiadiets.com/

EPA.gov: "Organic Farming | Agriculture | US EPA."
http://www.epa.gov/agriculture/torg.html

Sabrina Hernandez (@hummingwell) | Twitter.

Sabrina Hernandez, RD, LD/N, CDE Dietitian / Nutritionist:
http://www.hummingwell.com/sabrina-hernandez-cano/

PBS.org: "The Dirty Dozen and Clean 15 of Produce | Need to Know | PBS."
http://www.pbs.org/wnet/need-to-know/health/the-dirty-dozen-and-clean-15-of-produce/616/

U.S. News & World Report: "Traditional Asian Diet -- What You Need to Know."
http://health.usnews.com/best-diet/traditional-asian-diet

FDA.gov: "Trans Fat - Food and Drug Administration."
http://www.fda.gov/NewsEvents/Newsroom/PressAnnouncements/ucm451237.htm

US Environmental Protection Agency.

http://www.epa.gov

"USDA Nutrition Research Focuses on Cancer Killing Compounds." *Rodale's All-new Encyclopedia of Organic Gardening*. 1997. Print.

Duyff, Roberta Larson. *American Dietetic Association Complete Food and Nutrition Guide*. Hoboken, NJ: John Wiley & Sons, 2006. Print.

Elk, Ronit, and Monica Morrow. *Breast Cancer for Dummies*. Hoboken, NJ: Wiley Pub., 2003. Print.

Friedman, Rodney M., and Sheldon Margen. *Wellness Foods A-Z an Indispensable Guide for Health-conscious Food Lovers*. New York: Rebus, 2002. Print.

Koch, Maryjo. *Seed Leaf Flower Fruit*. San Francisco: Collins San Francisco, 1995. Print.

McKay, Judith, and Tamera Schacher. *The Chemotherapy Survival Guide: Everything You Need to Know to Get through Treatment*. Oakland, CA: New Harbinger Publications, 2009. Print.

Papale-Hammontree, Cindy, and Sabrina Hernandez. *The Empty Cup Runneth Over: Answers about Breast Cancer from the Experts*. Pittsburgh, PA: Dorrance Pub., 2008. Print.

Peto, Richard. "The Causes of Cancer: Quantitative Estimates of Avoidable Risks of Cancer in the United States Today." *The Use of Human Cells for the Evaluation of Risk from Physical and Chemical Agents* (1983): 587-93. Print.

Quillin, Patrick, and Noreen Quillin. *Beating Cancer with Nutrition: Combining the Best of Science and Nature for Healing in the 21st Century: Simple, Safe, and Effective Natural Methods to Improve Outcome for Cancer Patients*. Tulsa, OK: Nutrition Times, 2001. Print.

Rosenthal, Joshua. *Integrative Nutrition: Feed Your Hunger for Health and Happiness*. New York, NY: Integrative Nutrition Pub., 2008. Print.

Sawyer, Allie Fair., and Norma Suzette. Jones. *Journey: A Breast Cancer Survival Guide*. Alexander, NC: WorldComm, 1992. Print.

Servan-Schreiber, David. *Anti Cancer: A New Way of Life*. Melbourne, Australia: Scribe, 2008. Print.

Varona, Verne. *Nature's Cancer-fighting Foods: Prevent and Reverse the Most Common Forms of Cancer Using the Proven Power of Great Food and Easy Recipes*. Paramus, NJ: Reward, 2001. Print.

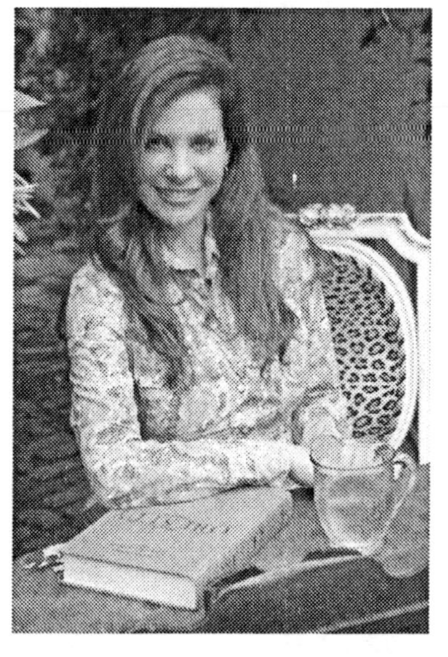

Sabrina Hernandez-Cano

is a Registered Dietitian, Nutrition Counselor, and Certified Diabetes Educator who graduated from Florida International University with a Science degree in Dietetics and Nutrition. Her training included Cleveland Clinic hospital and Palm Springs General Hospital. She also has a degree in Marketing and Merchandise from International Fine Arts College.

In 1988, Sabrina received the Miami Herald Silver Knight Award for dedication in community service. Sabrina continued her passion in helping others, internationally through her missions throughout the world. Speaking about malnutrition in countries such as Africa, Guatemala, Honduras and Mexico. She has spoken about the epidemic of child obesity in countries such as the Cayman Islands and throughout Miami Dade County Schools.

Her specialty in Cardiac and Diabetes education has positioned her as the Cardiovascular Nutrition Educator for Berkeley Heart Lab and the Miami Cardiac & Vascular Institute at Baptist Hospital. Sabrina became President of the Miami Dietetic Association from 1999 to 2000. She was also voted the Greater Miami Dietitian of 2000 by The Miami Dietetic Association.

She has appeared on ABC News, NBC, Telemundo, Univision and WLRN-TV for segments on nutrition, wellness and Diabetes. She is also co-author of the book "The Empty Cup Runneth Over" a book that gives expert advice on the subject of breast cancer. She is a member of the Academy of Nutrition and Dietetics and the American Association of Diabetes Educators.

Currently, Sabrina is in private practice counseling on all areas of Medical Nutrition Therapy with a specialty and passion for bariatric nutrition. She is the founder and CEO of Scientific Nutrition a company dedicated to developing nutritious snacks such as Hummingwell, wellness bar; made with balanced nutrition and designed to promote a healthy lifestyle. The company has

added the Latin line called "Que Flaca" a movement to educate, empower and promote wellness.

Chapter 16

Obesity and Breast Cancer.

Moises Jacobs, M.D.

Alex Fagenson

Results from the 2007-2008 National Health and Nutrition Examination Survey (NHANES) showed that 68% of United States adults age twenty and older are overweight and obese. This number is up 12% from the early 1990s and the trend is similar in regard to children. The burden this places on the health industry is significant. We have learned over the years that being obese puts an individual at increased risk for a number of chronic diseases including but not limited to: high blood pressure, joint problems, type 2 diabetes, heart disease, stroke, gallbladder disease, and some cancers. In recent years, it has been shown that there is a direct correlation between obesity and breast cancer (1).

Women who are overweight or obese after menopause

have a 30-60% higher chance of getting breast cancer than their counterparts who are lean (2). Many studies have shown that being obese is associated with an increased risk of postmenopausal breast cancer (3). The relationship between obesity and breast cancer may be influenced by the age at which the woman gains weight and becomes obese. After menopause the ovaries shut down and no longer produce estrogen, and at this point the main producer of estrogen becomes fat tissue. As we know, excess estrogen directly aids breast cancer in its growth and thus the more obese you are, the more estrogen you will produce. Additionally, obese people are in a state of ongoing, low-level inflammation that further increases their risk for development of cancer (4). The relationship between obesity and breast cancer may also vary by race; this is currently under investigation.

Thus it has been proposed that weight loss can help reduce the risk of breast cancer, especially once a woman has gone through menopause. One study showed that women who lost four to eleven pounds after menopause had more than 20% lower risk of breast cancer when compared to women whose weight did not change (5). Weight loss during pre-menopausal years should also have a similar impact with respect to reducing the risk of getting breast cancer; therefore, efforts to achieving a normal body weight should be the goal for all women. With obesity being such a problem, there has been a shift in thought to get the weight corrected as early as possible to avoid breast cancer and all the other negative health effects. Weight loss surgery becomes the best option for a woman once all diet and exercise regiments have failed.

There are currently two major weight loss surgeries offered by surgeons today. Known as the Roux-en-Y Gastric Bypass and the Sleeve Gastrectomy, both are minimally invasive. The Roux-En-Y is the older surgery and the first to become available. This surgery is a two-step procedure with the first being a restrictive phase to create a gastric pouch that reduces the size of your stomach. The second phase is known as the malabsorptive phase and this is where the term bypass comes into play. The surgeon reconnects the small intestine to the gastric pouch in a manner that shortens the distance the food travels. In doing so, the food no longer has the same distance to travel and thus fat and excess calories cannot get fully absorbed. In summary, this surgery creates a smaller stomach so the patient cannot eat as much, and the food that one eats doesn't get totally absorbed. However, there are many accompanying complications – the most common being deficiencies in key vitamins and nutrients simply because the body does not have enough time to absorb these essential factors. This requires the patient to take many supplements for the rest of their life, increasing the cost of life as well as putting the patient at risk of complications from a lack of satisfactory levels of the essential nutrients. Aside from deficiencies, the patient is at increased risk for constipation, diarrhea, nausea, bowel obstruction, and leaks from any of the connection sites of which there are three. All of the long-term complications from this surgery prompted surgeons to come up with a solution that resulted in a procedure known as the Sleeve Gastrectomy.

The Sleeve Gastrectomy is a one-step procedure that only consists of the restriction phase. The surgeon simply cuts the stomach in half, reducing the size of the stomach and quantity of food one can take in at any given time. The surgery is much shorter, straightforward, and carries less long-term complications. Since the surgeon is not reconnecting the small intestine, there is a much less risk of becoming deficient in the essential nutrients. Additionally, since there is only one section that is cut, there is a significantly decreased chance of any leaks, unlike the Roux-en-Y Gastric Bypass, which potentially has three sites that can leak. The time in the hospital after surgery is reduced with the Sleeve Gastrectomy and the patient no longer needs to spend all the money on the vitamins and nutrients that one would need to if they had the Roux-en-Y Gastric Bypass.

In conclusion, weight loss in an obese woman can reduce the risk of breast cancer. It is essential for women to maintain a healthy body weight and those who cannot should seek the option of weight loss surgery to prevent cancer and other long-term health problems. Of the surgeries available, the Sleeve Gastrectomy provides the patient with a simple procedure with minimal risks. This surgery has been adapted from the older technique of the Roux-en-Y Gastric Bypass that has many medical complications and increased financial burden on the patient in the long run.

Dr. Moises Jacobs would like to acknowledge Alex Fagenson, fourth year medical student at Florida Internatinoal University, for his assistance with writing this chapter.

REFERENCES

1. Nelson HD, Zakher B, Cantor A, et al. Risk factors for breast cancer for women aged 40 to 49 years: a systematic review and meta-analysis. Ann Intern Med. 156(9):635-48, 2012.

2. Huang Z, Hankinson SE, Colditz GA, et al. Dual effects of weight and weight gain on breast cancer risk. JAMA. 278: 1407-11, 1997.

3. Reeves GK, Pirie K, Beral V, Green J, Spencer E, Bull D. Cancer incidence and mortality in relation to body mass index in the Million Women Study: cohort study. BMJ. 335(7630):1134, 2007.

4. Key TJ, Appleby PN, Reeves GK, et al. for the Endogenous Hormones and Breast Cancer Collaborative Group. Circulating sex hormones and breast cancer risk factors in postmenopausal women: reanalysis of 13 studies. Br J Cancer. 105(5):709-22, 2011.

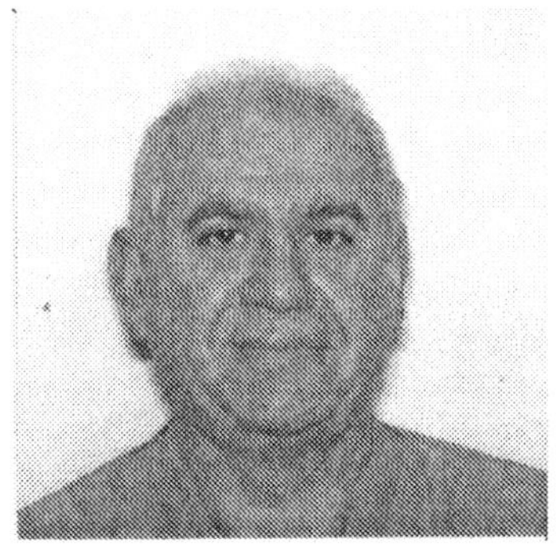

Moises Jacobs, M.D., F.A.C.S.

from the University of Miami Medical School in 1979 and finished his general surgery residency at University of Miami/Jackson Memorial Hospital in 1984. He has been performing advanced laparoscopic procedures since 1990 and is credited with performing the first laparoscopic colectomy in 1990. Dr Jacobs is world renowned as a pioneer in laparoscopy and has taught and mentored hundreds of surgeons throughout the world. In addition, he hosts a biannual "minimally invasive" conference where the latest and most innovative surgical techniques in laparoscopic bariatric surgery are presented by the world's experts. Dr. Jacobs has published several research articles and textbooks and has been awarded Unites States patents for his innovative surgical instruments.

Learn more about Dr. Jacobs at his website, www.gastricsleevecenter.com

Chapter 17

What Do We Know About Exercise and Your Health?

Don Torok, Ph.D., FACSM

GENERAL GUIDELINES: QUALITY OF LIFE

There are many factors that influence an individual's overall health. It is important to realize that our health is not just physical, but also has components that relate to our mental and social well-being. The crucial role that exercise plays in our overall health profile has expanded and gained greater credence over the years. We know that regular exercise is associated with many positive health outcomes. It wasn't until the 1990's that physical inactivity was identified by both the American Heart Association as a risk factor for heart disease and targeted by the American Cancer Society as preventive action measure.

While we understand that individuals are genetically different, there are some common risk factors everyone should be aware of; these are the things we can control in our daily lives. Here are some healthy habits you can adopt to help reduce your cancer risk:

1. Don't use tobacco products;
2. Limit inactivity;
3. Maintain a normal body weight;
4. Eat a healthy diet.

The American Cancer Society indicates that about one-third of cancer deaths are associated with tobacco use and another one-third of cancer deaths are tied to our diet and activity levels, which is also linked to our body weight (1). Making an effort to address these areas will not only reduce your cancer risk, but will also reduce your risk of developing cardiovascular and metabolic disease.

Let us look more closely at each of these areas and see what we can do to make a positive difference in our lives. The first one seems pretty clear: don't use any tobacco products. This includes cigarettes, cigars, pipes, hookah, chewing tobacco, snuff, blunts, cigarillos, bidis, electronic cigarettes, and other products containing tobacco. There are over 7000 chemicals in tobacco smoke and at least 70 that are known to cause cancer (2).

Be physically active – that is, engage in a minimum of 150 minutes of moderate intensity activity each week (in bouts of at least 10 minutes) with an additional 2 to 3 resistance training sessions/week (8-10 exercises of 10-15 repetitions per set, involving major muscle groups; avoid heavy lifting) and some flexibility or stretching exercises (3-4). The key here is to avoid inactivity. Many individuals revert to inactivity after diagnosis or treatments begins and this may result in the loss of muscle mass, decreases in fitness levels, and increases in body fat and other metabolic (Type 2 diabetes) problems.

Maintaining a normal body weight is in general terms having a normal BMI (body mass index-an index of ones weight in kilograms divided by the square of ones height in meters). There are many body mass calculators online, where you can input you numbers and get your calculated BMI (5). A normal BMI would be between 18.5 and 24.9. Anything below is considered underweight and anything over is considered overweight. Because being overweight is a cancer risk factor and a growing number of Americans' qualify as being overweight or obese, there is a real need to address our food selections and quantities, in addition to our level of daily activity. It is important to eat a diet that is high in fruits, vegetables, and whole grains, and avoid alcohol (limit one drink/day for women and not more than 2 drinks/day for men) and consume adequate water to remain hydrated.

Why Exercise?

Exercise is a free pharmacological aid available to everyone provided we engage in regular, sustained (at least 10 minute bouts) activity – preferably on a daily basis. Exercise has been shown to assist with improving fatigue, fitness, muscle mass, flexibility, appetite, and quality of life, while reducing depression and anxiety (6, 7). Studies have shown that regular physical activity may reduce the risk for breast, colon, and prostate cancer. As stated above, there are benefits to exercise done during treatment and there are additional benefits from regular physical activity after treatments have been completed. With all this in mind, let us examine how to best put our exercise program together.

Getting Started

As with any exercise program, it is always best to talk with your doctor to just be sure that there are no special concerns that you need to be aware of in planning your activities. Here are some of the factors to consider when you begin your exercise program and some special considerations for some types of cancers.

First, we need to know your present treatment status (before treatment, during treatment, or post treatment). Each of these conditions may require some modifications to the intensity and duration of your daily bouts and will be influenced by your prior exercise history. Always begin at a level where you can be successful and select activities that you find enjoyable. For additional support and encouragement, having an exercise partner adds immediate accountability. There may be times during treatment, where you may need to cut back or give yourself a little more recovery time. Keep in mind that your exercise program may just be that needed physical release to take your mind off your treatment and experience a good psychological boost. Even after your treatments are over, you may have some lingering side effects that may take some time to diminish. It will be important to keep your program going and to look at the specific aspects of your health that will continue to help improve your quality of life.

General precautions for some groups:

There are certain circumstances where special considerations need to be advised for some individuals (11).

Condition	Precaution
a) Severe anemia	Delay exercise until anemia is improved
b) compromised immune levels	Avoid public areas and pools until immune levels have returned to safe levels
c) severe fatigue	Limit activity to 10 minutes of light exercise until fatigue has improved
d) undergoing radiation	Avoid exposure to chlorine
e) indwell catheter or feeding tube	Avoid pools and other bodies of water where exposure may result in infections and be careful with resistance training of muscle groups that contain the catheter or feeding tube
f) significant peripheral neuropathies or lack of voluntary coordination of	Consider exercise equipment that provides more stability (recumbent bike, rowing machine, elliptical

muscle movements	machine). Consider supervision during activity.
g) multiple or uncontrolled comorbidities	Consult your physician for advice

TYPES AND DURATION OF EXERCISE

One should start with 10 to 15 minutes of aerobic (walking, biking, swimming, rowing, dancing, etc) activity if you have been sedentary and build up to 30 minutes or more per day. If balance is an issue, you can use a stationary bike or rowing machine. For those individuals that have been exercising, getting more vigorous exercise is fine as long as you do not overdo it to the point that you are still feeling fatigued the next day.

Getting some daily stretching or yoga and two or three session of weight training will help to maintain or build some muscle mass. Stay away from heavy weights and keep the reps to 15 to 20 per exercise for the major muscle groups of the body. Make an effort to record your activity with either a simple diary or use one of the fitness bands or pedometers. Reward your achievements and recognize that it is not a race for today, but a journey into the future. It is the constant small steps that we take each and every day that will help us reach our destination.

Here are some specific considerations that have been linked with exercise and different types of cancer:

Type of Cancer	What we know	Special Considerations
Breast Cancer	a) more fit have lower risk by 20 to 80% (8-9) b) normal BMI and regular physical activity has lower risk of breast cancer.	a) Individual experiencing lymphedema should consider using appropriate compression garments and

	c) 30-60 minutes of moderate to vigorous daily exercise has lower risk of breast cancer.	consult with their physician. b) Individual who had axillary lymph node dissection should refrain from upper body resistance exercises until given approval from their physician. c) Be aware of the risk for fractures for those treated with hormonal therapy or osteoporosis
Colon Cancer	a) more active have lower risk of colon cancer. b) 30-60 minutes of daily moderate to vigorous exercise may protect against colon cancer (8-9).	a) Avoid exercises that create excessive intra-abdominal pressure.
Endometrial Cancer	a) more active have lower risk by 20-40% (8)	a) Avoid exercises that create excessive intra-abdominal pressure until healed.
Lung Cancer	a) more active have lower risk by about 20% (8)	a) start slowly and be sure that the duration and intensity is tolerable for the individual.
Prostate Cancer	a) some evidence that regular vigorous exercise in older men (>65) may slow the	a) Be aware of the risk for fractures for those treated with androgen deprivation therapy

	progression of prostate cancer(10).	(ADT) or osteoporosis

Even though you may do all the "right things," there's always the possibility that cancer may strike. *How are you going to strike back and regain your quality of life?*

A crucial part of establishing a positive outlook is the knowledge that not every day is going to be like past times. What are some of the possible symptoms you may experience during your cancer treatment? It's not uncommon for individuals to deal with the following:

- Depression
- Anxiety
- Body image concerns
- Decreases in self-esteem and quality of life
- Difficulty sleeping
- Muscle weakness
- Weight loss
- Muscle loss
- Loss of aerobic fitness
- Nausea
- Vomiting
- Fatigue
- Pain

Exercise has been shown to assist with improving fatigue, fitness, muscle mass, flexibility, and quality of life while reducing depression (9, 10).

While the benefits of regular exercise are well documented, it's important to remember that there will be days when you'll have to adjust your individual program depending on how you feel. Realize that on any given day you may have to do a little less. The foundation of your exercise routine should be geared to a moderate intensity level and include both flexibility and resistance training.

Since cancer sites and treatments vary, it's critical to seek out an experienced professional to guide your program. While your tailored exercise program is good for your mind and body, it only works if you stick to it consistently. If at all possible, exercise with a buddy or in a group to help you maintain your motivation and adherence to the program.

When you include exercise as part of your daily activities throughout your life, you'll experience both mental and physical benefits. Think of exercise as your own special prescription for mind and body; each and every step you take will help you get closer to your goal of overall wellbeing.

REFERENCES

Nutrition and physical activity guidelines for cancer survivors. CA Cancer J Clin, 2012; 62:242-274.

U.S. Department of Health & Human Services: (July 31, 2015) Smoked Tobacco Products. Retrieved from: http://betobaccofree.hhs.gov/about-tobacco/Smoked-Tobacco-Products/.

Schmitz KH, Courneya KS, Matthews C, et al; American College of Sports Medicine. American College of Sports Medicine roundtable on exercise guidelines for cancer survivors. Med Sci Sports Exerc. 2010; 42:1409-1426.

US Department of Health and Human Services. Physical Activity Guidelines for Americans. Washington, DC: US Department of Health and Human Services; 2008.

Centers for Disease Control and Prevention: (August 3, 2015) Body Mass Index. Retrieved from: http://www.cdc.gov/healthyweight/assessing/bmi/.

Courneya KS, Keats MR, Turner AR. Physical exercise and quality of life in cancer patients following high dose chemotherapy and autologous bone marrow transplantation. Psychooncology 9:127-136, 2000.

Courneya KS, Friedenreich CM. Physical exercise and quality of life following cancer diagnosis: A literature review. Am Behav Med 21:171-179, 1999.

Lee I, Oguma Y. Physical activity. In: Schottenfeld D, Fraumeni JF, editors. Cancer Epidemiology and Prevention. 3rd ed. New York: Oxford University Press, 2006.

McTiernan A, editor. Cancer Prevention and Management Through Exercise and Weight Control. Boca Raton: Taylor & Francis Group, LLC, 2006.

Giovannucci EL, Liu Y, Leitzmann MF, Stampfer MJ, Willett WC. A prospective study of physical activity and incident and fatal prostate cancer. Archives of Internal Medicine2005; 165(9):1005–1010.

Rock et al., Nutrition and physical activity guidelines for cancer survivors. CA Cancer J Clin, 2012; 62:242-274.

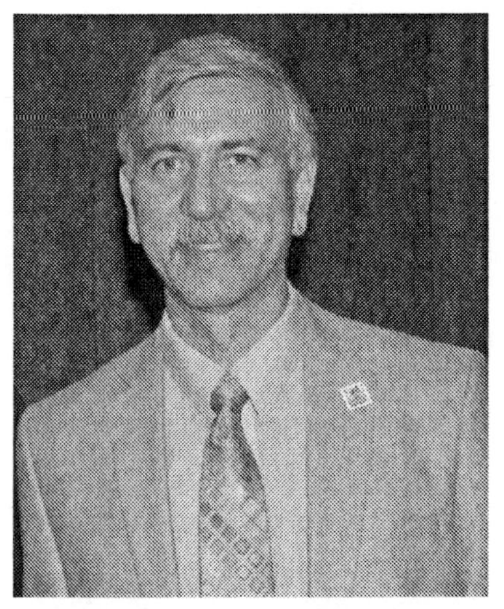

Don Torok, Ph.D., FACSM

is an exercise physiologist and fellow of the American College of Sports Medicine. He completed his MS in Exercise Science at Miami of Ohio and his Ph.D. in Exercise Physiology at the University of Tennessee in Knoxville. After receiving his degree in Knoxville, he spent almost two years at the Health Science Center of the University of Tennessee in Memphis before relocating to Florida to accept a position at Florida Atlantic University (FAU). While at FAU, he has been a faculty member, Department Chair of the Exercise Science and Health Promotion, and for the last nine years, Associate Dean of the College of Education.

Don is presently Chair of the Professional Education Committee for the American College of Sports Medicine, on the Executive Committee of the Southeast American College of Sports Medicine, Chair of the South Florida Asthma Consortium, and former Chair of the Tobacco-Free Partnership of Broward County.

Chapter 18

Nurture Our Breasts, Heart, Lungs, and Lymph Yoga Belly Dance Series

Michelle Alva, P.T., Intuitive Healer

According to the National Cancer Institute there is strong evidence that physical activity is associated with decreased risk of breast and colon cancers. Most studies suggest that 30 to 60 minutes per day of moderate-to-high-intensity physical activity is associated with a reduction in breast cancer risk (1.2). Research indicates that after a diagnosis of breast cancer physical activity may be beneficial to improve the quality of life, reduce fatigue (3), assist with energy balance and may be indicated and safe for lymphedema management.

Our bodies love to move! When we move we literally secrete the love, healing, pleasure, focus and connection hormone called Oxytocin. Oxytocin causes the release of Endorphins, our natural painkillers and evokes in us the feeling of a "natural high". Oxytocin aids in the release and processing of our trapped emotional energy. Movement also increases the circulation of blood and lymph fluid and the flow of energy in the body. We feel lighter, freer and more connected to who we really are when we move in ways that are rhythmical and repetitive such as in walking, dancing, swimming and making love.

Women healing through breast cancer may experience more emotional stress, physical stress, pain, inflammation, tension and tightness due to chemotherapy, surgery and other related interventions.

Learning to breathe with our diaphragm and engaging in daily nurturing and healing whole body movements in a rhythmical, pleasurable, repetitive way creates a supportive and healing inner environment which greatly benefits our body, mind and soul.

Nurturing Moves®, created by Michelle Alva, PT is a form of mind-body-therapeutic exercise that unites the movement science of Physical Therapy with the ancient wisdom of Yoga and Belly Dance. It allows us to nurture and bring out our feminine aspects to maximize self-healing, creative self-expression and provide a form of therapeutic exercise for the unique needs of women healing through breast cancer and other women's health related diseases.

Every moment and movement is an opportunity to celebrate life no matter what we are faced with. The diagnosis of cancer may bring emotions of fear, resentment, frustration, guilt, shame and anger to name a few. Movement and exercise benefits not only the physical body but also the emotional and spiritual body as it assists in the processing and releasing of stuck emotions in our tissues.

I learned firsthand how cancer impacts women, breasts and their family when my mother's sister was diagnosed with breast cancer. I saw how my aunt was treated as a body with cancer instead of a person with a soul that had a diagnosis of cancer. I was only a teenager when she was diagnosed and I remember her looking withdrawn and her spirit dull out as her cancer spread. She did not know how to activate her innate resources to heal or about the mind-body connection and the power of our beliefs and how that knowledge could benefit her body.

I learned from this experience how important it is to educate, empower and nurture women healing through cancer.

This experience coupled with my background as a holistic physical therapist, yoga therapist, belly dance teacher and intuitive healer has inspired me to create a scientific, sensual and spiritual approach to healing, energizing and living more fully alive.

Women diagnosed with cancer visit many different health care professionals for different reasons. Each expert addresses the different parts of the individual. The doctor examines the person's overall body-mind functions and prescribes different treatments, surgeries and drugs. The psychologist is trained to work with the person's mind, behavior and emotions. The physical therapist is an expert at working with the person's body and activities of daily living. The spiritual counselor offers support through prayer and meditation. However each of us is an integrated human being that is made up of energy and vibrating molecules constantly in motion. If we are treated as an integrated human being that is constantly moving, healing and growing, we can create new possibilities from how everyone views us. Movement exercise is an activity that causes us to integrate our whole self.

Movement experiences that support the integration of all our body systems for example singing while we are dancing, or consciously breathing while we are moving in and out of yoga postures, causes us to harmonize and align with all the parts of who we are. Our systems work in harmony for us when we integrate ourselves.

Our mind-set and intention when we exercise ensures we benefit to the highest degree. Yoga and belly dance combined offer an even more healing and gentler approach to exercise for women healing through cancer as we get to move in circular, gentle and rhythmical ways that embrace our masculine and feminine aspects.

The experience of combined breathing exercises, yoga asanas, conscious rhythmical movements, and mindfulness meditation facilitates the feeling of our whole-integrated human being. We learn how to quiet and calm the mind and body through these exercises which eventually leads to an even deeper and fuller experience of our true Divine and Feminine Nature that is always whole and complete. Healing is most efficient when we are present and connected to our authentic self and soul.

The following yoga and belly dance based exercises are opportunities to nurture, heal and connect to our multi-dimensional Human Being while also enhancing our immune system functioning and body-mind-breath-spirit connection. It especially helps to improve the flexibility, circulation, awareness, healing, and overall health to our chest, breasts, heart, lungs and lymph.

Research studies have found yoga to benefit breast cancer survivors by significantly lowering stress hormones, raising their vitality and decreasing inflammation and fatigue. Sleep also has been reported to improve as well as quality of life (Kiecolt-Glaser JK et al).

We can bring a loving intention to nurture, heal and honor your body, mind and spirit when practicing the following exercises. All these exercises are safe and promote major healing with minor effort.

Consult your physician before beginning any exercise program.

1. **Choose to feel safe, supported and grateful throughout the day**

Lay down on your back. Bring your arms out like a T, soles of the feet together, knees wide apart. Place pillows on the outer thighs if necessary for added support for your hip and knee joints. Invite into your being the feeling of safety, support and appreciation for everything AS IT IS. As you lay in this position, embody the feeling of full acceptance, of fully allowing your body-mind-spirit to BE supported.

Trust that everything in life is happening for us to grow and thrive. What are the opportunities and gifts that a diagnosis of cancer has given you? When we can shift our perspective of our cancer to one of full acceptance, we heal. Healing means to become whole. Can you see yourself and feel yourself as whole with cancer or without? Our soul is always whole and complete regardless of what our bodies are afflicted with. Feel your soul more and it will be easier to let go of the judgements and resentments that may have arisen from having a diagnosis of cancer.

Breathe IN gratitude for BEing alive NOW with a sense of amazement for the miracle that you are. Notice the breath that enlivens you and remind yourself how all that is green in nature creates oxygen and life force. Feel grateful for the beautiful harmony between you, mother earth and the whole universe. Breathe IN life to the fullest every morning and give lovingly back your exhalation to enliven nature. Notice your bodily sensations as you connect to your nature. Breathe in a violet healing light as you fill your heart and every cell of your body with a loving intention to nurture your whole-being through these following exercises:

2. **Breathe IN Life To The Fullest. (3 Part Sniff, Sniff, Sniff Diaphragmatic Breaths)**

While in that same position as in exercise 1, inhale through your nose for 3 sniffs. Inhale, inhale, inhale. Notice how sniffs cause a quick expansion in your rib cage, abdomen and chest. Feel the expansiveness to the end range of your center. Exhale the sound and sigh "ahhhh." Repeat this at least 5 times. Place your hand over your chest and abdomen to make sure your belly rises when you inhale. This ensures you are using your diaphragm to breathe in instead of your upper chest. When we breathe in with our diaphragm primarily, we relax our nervous system and this also makes us feel safe. This supports our healing, regenerative and restorative functions in our bodies which is ideal for healing through cancer.

Inhale, inhale, inhale and this time hold your breath for as long as you can with minimum effort. Notice how it feels to be expanded fully at your center and hold your breath. When we slow down our breath, we slow down our mind and experience a more profound sense of peace and calm. Exhale the sound "Ahhhh" and as you do this think of all the stress and tension you may be feeling in your body and allow that body part to release by making a sound. This is called toning and it is something children naturally do when they stub a toe. Animals in the wild also use sound repeatedly to release tension and stress. When we create sound, we vibrate our bodies and vibration causes the release of the love and healing hormone.

Play with your sounds throughout the day and express your stress. It liberates us.

3. **Rhythmical Chest Waves with a Smile.**

Lay on your back, sitting and standing. Inhale to arch your head, neck and upper spine while raising your chest upwards. Press your elbows and forearms downwards along your sides to allow your chest to rise up even more. Bring your shoulder blades down and backwards. Smile and feel grateful for your expansive heart. Exhale bringing your low back down returning the spine and head back to neutral. Inhale to arch your upper body, exhale to lower your body back down to supine. Continue to create at least 10 rhythmical waves of inhale/exhale.

4. **Shoulder rolls backwards with rhythmical arm movements.**

This exercise can be done while sitting or standing. Inhale to move your right shoulder up, back, down and then forward.

Alternate with the opposite arm and movement. Roll one shoulder backwards at a time and notice how this rhythmical movement helps you to relax your shoulder and neck muscles and loosen up your rib cage and chest.

5. **Arms reaching up over head.**

Do this repetitive and rhythmical arm movement while sitting, laying down, and standing. It also feels great to do while in the shower, in a pool or at the beach. Inhale reach your arms up over your head as far up and out as possible. Feel the expansion and elongation of the front and sides of your body and armpit area.

Look up at the sky and ceiling feeling grateful for the range of motion that is available to you. Stretch your 10 fingers out splayed in all directions with your palms facing forwards. Feel the fullness of reaching your arms upwards and outwards. Feel fully this exercise. Exhale to bring your arms back down along your sides. Repeat this motion allowing your breath to guide the movements. Inhale to bring your arms up, exhale to bring your arms back down. Become aware of how soothing rhythmical and repetitive movements feel. Repeat this movement with full presence and the intention to reach your arms up as high and spread out as possible. When we allow our breath to guide our movements, we ensure our soul is also engaged fully and integrated in the present moment with our body and mind.

6. **Side bend expansion of the spine and ribs with maximum lengthening.**

Do this exercise while sitting with legs wide apart or standing with legs wider than hip width apart. Breathe IN and raise your left arm upwards and to the right side. Lengthen and laterally bend your spine. Keep your shoulder blades down and backwards. Exhale to move your body and arm back to center. Inhale to laterally bend to the other side, exhale to return to the center for 10 breaths. Once again feel the expansion and elongation as your breath guides the movements.

7. **Arms out like a T with spinal twist.**

Sit or stand for this exercise. Inhale and bring your arms up so they form the shape of a T. Keep your palms facing upwards towards the sky. Inhale to twist to one side. Exhale twist to the center. Repeat to each side coming back to the center 10 times. You can inhale and create your sniffs to make it easier to rotate and twist your shoulders. Focus on rotating at the shoulders while keeping the shoulders down and back.

Nurturing Moves Belly Dance Basics.

Belly dance is the oldest form of dance. It was designed for women thousands of years ago while the men were creating yoga. This dance is unique in that we get to create isolated movements of our belly, pelvis, rib cage, head, arms and spine while our feet are grounded to the earth. We get to feel stable through our own two feet while creating fluidity and lightness with our upper body.

This feminine dance is graceful and grounding. The movements are rhythmical, repetitive and hypnotic thus promoting a healthy circulation, a calm and alert mind and freed up emotions while integrating all our body parts. The combination of isolated movements that focus on the pelvis, rib cage, spine and arms makes for a very fluid, fun and healing experience for breast cancer survivors. Belly dance evokes feelings of pleasure, safety, gentleness, ease and grace.

1. Basic Stance.

Feel yourself standing tall with your heart and chest lifted. Feel yourself as a divine body temple that houses your soul. Your unique essence permeates through your body and is animated by your breath. Take a deep breath in and allow the feeling of fullness, richness and abundance to overtake you. Feel fully expanded and elongated as you stand owning your full and whole self.

Each woman is a goddess; a divine miracle of life, a unique creation. When we dance, we dance from this place of knowing and awareness. The dance is a celebration of our bodies, our minds, our souls. We dance as a way of saying "thank you" to our creator and ourselves. The dance is a way of loving ourselves and making time to celebrate through gentle and rhythmical movement. We get to experience our bodies as a source of peace, pleasure, lightness, ease and flow. Regardless of how we look or feel, we can begin with the smallest excursion of movement and move within the comfortable range to eventually create a wider excursion of movement. It is important to only move within a safe and comfortable range so the body continues to feel relaxed and soft. This dance is not meant to be forced or pushed as the body actually allows and surrenders into the movements.

1. Hip slides.

Stand with feet hip width apart. Your arms are placed softly about 80 degrees upwards and way from your center with your palms facing down and your thumb and middle finger touching with the wrists in a slight extension. Connect to your diaphragm as we did in the beginning of our yoga postures. Breathe deeply and fully while you slide your pelvis and hips in the transverse plane as far as comfortably possible to the right side. Slide your hips fully to the left side now. Continue this repetitive pattern of sliding your hips to the far right and then to the far left. Notice how the sensations that arise as you slide your hips to the right and then to the left at least 10 times.

2. **Hip Circles.**

Stand with feet hip width apart. Your arms are placed softly about 80 degrees upwards and way from your center with your palms facing down and your thumb and middle finger touching with the wrists in a slight extension. Slide your pelvis forward in the transverse plane, then to the right, then backwards and then to the left creating clockwise circles of your hips and pelvis while keeping your arms raised. Move rhythmically in circles at least 10 times. Then move your pelvis and hips counterclockwise 10 times. Notice how this movement feels.

3. **Hip Shimmies.**

Stand with feet hip width apart. Your arms are placed softly about 80 degrees upwards and way from your center with your palms facing down and your thumb and middle finger touching with the wrists in a slight extension. Move your tailbone right to left in the frontal plane and then left to right quickly and repetitively moving slowly at first and then move quickly. The quicker we "wag our tailbone" the more our buttocks and thighs seem to shake. This is a great sign as it means your core muscles are working while you relax your thighs. This vibrational movement is excellent for circulation and to feel more energized and lighter. It is a great movement to integrate with the sniff, sniff, sniff breaths we did in the beginning of our yoga postures. You can also shimmy while you tone. Create the "ahhhh" sounds to release any tension in the body or emotions. I love to do this in the shower as it feels wonderful to release.

4. **Heart-Rib Cage Slides.**

Stand with feet hip width apart. Your arms are placed softly about 80 degrees upwards and way from your center with your palms facing down and your thumb and middle finger touching with the wrists in a slight extension. The pelvis does not move for this exercise. The rib cage and chest-heart are the only thing that slides side to side in the transverse plane. Connect to your diaphragm as we did in the beginning of our yoga postures. Breathe deeply and fully while you slide your heart and rib cage as far as comfortably possible to the right side. Slide your heart and rib cage fully to the left side now. Continue this repetitive pattern of sliding your heart and rib cage to the far right and then to the far left. Notice the sensations that arise as you slide your heart and rib cage to the right and then to the left at least 10 times.

5. **Heart-Rib Cage Circles.**

Position: Stand with feet hip width apart. Your arms are placed softly about 80 degrees upwards and way from your center with your palms facing down and your thumb and middle finger touching with the wrists in a slight extension.Slide your heart and rib cage forward in the transverse plane, then to the right, then backwards and then to the left, creating clockwise circles of your heat and rib cage while keeping your arms raised. Move rhythmically in circles for at least 10 times. Then move your heat and rib cage counterclockwise 10 times. Notice how this circular movement feels.

7. **Snake arms.**

Place your thumb and index fingers together. Inhale and raise your right hand along your side. Lead with your shoulder, then elbow, then wrist and then hand while you extend your wrist upwards. Exhale and lower your arms beginning with the shoulder, then elbow, then wrist and then hand while you slightly flex your wrist. Do this 10 times consecutively and alternate arms. Notice how it feels to move your arms rhythmically. This is a great way to lubricate your joints, decrease swelling, reduce muscle tension, reduce pain and increase circulation.

8. Arm Shimmies.

Shake your arms. Allow your arms to vibrate first slowly then gradually pick up the speed. You can set a timer for up to 1 minute.

Continue shaking. You can start with one arm at a time and then build up to shaking both arms at the same time. Shaking the body is a great way to increase circulation and to feel lighter and freer. Combine this exercise with the 3 part sniff, sniff, sniff breaths and the toning "ahhhh."

9. Proud Walking with an Open Heart.

Get a silk veil or scarf and hold the scarf behind you with your arms outstretched so the veil is taut. Walk with your chest lifted and expanded. Allow your breath to be diaphragmatic and full. Think of yourself as the goddess and empress that you are. Feel yourself as royalty and taller. Allow yourself to walk fully present and available to your greatness. You are brilliant and magnificent because you are you! Make time every day to appreciate and walk yourself as a fully embodied goddess and empress. Just as we take our dogs for a walk a few times per day. Honor and appreciate yourself by walking fully aware and awakened to your greatness.

When we feel divine and magnificent just as we are, our body and mind benefits. You are a gift to the world when you are present and authentically you. Feel your chest and heart open and completely present to the experience of "feeling" your conscious walk as you move throughout your day. Play music and walk with your veil around your room. This is a gift that you give to yourself of your own full undivided attention.

Make time throughout your day to dance, to breath and move guided by your breath. Whenever you feel stressed or tired, take a deep breath in and come back to your feeling expanded and centered with our sniffs and "ahhhh" breaths. This quickly re-boots your nervous system and connects you to your body, mind and soul in the present moment. It also quickly assists you to process and release emotions that many times stay contracted in our bodies.

Thank you for making time to nurture yourself with your nurturing moves. When you do these exercises you benefit yourself, your family and everyone on the planet. When we raise our vibration to love and acceptance, we effect the world in a positive way!

Email me at info@michellealva.com if you would like to receive a free guided meditation and also for a playlist of my favorite belly dance music. There are also free guided audio downloads at www.michellealva.com and www.sexysacredsensualyou.com

I am here as a resource for you and I can work with you via Skype or in person.

REFERENCES

Bicego, D. et al. Exercise For Women With or at Risk for Breast Cancer-Related Lymphedema. Physical Therapy October 2006 vol. 86 no. 10 1398-1405
http://ptjournal.apta.org/content/86/10/1398.full

IARC Handbooks of Cancer Prevention. Weight Control and Physical Activity. Vol. 6. 2002.

Lee I, Oguma Y. Physical activity. In: Schottenfeld D, Fraumeni JF, editors. Cancer Epidemiology and Prevention. 3rd ed. New York: Oxford University Press, 2006.

McTiernan A, editor. Cancer Prevention and Management Through Exercise and Weight Control. Boca Raton: Taylor & Francis Group, LLC, 2006.

Lane K, Worsley D, McKenzie DC. Exercise and the lymphatic system. implications for breast-cancer survivors. Sports Med. 2005; 35:461–471.

Kiecolt-Glaser JK et al. Yoga's impact on inflammation, mood, and fatigue in breast cancer survivors: a randomized controlled trial. J Clin Oncol. 2014 Apr 1;32(10):1040-9.

Michelle Alva BIO www.michellealva.com
www.sexysacredsensualyou.com

Soul Connector Michelle Alva, Holistic Physical Therapist and Intuitive Healer, is a woman on a mission to uplift our world and remind us of our essential nature, that we ARE love. She does this by integrating her over 20 year background sharing an approach that unites modern movement science with ancient wisdom and includes holistic physical therapy, yoga therapy, belly dance, massage, emotional release bodywork, PSYCH-K®, Therapeutic Touch® and Vibrational-Sound Therapy.

Michelle creates a sacred space where clients learn how to easily and effectively release and process old repressed physical and emotional traumas and tensions. She intuitively guides us through a process that leaves us feeling lighter, connected, fully alive and aligned to your true, authentic essence! Michelle has created a "life fulfillment enhancement program" for women to embrace and embody their wholeness called Sexy, Sacred Sensual You.

Michelle's passion is expressing her mission through videos, writings, her blog, one-on-one emotional release bodywork session, retreats and professional speaking. She is a catalyst for individuals to heal, de-stress, energize and align with their authentic self and soul. Michelle recently released a new album of guided meditations called "YES! YES! YES! Guided Meditations To BE The Love We Wish To See In The World" to create a new mindset for each one of us to BE an embodiment of uplifting change on our planet.

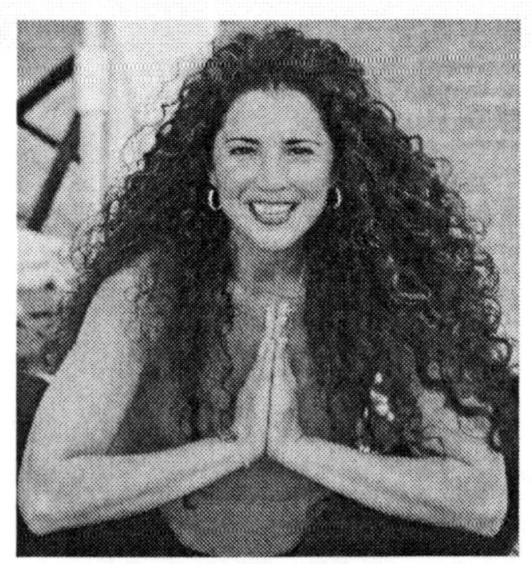

Michelle Alva

is an intuitive channel of Divine Love and Healing Light. Her life's mission to share the safest, easiest and most effective healing and wellness approaches to align with one's True essence of who they are.

Her intention and passion is to teach people how to learn in practical and experiential ways how to harness one's natural energy, vitality and self-repair, self-healing resources. She does this by integrating the modern science of Physical Therapy with mind-body-spirit medicine and ancient wisdom approaches.

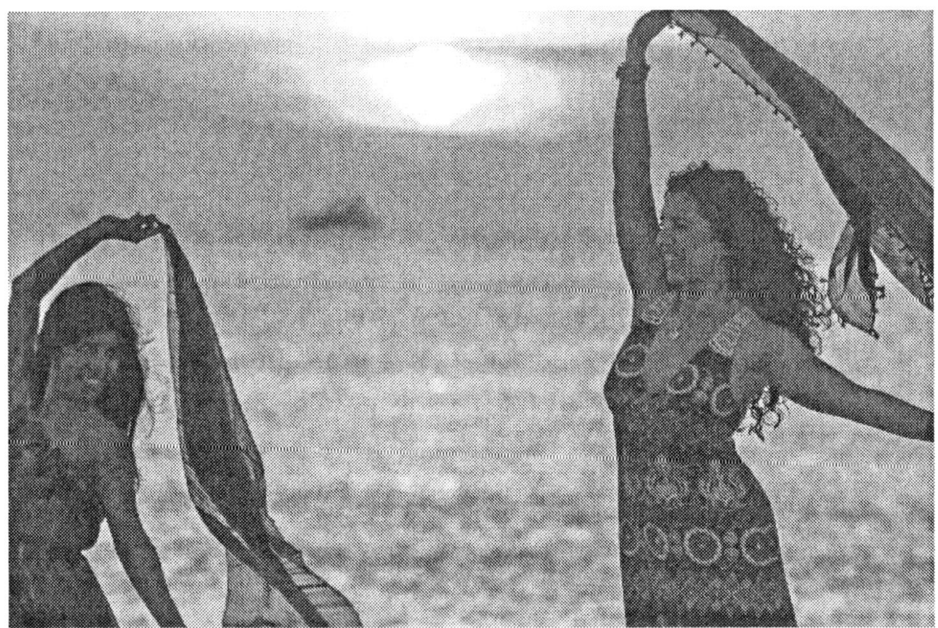

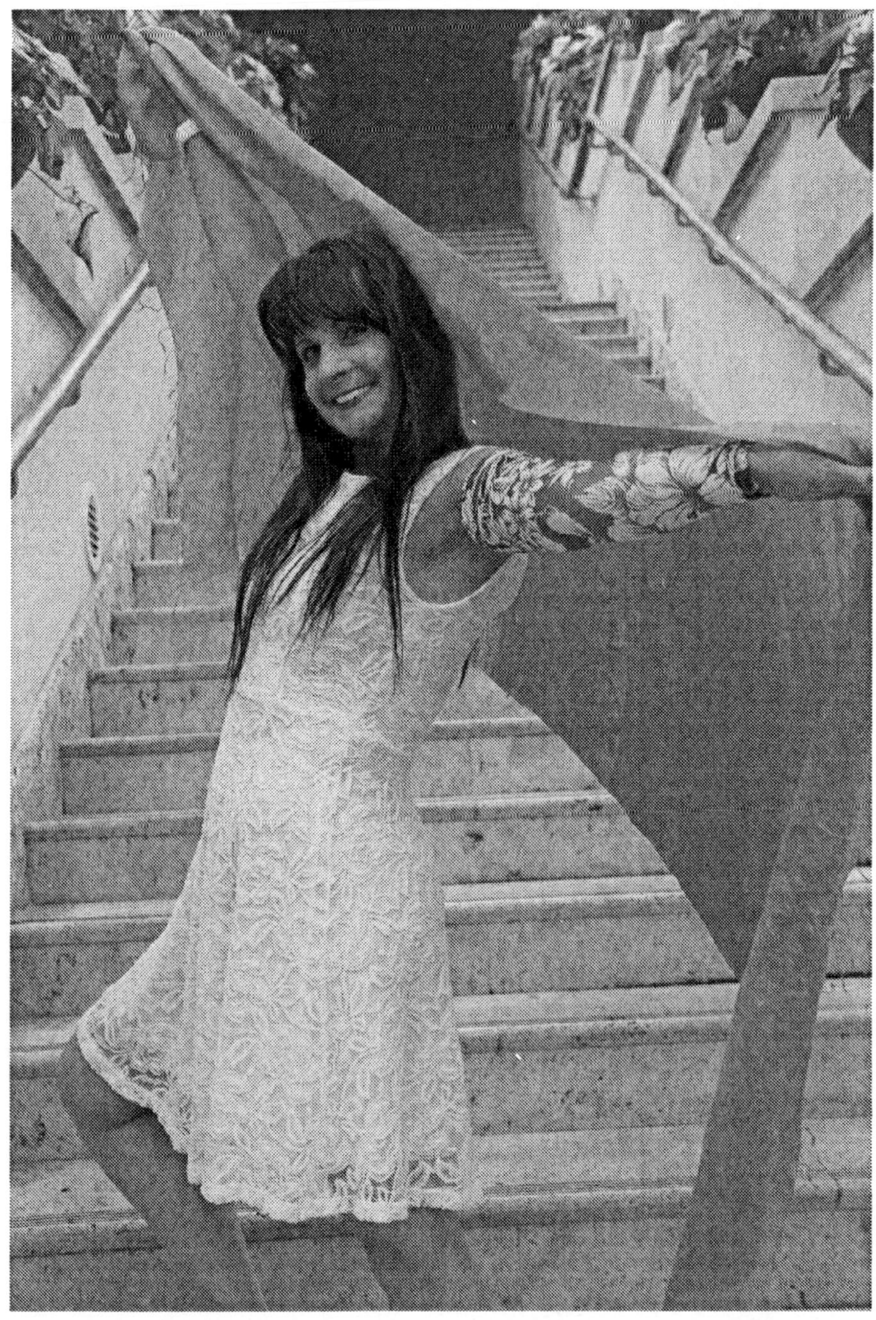

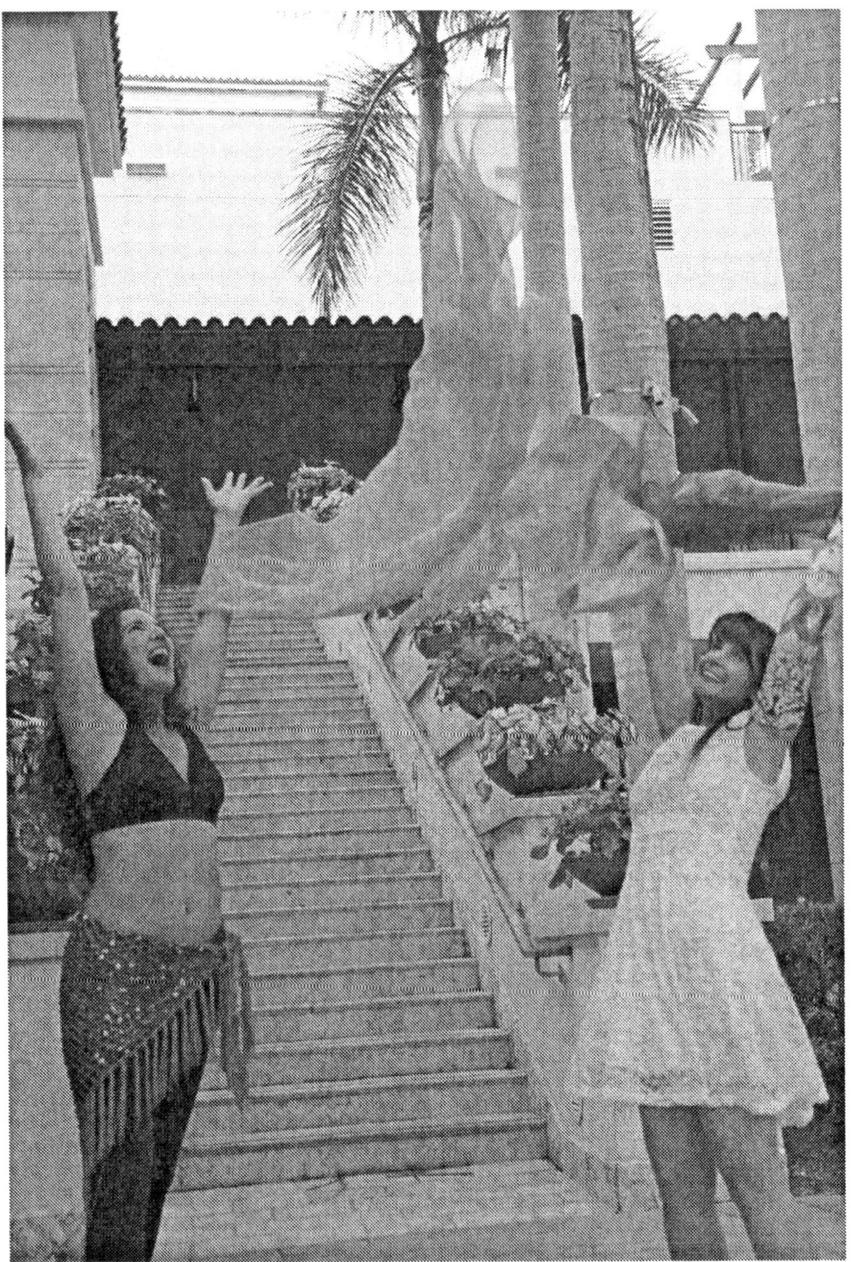

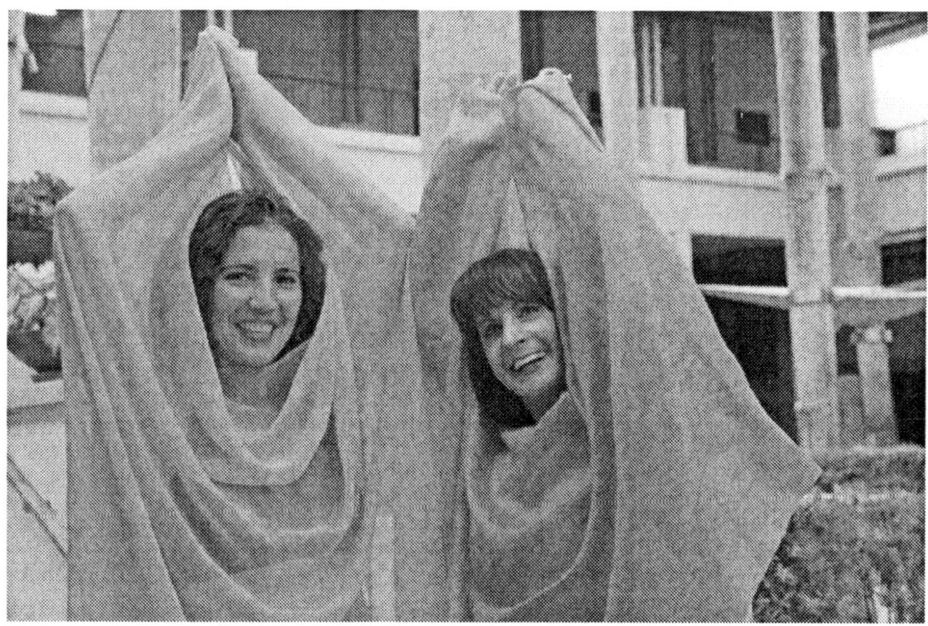

Chapter 19:

On The Other Side of the Couch

Nicole Eldridge Marcus, Ph.D.

I remember Friday, April 15 2005 as "Diagnosis Day" – an emotional rollercoaster of a day. The morning has now become "before" – before we learned about my mother's breast cancer diagnosis. I went to Pilates, chatted with a friend in the parking lot about eye doctors and the licensing exam, uncharacteristically bought candles and challah for a rare Shabbat celebration, and made dinner plans with our friends to come over in the evening. At my afternoon haircut appointment, I told the stylist I was awaiting a phone call to give us the news of my mom's biopsy.

My cellphone rang midway through the appointment and away we went...crossing over in an instant from one world to another; from the world of good health to the world of cancer; to trying to absorb what all of this meant.

In that initial hour of learning the news, I spoke with my mom and sister while still at the hair salon, trying to be strong and proactive. I hung up the phone depleted and a bit scared. At Barnes

& Noble that afternoon, I tried to find an appropriate book to educate me, but they all looked too dense and overly comprehensive at this initial moment.

Instead, in information-seeker mode, I began reaching out to friends in the medical world to obtain a translation of the doctor's oral report – medical lingo that was all Greek to me: "moderately differentiated invasive ductal carcinoma; confluent intermediate nuclear grade cribiform ductal carcinoma in situ; Ductal focus – majority is in ductal system with comedo necrosis and micro calcification; 1.5 millimeter focus; lumpectomy and radiation are likely."

That evening, purely by coincidence, we entertained friends in our home for dinner who were connected to the breast cancer world – one ran a support group for breast cancer patients and the other was an acupuncturist who often worked with this population as well. Speaking with them and listening to their perspectives as we sat on the hardwood floor making wines was comforting, as was the distraction of our sons struggling and laughing and playing with one another.

However, I couldn't fall asleep that first night. Instead, I read through my first breast cancer book, beginning to get a sense of the road we all had ahead of us. In my work as a clinical psychologist, I had been trained to view traumatic events as those that were sudden, unexpected, and uncontrollable, and that could produce ongoing effects. I realized on that first night that my mother's diagnosis did indeed constitute a family drama.

To back up just a little, my mother's biopsy had been scheduled as the result of a routine mammogram screening. My dad had written to me just two weeks prior, immediately following the mammogram:

"As I understand it from the way she presented it to me, they found some calcification (not sure what that is) and thought they should check it out, although the chances of it being anything really threatening or serious were very low. Pretty much a case of just being extra careful, I think.

"The procedure she's having isn't a 'real' surgical biopsy, but just some sort of 'mini-biopsy' they do first in the hopes that this will be enough. Which hopefully it will be, so I don't want you to worry unduly. Of course, despite my ever-optimistic nature, I realize there's always a chance of a problem. That's why they have these exams in the first place, and why they follow up on them if they see anything at all out of the ordinary. So of course it would turn out that there's a problem. But the chances appear to be low, so I think we should all be optimistic and try not to worry unduly unless and until there is something to worry about."

With the family focused on being optimistic, the news itself on that Friday afternoon in April caught us all unprepared. My first goal was to understand the diagnosis and prognosis as clearly and realistically as possible.

Since medical offices were closed over the weekend, friends and family connected both my sister and me to a number of colleagues in the medical world who generously took the time via email or phone to help decipher the findings. Their encouraging responses indicated we were fortunate – that the cancer was caught early and there was a very good chance of recovery.

I remember being grateful that these medical professionals were so generous with their time as to translate the dictation for us, and feeling reassured by their optimistic assessments. Obtaining their input was valuable.

And from that point forward, it seemed to me that my entire family spread its wings to each play a role in rallying around my mother, her treatment, and her recovery. My husband was the first to set a positive tone on the email front, in what would become a long chain of family emails.

Identifying himself as a proud member of "Team Joyce," he encouraged us to "stay positive and proactive," found websites that could educate the entire family, and began providing his own informal legal counsel:

"If the radiologist refuses to give you the med report tomorrow, inform him or her that under HIPPA you have a federally protected right to your medical information. [Feel free to inform them that you have attorneys in the family who don't take kindly to doctors who give cancer patients incomplete medical information before a long weekend over the phone, refuse to fax the actual report, and then expect the patient to scribble down contents of the report after they just learn they have cancer!]."

On April 18, 2005, three days after we received my mom's breast cancer diagnosis and begun researching the treatment options, I composed this letter and sent it to my mom and immediate family:

Dear cancerous cells in mom's left breast, I feel it's my obligation to let you know that you have no idea what you are up against. My sister Robin used the excellent analogy that the cavalry is coming in, and so I think it is only appropriate that you know with whom you are doing battle.

It is not just Joyce Leffler Eldridge, our most spectacular wife/mom/sister/friend. It is also Team Joyce, which includes the seven of us (my dad Larry, my sister Robin, my brother Ross, my husband Jeff, my uncle Stu, and me) and about a trillion others – close friends who love my mom enormously, extended family who will be there for her, and all of our little munchkins who are too young to understand what's going on, but adore their Nana and will not put up with anyone hurting her. There are even a couple of four-legged little ones who like nothing more than snuggling in her lap and – while it's not their natural temperament – can be very fierce when necessary.

This is to say we're united and strong – all of us here for my mom at every single moment of this battle with you. And we will each bring our own contributions to this fight to ensure that the different pieces – the medical knowledge, the logistical plans for treatment, the emotional support, and the pieces we cannot yet anticipate, will be fully covered.

We want you to know that we are all in this together. We want you to know that we are very strong fighters. And we want you to know that we are going to win.

Sincerely,
Nicole, Robin, Ross, Larry, Stuart, Jeff, and all of Team Joyce.

With my immediate family scattered all over (New York, Miami, Boston), I was touched that on the same day I sent this letter out, my sister-in-law and her husband wrote me to indicate they were planning to visit my mom that weekend. Knowing she was being looked after and supported when we were all at a geographical distance was reassuring.

As we continued writing to one another, the positive energy within our family became palpable, as evidenced by a note from my sister on April 20:

Just wanted to quickly say that I feel really (almost overwhelmingly) fortunate that this is our Team Joyce. I've known what an amazing, intelligent, resourceful, loving, fun(ny) group we (!) are, but I have never before felt so forcefully confronted with its solidarity and power. I LOVE YOU and if I were a kickball captain picking teams, I WOULD not and COULD not possibly choose a more KICK ASS one.

We were most excited when my mom was able to obtain an appointment with Dr. Susan Troyan, a surgical oncologist in the Boston area highly recommended to us. As Mom informed us:

The meeting will involve Dad and myself and whoever, plus the radiation oncologist, breast surgeon, medical oncologist, and then afterward the pathologist and one other. In the middle of this meeting, which will last 3-4 hours, the doctors will go off and conference and we'll talk to some miscellaneous people. Then they'll present my alternatives and we'll select a course. That's all for now. Love you all immensely.
XXXX Mom J.

In preparing for the medical appointment, I sent my family the following information:

Hi everyone,

Spoke with a support person who had some great thoughts for Mom's upcoming appointment.

- *Bring a tape recorder to tape the session*
- *Try to do it on a conference all if possible, so that perhaps one of more of us who aren't there physically can still be*

involved (if this is something Mom would even want, it probably involves her clearing it with them first)

- *Have at least one family member with you and perhaps also a friend if possible*
- *Ensure all the right questions are asked*

"On that last point, she recommended Dr. Susan Love's book, which is highly popular and respected. At the end of this book and other breast cancer books, there are usually suggested questions for these meetings including the following:

- *What did the biopsy show exactly?*
- *What stage and grade?*
- *Estrogen/Progesterone, DNA analysis, F-phase testing, Her2neu, proliferative markers?*
- *Tumor markers clean?*
- *Alternatives prior to surgery?*
- *Lymph nodes under arm checked?*
- *Sentinel node procedure?*
- *Tests before surgery?*
- *How long in the hospital and after surgery, what restrictions?*
- *Should family members (e.g. Nicole, Robin) consider genetic testing?*
- *Hormone therapy?*

I'm not even sure what all that means....just some stuff to start digesting. Love, me.

By early May, my sister was working on improving my mom's nutrition and refusing to allow this piece to slide.

"You guys have a Whole Foods right near you. Please, can I have a PROMISE that one of you will get veggies TONIGHT? I'll say I love you when I hear a PROMISE FROM SOMEONE. And then, MOM, a PROMISE from you (and I'd love one from you too, Dad) that you will eat two handfuls (at LEAST) a day of combined veggies – Brussels sprouts, broccoli, cauliflower...are we clear and are we on????"

And then, following my mom's treatment planning session with her medical team, we began planning for our whole family to come together for her surgery. She had her lumpectomy on Wednesday, May 11 and the entire family was at the hospital the whole day (this despite my sister's accidentally slamming her hand through a glass window five minutes before our departure for the hospital in a well-meaning attempt to kill a hornet). As I wrote to far-flung friends and family the next day:

"My mom had her surgery at Beth-Israel Hospital here in Boston and it seems to have gone really well. She was a total trooper, having to withstand all kinds of injections in Nuclear Medicine prior to the surgery, and then during the surgery itself. My whole family has really pulled together on this one and is has been tremendous having all of us here at home together for her – and she seems to be doing just great one day post-surgery."

An array of different friends came over in the following days of recovery, buoying not only my mother's spirits but our entire family.

Over the summer, she completed a course of radiation. She did not complain, she just made it a part of her morning routine prior to work each day. At the end of the treatment course in August, we surprised her with a luncheon in Brookline with five of her best friends – a chance to celebrate her coming through the treatment and reaching this longed-for finish line. One of her best friends was not in attendance; she had died from complications related to breast cancer over the summer. A picture of her and my mom proudly holding their infants together (one of which is me), proudly hangs in our home.

Nearly a year later, I had my own first mammogram – just as a routine procedure to obtain baseline information. It went smoothly and I will now continue to follow up as recommended by my doctor. My mother is doing beautifully; she continues to take the Tamoxifen, gets checked on a regular basis, and maintains an optimistic outlook.

In October, my husband and I helped our three year-old son Zachary to run in his first "Race for the Cure." Below is the email we sent to his supporters on his behalf:

To All My Generous Family and Friends,

Wow. The support that all of you gave me for today's 2006 Miami Race for the Cure was just overwhelming. Thanks to each and everyone one of you – I was blown away by the response.

Thanks to all of your generosity, my race today raised an astonishing $1,750 for the Susan J. Komen Breast Cancer Foundation. This contributes to the nearly $131,000 current total raised by all of today's committed runners and walkers in the unseasonably hot October sunshine of downtown Miami.

Although my toddler race was short, I ran my little heart out this morning (see picture on the left) and – through all of you – hopefully helped to make an impact in the fight against this formidable disease.

With much love and enormous thanks to each of you who made today that much more special,

Zachary Eldridge Marcus.

Our family will continue to participate in this race on an annual basis, in tribute to my mom and all the women we know who have struggled with breast cancer. Tedeschi and Calhoun (1995) define "traumatic growth" as the experience of positive growth following traumatic life events. Perhaps through this annual race, along with a sense of living for the moment and reordering our lives' priorities, we are a family moving toward this growth every day.

Re-reading this chapter is a bit like opening a carefully preserved time capsule—all of the details are vivid and real, but they also emanate so notably from another lifetime. Since the writing of this chapter, many memorable years have passed, filled with countless moments of exquisite beauty, none more so than the birth of our second son. And yet with so many joys and blessings to appreciate, including the continued excellent health of my own mother (about whom this piece was written), my family and I have also gone through the challenges of supporting various good friends (often young mothers themselves) as they cope with the treatment ramifications of both BRCA-positive and breast cancer diagnoses; we have taken an emotional journey over the past year and a half with a particularly close college friend (and spectacular young mother of two daughters) as she moves as courageously as possible through terminal cancer; and we have experienced the brutal and devastating sadness in taking that same journey with a most beloved family member, whom we ended up losing far too early to yet another form of cancer.

There is a quote that I often give to my therapy patients, in part because I personally have found it so helpful along the way. I share it now, with the hope that it kindles a sense of strength and bravery during those times of darkness.

In the midst of winter, I found there was, within me, an invincible summer."

-Albert Camus

May the invincible summer be always within our reach.

REFERENCES

Tedeschi, R.G. and Calhoun, I.G., Trauma and Transformation: Growing in the Aftermath of Suffering, Thousand Oaks, CA: Sage, 1995.

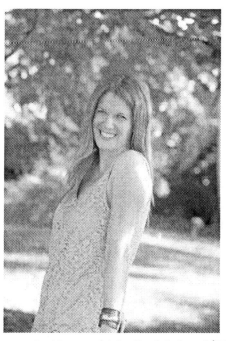

Nicole Eldridge Marcus, Ph.D

Boston native Dr. Nicole Eldridge Marcus is a magna cum laude Phi Beta Kappa graduate of Yale University. She earned both her master's and doctoral degrees from the University of Miami's five-year Clinical Psychology program, a rigorous and highly-regarded scientist-practitioner doctorate program which emphasizes the clinical science component of psychology.

At Harvard Medical School/Children's Hospital Boston, one of the top training programs in the country, she completed both a predoctoral internship and postdoctoral fellowship in child and adolescent psychology. Upon invitation, Dr. Marcus completed an additional postdoctoral fellowship at the University of Miami.

Dr. Marcus is presently in private practice in Pinecrest, Florida, having developed a boutique family practice that specializes in child, adolescent, young adult, and parent-focused therapy and consultation. Learn more about her at her website: www.NicoleMarcus.com.

Chapter 20

Coping with Breast Cancer

Sameet Kumar, Ph.D.

A breast cancer diagnosis can present a set of unique challenges for every patient who receives one. No two people will process the experience the same way emotionally; it may be the hinge upon which your life begins to revolve, or it may feel like just a bump in the road. While it's tempting to think there is a "right" way to go through breast cancer, the truth is there are as many pathways as there are people diagnosed. Although each path is unique, there are some commonalities that this chapter will illuminate.

What to Expect From Yourself

For many patients with breast cancer, questions arise in the middle of the night that can seem too difficult to even speak out loud – trying to figure out why you got sick; the statistics you read on the Internet; an off-handed comment your oncologist made –

there's no end to the uncertainties your mind can dwell on. Even though most women with breast cancer are living longer and better lives, the hardest questions still have to do with uncertainty and thoughts of death and dying.

Nights like these are quite common for breast cancer patients. If you find yourself pondering these questions over and over again, you've probably discovered there are no easy answers. I've come to believe that these are attempts by the mind to try to establish some sense of control amid the ambiguities and uncertainties created by a cancer diagnosis.

The first question most people ask is "Why me?" Even with the best medical knowledge, this is a difficult question to answer. A perfect storm of genetics, environmental factors, lifestyle, and bad luck does not offer an easy solution, nor does it fit into an easily digested sound bite. Surely, with all of our impressive scientific progress and medical knowledge, there must be a simple explanation?

Unfortunately not. It seems that the more we learn about breast cancer, the more questions we learn to ask that we didn't know before. Rather than obtain the elusive answers, a much more realistic proposition is to figure out a way to live and thrive with uncertainty. The problem of sickness, suffering, and mortality is one that has been the focus of humanity for millennia. Our current scientific advances seem to have contributed to the mystery instead of solving the riddle. The world's great spiritual traditions have traditionally been used to help us understand the mysteries of our existence. More recently, many popular self-help authors and thinkers have also attempted to answer these questions.

In the popular culture, there's a general belief that cancer can be caused by negative emotions, stressful life events, etc., much like with the flu or heart disease. Research in this area consistently finds that this is not exactly true for cancer, at least not directly.

Many people believe that life's stressful and negative emotions wear down the body's immune system, thereby weakening the ability to fight off cancer cells. Therefore, it is seen as paramount to surround yourself with positive emotions, supportive relationships, and a stress-free lifestyle. These are ideal goals for anyone, with or without cancer. However, as we all know, life is not very predictable, nor is it always pleasant.

Bad feelings, relationships that turn sour, daily stress—these are universal experiences that color all of our lives; to place the cause for illness on things over which you have little control over doesn't seem all too helpful. Furthermore, in my experience the belief that stress causes cancer doesn't exactly facilitate relaxation in most people. Stress is inevitable; no one holds the key to turning off that aspect of life in a comprehensive way. I think it's much more helpful to know how to manage stress than to try and pursue an unrealistic life without stress at all.

How Do I Cope?

Over the years, I've observed that people who are involved in their treatment in a deliberate, active way are typically better prepared psychologically for the roller coaster ride that is cancer. However, active involvement means many different things. For some, it means learning all there is to know about breast cancer diagnosis and treatment. For others, it means delegating this knowledge to a caregiver or friend who accompanies them to appointments. For others still, it means focusing on healthy behaviors, or some combination of all of the above.

Although many people find it helpful to research their cancer, not everyone needs to be an expert to be actively involved. Some people choose to become experts in breast cancer; others choose to let their doctors make all the choices, preferring not to know the details. In most instances, you are going to have to decide based on your own comfort level what works best for you. What I frequently tell my patients is to set aside a few hours to learn what you want to know. Generally, the Internet is a decent source of information, but it is frequently discouraging and sometimes irrelevant to your particular disease variant. Like a local newspaper or the evening news, I've found that generally bad news about cancer is much more frequent on the Internet than good news. If you find yourself feeling better by learning more about the disease, keep educating yourself. If you find yourself becoming discouraged, demoralized, and depressed, perhaps the information-based approach is not for you. Stick to other areas of self-advocacy, like taking notes during doctor visits, or appointing a willing caregiver as your go-to person for information.

There's one area in which I advise everyone to be equally informed about: pain management. If you are experiencing pain related to your cancer or cancer treatment, it is imperative that you discuss this with your doctor. Adequate and appropriate pain management is the corner stone of psychosocial well-being. If you are in significant physical pain, it will be nearly impossible to do anything else or feel very good until it's under control.

When it comes to emotional pain, most cancer centers utilize a psychosocial team consisting of psychologists, psychiatrists, and/or oncology social workers. You can ask your oncologist's office for guidance in how to connect yourself to these services. Many people also choose to join a support group. In these settings, people of different backgrounds and knowledge bases can share feelings and compare notes on their doctors and treatment options. It often feels better to talk to someone who is going through the same thing you are, or has already finished.

Additionally, we now know that not all coping strategies are created equally. The combination of exercise and healthy nutrition can not only help you cope with the stresses of diagnosis, treatment, and uncertainty, it can also reduce the risk of breast cancer recurrence! Studies have shown that women whose breast cancer was hormone- positive face increased risk of recurrence based on alcohol consumption (Zhang et al., 2007). Studies also show that post-menopausal women whose tumors were hormone-negative who exercise more than five times a week can reduce the risk of recurrence by as much as 13% (Peters et al. 2009).

Finally, if you have found that your religious or spiritual beliefs have been helpful to you in the past, use them now. If you are not this type of person, use what has worked before, but only if it promotes health and well being in you and your relationships.

You can also explore spiritual teachings that work to help soothe you or give your suffering meaning. Don't hesitate to reach out to close friends or family, or to talk to other survivors. You don't have to go through this alone.

Be Positive or Get Real?

Another prevalent pop culture belief is that being "positive" will aid healing and "negativity" in any form will sabotage your treatment. I find that whenever there is someone talking about how negative emotions can be physically toxic, the atmosphere in the room is decidedly tense – exactly the opposite of what the speaker intended. Similarly, when cancer patients begin to feel that the negativity in their lives has made them sick, this insight generally is accompanied by feelings of guilt, anger, and shame. These are precisely the emotions you are being told to avoid!

In many ways, the pressure to be a positive cancer patient can a self-defeating strategy. Jimmie Holland (2000), one of the pioneers in the field of psycho-oncology, calls this the "tyranny of positive thinking." To sum it up, the journey through cancer, in all of its phases ranging from diagnosis to treatment, is likely the most difficult physical – and perhaps also emotional – task that you will ever face. Isn't it unrealistic to force yourself to be the most positive you have been during the most grueling journey of your life? Of course, it always feels better to be hopeful, happy, and driven. But feeling pressured to feel happy rarely results in genuine joy.

The challenge is not to be a positive cancer patient, but an emotionally healthy human being who is experiencing cancer. In my practice over the years, I've found that those individuals who are willing to face their frustrations, anger, shame, guilt—all their very human negativity—are the ones who tend to be happier years later. Denying these essential human emotions and states of mind only stifles the capacity to feel along our emotional and spiritual continuum. The majority of us need to experience temporary distress to find a more lasting happiness. The key word here is *temporary*; just as trying to only be happy on positive can be stifling, so to can wallowing in all of the frustrations, uncertainties, and misery that cancer can bring.

Remarkably, there is as yet no credible research or evidence to substantiate the idea that the way in which your emotions navigate breast cancer will determine how long you live; to the contrary, research finds that there really isn't an overall effect of how you feel on your long-term health outcome in the face of cancer (Coyne and Tennen, 2010). I find this very liberating to consider; you may experience a ton of pressure to feel one way or the other, e.g. to try to always be positive and grateful. While it may feel better to be positive, it's not always realistic or possible, especially when you're feeling sick or experiencing some painful side effects. Now we can say with some certainty that if you can't feel positive all the time, it really doesn't matter too much in terms of your cancer risk.

Rather than control thoughts and feelings, most psychologists and other mental health practitioners place an increasing importance on accepting them instead as a way to dissolve the power of negative emotions (see Kabat-Zinn, 2005). This approach is in sharp contrast to the repressive, selective attention touted by the "be positive" approach. In my professional experience, repressed feelings don't go away, they just learn to wear masks and re-surface in unexpected areas. Since you can't turn your feelings off, you can give yourself permission to feel them, especially if you know that this is part of a larger process of getting better. Also be re-assured that distress, like any other emotion, tends to be temporary. One of our gifts as human beings the variety of emotions we can feel; we can't feel the good without the bad.

What to Expect From Others

You may have certain expectations of how people around you will react to your illness and you'll quickly learn who's really in your corner. Or you may have already learned this lesson. Don't be surprised if people you had assumed would be there to help seem to disappear, and people whom you'd taken for granted become priceless.

The diagnosis can amplify aspects of relationships, bringing out the best in some and the limitations of others. The happiest breast cancer survivors tend to focus on the relationships that work rather than in disappointment or anger about those that don't. Again, everyone experiences breast cancer differently. There is also a range of how caregivers experience people with breast cancer.

What to Expect in the Future

Most people assume that the day you are told you have cancer is the hardest emotional part of the experience. However, my professional experience tells me that there are actually three peaks of distress which are fairly universal.

Of course, the first of these is the day of diagnosis. This might be the day your radiologist tells you your mammogram or ultrasound was highly suspicious. It might be when your physician called you to tell you he or she had some bad news to share. It might be the day you felt a strange lump in your breast. Or, it might be when you first met with an oncologist and discussed the specifics of your disease and the treatment options available to you.

Whichever of these examples resonates with your experience, this moment is when you began to grieve the loss of a healthy future. This is not to say that your future won't include health; most of us assume it will. But the day you knew you had cancer, you also learned that this universal assumption is a fantasy. We grieve the loss of that fantasy. I've written extensively elsewhere about how to cope with grief (Kumar, 2005).

The second peak of distress is the day before or the day of your first treatment. This can mean surgery, chemotherapy, or radiation. Whatever treatment modality is indicated for your disease, the day it begins is often filled with a complex mix of anxiety, fear, impatience, and reluctance. Furthermore, if you are receiving steroids like dexamethasone or prednisone as part of your chemotherapy treatment, you may have slept poorly, or feel energized, irritable, or anxious from the medication in addition to the normal stress of treatment. In many ways, the kinds of emotions that emerge on that first treatment day is analogous to the first day of school: deep down, you know this is going to be helpful, but you're reluctant to leave the sheltered, safe, and familiar world behind for this new room full of people you've never met before.

There is no "right" way to feel for these momentous occasions. Truly, the best strategy is to simply get through the day. For many of us, the complex emotions of this first treatment day are fed by another step into the unknown. You wonder what it will be like, how it will feel today and tomorrow, and if it will be like everything you might have heard.

The third peak of distress often occurs shortly after treatment is completed, or shortly before the first follow-up appointment after finishing treatment. Sometimes, there is a peak after treatment is finished, and another one at the three-month or six-month follow-up visit.

You might ask, *"Why would I be distressed about finishing my cancer treatment?"*

I think of the answer to this question as a tendency of our mind to want what is familiar in our lives, no matter what the content of that familiarity might be. When you first started cancer treatment, it may have felt distressing in part because it was new. It felt better as time went on because it became familiar. When you are no longer in treatment, this familiarity to which you've grown accustomed disappears.

Furthermore, when you are receiving treatment, you are actively engaged in a fight against breast cancer. Finishing treatment in many ways can open up issues of uncertainty and vulnerability that you didn't realize were being managed by active treatment. Follow-up visits can only open up this uncertainty by the unexpected news they might bring. It is not uncommon for people to experience increased general symptoms during the week of the follow-up: exhaustion, aches, anxiety, and depression. I am not sharing this with you to help you feel that way. Rather, knowing that this is normal can take quite a bit of the edge off if you should find yourself wrestling with some of these uncomfortable feelings.

What Next?

What do I most hope for when I meet someone with cancer? That they will eventually develop an appreciation for each of life's precious moments after having experienced one its most difficult twists and turns. That is, by experiencing physical illness, you develop an ability to cherish the here-and-now of life's moments rather than dwelling on the failures of the past or the uncertainties of the future. I have found that this focusing on the moment is the only reliable antidote to the unpredictability inherent in human existence. This profound uncertainty about "what if" is at the heart of the fear that most people develop with cancer, or any life-threatening illness.

There are many ways to bring your mind back from the fear and into the reality of today. Many people engage in meditation. I've written a book you might find helpful about how meditation and other techniques can be used to help your mind and body cope with anxiety (Kumar, 2010). Others find artwork to be soothing and comforting. Other people devote more quality time to family and friends. What matters most is not what works for other people, but what works for you. The one thing to remember from the day you are diagnosed is that although you did not choose cancer, you do have choices in how you live, and what you make of the experience.

References

Coyne, JC and Tennen, H. (2010). Positive psychology in cancer care: bad science, exaggerated claims and unproven medicine. *Annals of Behavioral Medicine*, 39, 16-26.

Hewitt, M., Herdman, R., and Holland, J. (2004). *Meeting the psychosocial needs of women with breast cancer*. Washington, D.C.: The National Academies Press.

Holland, J. and Lewis, S. (2000). The human side of cancer: Living with hope, coping with uncertainty. New York, NY: Harper Collins Publishers, Inc.

Kabat-Zinn, J. (2005). *Wherever you go, there you are: Mindfulness meditation in everyday life*. New York, NY: Hyperion Books, Inc.

Kumar, S. (2005). *Grieving mindfully: A compassionate and spiritual guide to coping with loss*. Oakland, CA: New Harbinger Publications, Inc.

Kumar, S. (2010). *The mindful path through worry and rumination*. Oakland , CA: New Harbinger Publications, Inc.

Peters, TM, Schatzkin, A, Gierach, GL, Moore, SC, Lacey, JV, Wareham, NJ, Ekelung, U, Hollenbeck, AR, and Leitzmann, MF. (2009). Physical activity and post-menopausal breast cancer risk in the NIH-AARP diet and health study. *Cancer Epidemiology Biomarkers Prevention*, 18: 289-296.

Zhang, SM, Lee, I, Manson, JE, Cook, NR Willet, W., and Buring, JE. (2007). Alcohol consumption and breast cancer risk in the

Women's Health Study. *American Journal of Epidemiology*, 165:667–676.

Sameet Kumar, Ph.D.,

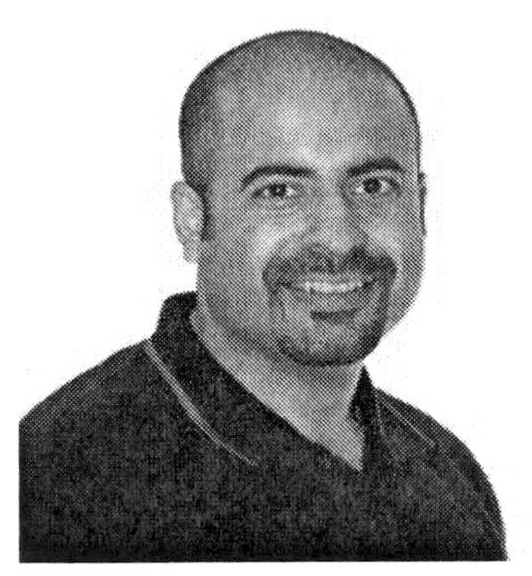

is the clinical psychologist for the Memorial Cancer Institute in Broward County, Florida. He specializes in working with cancer patients and their caregivers. In addition to his training as a psychologist using mindfulness-based therapies, he has also studied with many leading Buddhist and Hindu teachers. He is the author of Grieving Mindfully: A Compassionate and Spiritual Guide to Coping with Loss, The Mindful Path Through Worry and Rumination: Letting Go of Anxious and Depressive Thoughts and Mindfulness for Prolonged Grief.

Chapter 21

Mindfulness and Positive Rewiring of Our Thoughts

Cynthia Dougherty, BCC, M.F.T., Ph.D.

We are constantly climbing a challenging journey that at times feel as though life is a struggle and just plain hard. Even when our lives feel balanced and in a good place, we can always find something for us to worry about and stress over. It's in our DNA. During difficult and overwhelming times personally or collectively, it is human nature to question ourselves and wonder how we are going to get through this difficult patch and painful time.

Going to a doctor and receiving an unexpected diagnosis of breast cancer, one can only imagine the emotional rollercoaster that follows. Fear, confusion, self-doubt, inner conflicts, anger, frustration, sadness, hopelessness, dread, loss, grief and other turbulent emotions surface immediately.

Believe it or not, when encountering such shocking news, it is often our mind that causes us the most difficulty. Our minds immediately shift into what is familiar to us. The pre-recorded message kicks into gear and we remind ourselves about our previous pains, suffering and trials from our past. Immediately, the most negative thoughts enter our mind. We visualize the worst scenario possible. We feel that we are in this battle alone. "This must be a mistake, I need to avoid this and run". Denial becomes powerful. Why me???

Our thoughts, feelings and behaviors are all packaged together. When we are feeling sad, frustrated or anxious, our minds kick into a negative mode. Then we behave in ways that can set us up for a failure. We think it and we bring it! Throughout our experiences in life we typically develop a negative cycle of feelings, thoughts and behaviors which result with negative consequences. These consequences can reinforce the negative cycle. Over time as we repeat a cycle over and over, the feelings, thoughts and behaviors kick into drive and become an automatic response. The neural patterns and experiences of that specific cycle become hardwired into our brains. For example, the doctor recommends a blood test. Because of previous bad experiences having blood drawn, our brain learns blood tests equal something negative. This automatically brings anxiety and thoughts of dread. The neuropathways are telling our brain this too will be a bad experience so be prepared for the worst. "They will never find a vein, this will be painful or I will faint just like the last time". By the time we reach the blood lab, we are so stressed and on the defense we lower the chances of having a positive outcome.

It's curious to many people why certain individuals are more positive than others. While conversely, why certain people we know live in a negative cloud always expecting doom and gloom. Facing our situations and learning how to work them is the best way to emerge stronger, happier and wiser for the next challenge. Throughout life no one scathes adversity. Grief, loss and darkness are all a part of our life's journey. Why do some people maintain a positive attitude and forge ahead while others are unable to see past their darkness?

Let's take the pressure off; you are not alone. Everyone's brain is predisposed to negative thoughts and negative cycles. You can blame negativity on your previous ancestors! So stop beating yourself up; it's in your cells. The brain is the most important part of our body. It's responsible for all of our thoughts, feelings and behaviors. A heavy load for something that only weighs two percent of our total body weight! Neuropsychologist, Rick Hanson (Hardwiring Happiness, 2013) describes the brain as having a "Negativity Bias." We have a tendency to bring in bad experiences and to repel the good ones. The bad is always stronger than the good. People tend to be more upset for losing a bet with money than they are happy for winning a bet. A bad recommendation about someone is more memorable than a good one. A bad mood is more likely to extend to the next day, however a good mood will dissipate faster. Childhood traumas are more enduring and can last a lifetime. The brain evolved the "Negativity Bias" mostly because negative experiences have more of an impact on our survival in comparison to the positive ones (Baumeister et al. 2001). In essence, negative experiences are fast memory systems that convert into negative mental states then into enduring negative neural traits. While positive experiences which is the source of our inner strength, take longer to transfer into a long term memory storage. Therefore, our positive experiences have a tendency to wash away while the negative ones stick like glue. We over-learn the negative and under-learn the positive. Our brains are good at learning from the bad and bad at learning about the new experiences.

Back in the cavemen days the brain was developed to respond to many external threats and extraneous variables. Life appeared to be more simplistic, however the cavemen were faced with daily survival challenges which included being eaten by a predator or running very fast. They also faced starvation, sickness and conflicts between groups. It became self-preservation to expect the negative stimuli and be prepared to react to them quickly. We have carried this need to look for the dangers, fears and interpersonal problems in our daily lives. When the caveman brain is on alert it can cause us to become fatigued which reduces our immune system and leads to never ending stress. Think about your daily routine. Our lives are so much more complicated and our brains are still on high alert for threats. We are scanning for potential dangers, problems and unpredictable situations. When we walk into a new situation, our attention is pulled to the negative or triggers which help us decide whether to fight or run. We are trained to survive.

Within the middle of our brain there are three parts forming the over reactivity section. These include the amygdala, the hippocampus and the hypothalamus. The amygdala is activated by both positive and negative emotions, however it prefers the negative. It's the amygdala's job to signal the hypothalamus and our sympathetic nervous system. The hypothalamus alerts our stress hormones which include adrenaline, cortisol and norepinephrine. This causes our mind and body to speed up. We begin to feel anxious or upset. The hippocampus takes the experience and how we responded and felt and stores it in cortical memory networks. This allows us to learn and recall the experience later. When we are exposed to repeated negative events, our amygdala kicks into high alert and is strengthened by the increased amounts of cortisol. Higher levels of cortisol can have several negative effects. It can overstimulate and destroy cells, therefore shrinking the hippocampus. This can lead to a decrease in our ability to put things in proper perspective and reduce the signal to the amygdala to alert the hypothalamus to stop the stress hormones. Our minds are on overdrive and we then have difficulties perspective taking, seeing the entire picture and thinking clearly. Our emotions feel overwhelming and are all over the place and we are stressed and frustrated. Hello negative cycle.

As we enter this negative cycle, our thoughts, behaviors and emotions result with consequences. We the have a tendency to repeat the cycle over and over most often resulting with the same consequences. These neural experiences become hardwired into our brains. For example, we may associate having blood drawn as a negative experience and we automatically associate this with feelings of anxiety and self-doubt. A negative bias is formed and packaged together based on past experiences. Our inner strengths that are needed for the development of our well-being, coping and success are at times compromised by the negativity bias that we have created. However, if we can identify our triggers or threats then we can recognize our patterns in the way we respond.

Current research recognizes the neuroplasticity of the brain and its ability to change. The brain is like a muscle that we can build up with new capabilities. It just takes practice. We can learn to take in the good and we will become calmer and see the strength in ourselves. This is about transforming fleeting experiences into lasting improvements in our neural net worth. It is learning to change our brain for the better. This involves building effective ways to take in the good and become skillful.

How can we hardwire our brains to think and respond positively against the negative bias upon receiving the news we have cancer? And why is this mindful approach helpful with our recovery? Our brains like to stay rested, at equilibrium and like to feel good. When we hear the word cancer it's only normal that our "Negativity Bias" will kick in. We are vulnerable to a new threat that is coming into our brains. Once in the reactive mode, it sensitizes the brain towards future reactivity. We start to get caught up in our established patterns of worry, irritation and loneliness. We immediately bring our attention to endless worries about the future and negative reruns of the past. Being overwhelmed by the challenging emotions is normal and a part of the journey. So we shouldn't beat ourselves up on how we "think" we should be feeling and acting as we will only add to our confusion and suffering. However, staying in the present will ultimately help us heal. The present, although difficult to do, will open a doorway of calmness and a healing refuge. The future is a mystery. But living a day at a time in a mindful way will strengthen our survival instinct that is inborn in us. Staying in the present allows us to acknowledge the ways things are and to love and trust no matter what we are facing. It will help us to see the bigger picture. Being mindful and resting our brain is the not the end all or a magical cure. However, mindfulness lowers cortisol levels and builds stronger immune systems. The effects of mindfulness are substantial for both mental and physical health. Additional health benefits of mindfulness practices include a decrease in stress, anxiety, depression and an increase in mood, well-being and compassion. Healing also involves relying on our own innate courage and wise heart. This is a part of our journey and will be an important part of who we become. Difficult times always bring us face to face with great pain, fear and a whole lot of loneliness. However, mindfulness can bring healing and transformation. Mindfulness, simply stated means having good control over our attention. When we are mindful we can place our attention wherever we want and stay there. If we want to shift our attention, we can. The control over our attention is the most powerful way to reshape our brain and our mind (Hanson, 2013). A person can train their brain by strengthening their attention. According to Hanson (2013) brains are like vacuum cleaners; it lights up what it is resting on and then it sucks it up to the brain. So what our attention is focused on whether it is self-criticism or recognition of our best qualities, the brain is taking shape on what it is resting upon. Mental activity also shapes neural structure, so changes in our mind can lead to lasting changes in our brain. Mindfulness is bringing awareness into an experience without judgment, expectation or distraction. It's not the same as a religion or spirituality. Mindfulness practices foster the development of new mental skills through purposeful attention, focus and concentration. Mindfulness training provides a means to experience greater balance, regulation and equanimity.

Being mindful allows us to enter a more receptive state and stay present. One trait of mindfulness is being aware of what's happening as its happening. So when negative evaluations are entering our mind, we can pause and be non-reactive. We do not allow ourselves to get lost in our actions. We can also name or label what is going on inside of us. Therefore, we can distance ourselves from the here and now emotional experience.

Let's examine the area of self-compassion and mindfulness. This is an area that is so important when we are facing a tough time in our lives. Self-compassion involves several factors. First, we should always remember that we are a friend to ourselves and should treat ourselves with care, patience, love and understanding.

Do we have a mindful awareness to how we are addressing ourselves? Are we reacting in a negative manner? Are we self-judging or self-critical? "I am worthless"; "I deserve bad things to happen to me". Secondly, when things are not going well and life is stressful, we have a tendency to feel responsible as if we failed. We then isolate ourselves from our friends and family who we perceive as having a better time or life. We need to be mindful of our need for interconnectedness with the people around us. They are in our lives to offer us support. Self-compassion includes the reminder that life is not perfect for anyone. No one is perfect. Finally, mindfulness allows us to see things as they are happening. We can open ourselves up to self-compassion by allowing ourselves to tune in on our pain and our fears. "I like myself no matter what"; "I am strong and will get through anything."

Self-compassion mindfully accepts whatever we are experiencing no matter if it's positive or negative. Self-kindness involves being supportive with encouragement, patience, and understanding verses harsh judgments and negative feelings. Having a sense of connection to ourselves and others is key. Mindfulness helps us accept what is happening as it is, no exaggeration and it gives us the ability to respond to the experience with compassion. There is a difference between, "I am the only person who is angry that I have cancer" and "I am angry that I have cancer and I know that many people with cancer feel the same anger that I do." This is normal in a collective way despite the negativity.

Mindful self-compassion includes giving ourselves emotional support; being there for ourselves. We should give ourselves what we need and want. This will make us less dependent on someone else to fill those needs and respond in the manner that we want. Self-compassion provides a calmness that we provide to ourselves when we are upset. Therefore, it make it easier for our loved ones to help us as well. We should acknowledge that we are suffering and see if we can treat ourselves with as much kindness as we would a dear friend or a relative that was suffering. We need to give ourselves permission to adopt a physical gesture of compassion as in the following example: Place both hands over your heart and add a little pressure. Think of someone who loves you unconditionally; someone who makes you feel safe. Savor the feeling of warmth and love. Hold on to it for 30 seconds. Place your hand on your belly or the side of your face and feel the warmth. Sometimes, I hold my hand and feel the warmth. I visualize my dad reaching out to touch my hand. Be compassionate and remember that you have a kind, warm heart no one can take that away from you. Remember the saying, "Give yourself a hug"?

Ok, you are asking yourself, how can I start to be mindful? You can start by knowing it takes time. No one is an expert at mindfulness overnight. Just increasing your awareness and attention to the present is a beginning. Regular practice is required of mindfulness. The brain is an organ that needs to be exercised. It will take time to rewire the brain to replace the "negativity bias" with a "positive bias".

One way to think about rewiring the brain in a useful way is to understand whenever a difficult situation arises, we have already developed a pattern. This pattern involves our thoughts and feelings that is cycling and fueling this uncomfortable experience in our body. Think about Gandhi and his quote, "Your beliefs become your thoughts. Your thoughts become your words. Your words become your actions. Your actions become your habits. Your habits become your character. Your character become your destiny." When we experience sudden bad news, we head right for the memory bank of thoughts and emotions. We go to patterns from the past that made us feel sad, angry and a fearful self. Real power of mindfulness allows us to undo our repetitive patterns. We do this by taking a pause. We think about the chain reaction. "Is this the usual way that I react"? How can I stop and think and undo this pattern to help me find a more positive outcome"?

Visualize a good day. You are feeling good. Think about your wins for the day. How would that day change for you if you were stuck in traffic in the pouring rain and your window wipers broke? When you finally arrive at home, you are tired and frustrated. How will you deal with the stressors when you enter your home? Think about how you react when you are irritable and are faced with more stressors. Are you thinking effectively? Are your emotions in check? Is your negativity bias creating a vulnerability that is triggering the reactive mode of your brain? Are you focused on the present or are you still stressed long after your challenge of getting home? Holding onto the negative triggers is just bad for your well-being. It weakens your immune system, wears and tears on your body and effects your relationships.

If we learn to take in and focus on the good experiences and take a pause, we will become calm and begin to see the strength inside ourselves. An effective way to become skillful is to take a positive experience, enrich it, absorb it, then think about the negative challenge so that it becomes positive and replaces the negative feeling. When the doctor gives you the good news that your cancer treatment is working hold on to that feeling in your heart and the emotions you feel. Pair these positive feelings with the negative thoughts of having more tests and treatments to endure.

The mindfulness used in meditation is useful everywhere. Meditation can be an amazing tool. There are many ways to mediate. A good mediation practice helps to develop an awareness or mindfulness of our body, our senses of our mind and our heart. A technique that works for you, may not work for me. No judging remember? Mediation takes practice and consistency. Pick a type of meditation and work on it every day. Find a teacher, coach, take a class or even buy and application for your phone. With time you will be able to allow yourself to be open to the present moment. Meditation teaches us to let go and how to stay centered in the midst of change. When we sit and meditate we feel the current state of our body. Sometimes it will feel good and other times it will feel painful. We develop over time, a relationship between our minds, our bodies and our hearts. Mindfulness is a caring and respectful attention.

Find a quiet place. Then find a stable, comfortable posture. Sit up, tall in a chair with your feet placed on the floor. Be as awake as you can be. It's important for you to feel comfort, ease and stability. Allow your shoulders to drop and place your hands in your lap

Close your eyes.

Bring your awareness to the present. Become aware of your surroundings and the sounds around you.

Begin by taking a few full breaths. Try to exaggerate the in-breath so that you fill the chest and lungs. Then take a slower out-breath. Repeat this several times, inhaling deeply, filling the lungs and exhaling slowly your out-breath. Let go. Slowly allow your breath to resume its natural rhythm.

Be aware of your body; the sensations and tensions. Try to feel your body relax.

Feel the energy going through each and every part of your body: down your face, into your neck through your arms and hands, down your navel area, the belly. Breathe and feel the loosening and relaxing through your sides, your back and into your legs. Imagine a sensation or tingling into your feet and toes.

Take a deep breath, relax your legs, breath out. Deep breathe in and relax your arms, breath out. Connect with your breath. Feel the coolness in your nose and with your breath.

Feel the movement in your chest and the rise and fall in your body.

Breathe through your nostrils.

Notice if your mind wanders off, tell your mind to just concentrate on your breath. Each time your mind wanders off, try to bring it back. Let go of the thought and return it to the breath. Let the majority of your awareness be on your breath.

If it helps, count each breath in your mind from one to ten.

Start again if you lose track of your count.

Let the majority of your attention be on your breath and the energy inside of your body. Then widen your attention and feel the entire body at once. Can you feel your inner stillness?

Your patience is in the willingness to keep coming back again and again.

Thank yourself for all of what you have released. Open your

eyes.

It's natural for your mind to wander. It's not an easy process. Most people tend to start thinking about their plans, worries and stress over why they can't stop thinking. Your mind has been wandering all your life. Just acknowledge it and keep breathing. Gradually you will start to live more in the moment and less in the mind wandering space. Get a sense of how you are feeling in that moment. Is your mind calm or busy? Try to tune into your emotions and your body.

If you cannot calm down your thoughts as you breathe and you feel your body and mind clearer, you can repeat simple sentences following each breath. For example: breathe in and repeat "Calm my body", breath out and repeat, "Calm my body". Repeat, "May I find peace", "May I quiet my mind". Take your time repeating these phrases. Let your body rest in stillness and the calm.

If initially sitting is not working for you, take a long walk. Be mindful of your body and your breathing. Set an intention, saying; "Allow my body to be steady".

Everyday mindfulness can include: slowing down, reduce multitasking, focus on your breathing when doing daily activities, relax-practice feeling calm and simplify your life. In addition, you can learn how to find a place of refuge. Sometimes when we are faced with a challenging time, we search for a place where we feel safe, at peace and a sense of connectedness. It feels as good as that transitional blanket. It could be a specific place, a memory, activities, a favorite person, or even an emotion. This refuge helps us know that we can handle what is coming our way. I personally find this refuge at the Chesapeake Bay. I feel centered and safe. I feel an inner connectedness and an inner wakefulness. I feel a warmth wrapped around me that touches my soul. You can also have more than one refuge. Pick something that inspires you or lifts you up. When you have a sense of refuge you regularly take it in and internalize it. Most likely you already have a refuge already inside of you. A gentle current you carry with you that you find when you are challenged or upset. As you become more aware of this refuge, it will automatically activate itself with little effort. You will feel secure in the fact that there is a reliable resource stored internally within yourself that is a reliable sanctuary. Mindfulness can reduce your stress through breathing practices. You are training you brain to learn new ways to shift your whole orientation toward what matters in life. Split attention and distractions add to your stress and can reduce the quality of your life. Slow your life down, stay in the present. Remember, you do not have to respond right away to the demands on your attention. When your life in the present, you will feel more connect with the things around you.

When we are stressed out and worried about our health, sitting and being still even if it's for a short period of the day, will bring your mind to the present. So a few times a day, pause. Feel your body and breathe in that wonderful feeling of aliveness. Take pause when you pause. For example, I take several deep breaths and pause at red lights, during traffic jams, before I enter an appointment, when I brush my teeth or at night when I am closing my eyes to sleep. I have established a little voice inside my head to remind me to take a pause throughout my day. Be kind to yourself. If you miss a day, begin again.

Another tool for you to consider to practice your mindfulness would be keeping a daily mediation journal. Mindfulness journals can help us reflect about being in the present, where we have been with our reflection and where we would like to go. You can record your observations, thoughts, feelings, emotions, images, creative ideas and weaknesses of your meditation session. This will allow you to develop a better understanding of what you will need to work on next time. Keeping a journal will also provide you with the opportunity to review your progress and see how you have changed over time and help you to continue to develop your goals. For example, are you looking for more calmness? Are you trying for more persistence? Do you find reinforcing your habitual thinking and feeling patterns? Meditation will help you to sort out the laundry in your head as you observe what your mind generates. Holding on to the stories in your mind will not only hold you back from reaching your happiness but also your chance at making a positive change to your life and healing.

Finally, as we are striving for mindfulness and positive thoughts, try the "Yes" technique. Sit quietly and close your eyes. Think of a stressor like a pending medical appointment. What reaction are you having in your mind? What about the cancer provokes the strongest feelings? What belief are you thinking about and what does this mean to your future? What sensations are you feeling in your chest and belly? When you connect with your hurt, pain and the fear of the situation repeat to yourself, "No." No to the fear, no to the stream of feelings or grief. What sensations are you feeling in your body? Say no to any feelings that are painful. Think of how different your life would be if you kept saying no to painful thoughts and feelings.

Now, take a brief break. Reposition yourself. Relax your body and take a few deep breaths. Try to remember the feelings and thoughts that were so hurtful as well as the beliefs that you can connect with the experience. This time say, "Yes". Say yes to what is happening inside you at this moment in time. Remember you are not saying yes to another behavior. Just keep repeating yes. Feel the thoughts freely and moving along. If you feel angry or fearful that is a normal response. Just say "Yes". Yes, to the pain, yes to the fear, yes to the sadness. Yes, to the pain or the situation that you want to end. Yes, yes, yes. Yes, to the pain that you want to go away. Do you feel a difference in your body when you say yes? Do you feel a softening or relaxation? What happens to the sadness or your painful feelings when you say yes? Do your feelings become more intense? Practice this exercise daily. Your intension should be yes to whatever comes into your awareness. Over time the sensations in your body will keep getting better and so much more positive and peaceful. Just remember, mindfulness is really paying attention to your senses as well as what is happening right here in the moment.

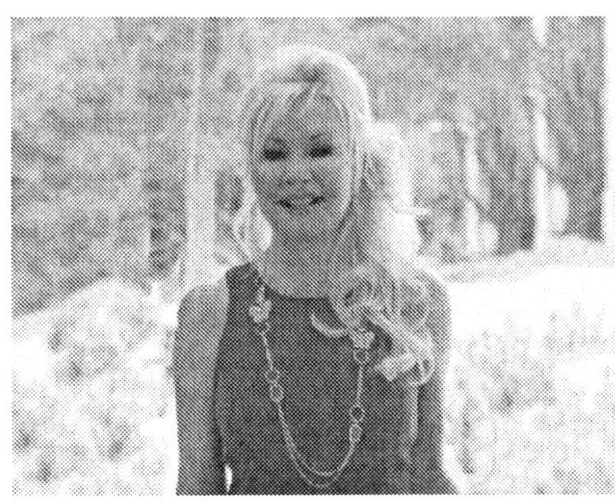

Cynthia L. Dougherty, BCC, M.F.T., Ph.D.

is a Board Certified Wellness Life Coach and Certified School Psychologist. She has a Master's Degree in Family Therapy, Ph.D. in Human Development and a Certificate in Neuropsychology. She has worked both in clinical and corporate settings. Currently, Dr. Dougherty is an international lecturer and trainer in the areas of Meditation and Mindfulness. She has offices in Washington D.C., Miami, and St Michael's, Maryland.

Chapter 22

Therapist, Wife, Mother, Survivor

Mary Darling Montero, Ph.D.

I was diagnosed with breast cancer after a decade of working in the mental health field, most recently as a psychotherapist in private practice. I'd pursued specialized training to work with people who'd experienced traumatic events, and I've looked at and dealt with my cancer experience through that lens: facing, experiencing, and healing from trauma. As a therapist, I was amazed by the resiliency of the human spirit and by a person's ability to heal. For me, healing from breast cancer – which is ongoing both physically and emotionally – is the most difficult, meaningful, and transformational experience of my life.

In talking about the effects of cancer trauma, I'll be focusing on early-stage breast cancer, as that is what I know. Metastatic breast cancer (breast cancer that has spread to other parts of the body) presents unique challenges, including ongoing medical intervention and end-of-life issues. I'd also like to note that although I will be writing about women with breast cancer, it's important to remember that men also deal with the disease. **The Trauma of Breast Cancer**

As a therapist doing trauma work, I encountered the types of trauma we tend to think of: abuse, rape, car accidents, and natural disasters. All of these situations can result in anxiety, depression, worry, feeling on-edge, intrusive thoughts, flashbacks, nightmares, and avoidance of situations and people that trigger memories of the trauma. When I was diagnosed with cancer and subsequently endured treatment and surgeries and met other patients and survivors, I saw varying degrees of these reactions in others, while experiencing many of them myself.

Simply defined, a traumatic event is one that causes us to fear for our physical safety and feel highly distressed. A typical first thought after hearing the words *you have cancer* is: "Am I going to die?" Talk about highly distressing!

The trauma doesn't end there. It continues with events such as scans, surgeries and other invasive procedures, losing breasts, or finding out that treatment is not working or that the cancer has spread. Every woman reacts in her own way to these stressors based on how she has coped with crises in the past, her innate or learned coping strategies, and the extent of her support system. Some want to know every detail of their biopsy report and research everything they can about their type of cancer, while others prefer to leave the details to the doctors. Some feel a profound loss of control, while others feel empowered and adopt a "fighting" spirit. Some reach out to family, friends, and strangers for support, while others feel most comfortable dealing with their situation in private. The important thing is to cope, in whichever ways work, in order to avoid intensifying feelings of anxiety, depression and stress – all of which can negatively affect sleep, relationships, and the ability to carry out tasks associated with treatment or everyday life.

In my work as a therapist and during challenging times in my own life, I've come to believe that during a crisis, a support system is profoundly important. For some people, a support system casts a wide net to encompass family, friends, acquaintances, professionals, and even strangers. For others, it includes just a few people. The size of a person's support system depends on his or her personality, culture, and exposure to other people. In my opinion, the number of people in a support system is less important than the support itself. Quality over quantity!

We are a social species. Since the beginning of time we have relied on each other to meet our physical, practical, and emotional needs. It makes sense, then, that social support plays a crucial role in how a woman copes with breast cancer. Trusting her medical team, having someone she can rely on for help with practical tasks such as getting to appointments or picking up prescriptions, and being able to confide in someone when she feels distressed are all central aspects of that support.

For some people, another level of social support is connecting with other patients and survivors. Support groups offer women a chance to relate to others in similar situations, learn about the disease, and share coping strategies. According to the American Cancer Society, "research has shown that people with cancer are better able to deal with their disease when supported by others in similar situations," and "evidence suggests that support groups can improve quality of life for people with cancer." http://www.cancer.org/treatment/treatmentsandsideeffects/complementaryandalternativemedicine/mindbodyandspirit/support-groups-cam

Aside from in-person support groups, many women turn to the internet to connect with other breast cancer patients and survivors. This approach has unique benefits and downsides. For someone who is isn't able to attend an in-person support group due to extreme illness or geographical location, online groups can provide similar benefits such as emotional support, validating feelings, and sharing coping strategies. An aspect of in-person support that isn't always available online, however, is the presence of a trained professional. In-person support groups tend to be run by mental health professionals trained in the unique dynamics of a group therapy setting. Oftentimes support groups include psychoeducation (again, presented by a trained professional), which is tricky to navigate online. Googling for information about a certain aspect of cancer or cancer treatment can lead a person down a path of misinformation or scary stories. There's nothing like looking up a side effect of a cancer drug and ending up reading worst-case scenario cancer stories. Certainly the information available on the internet can empower us, as we have access to articles, research studies, and others dealing with a similar situation, but it's a good idea to stick to reputable sources such as well-known cancer hospitals and organizations.

Many early-stage breast cancer patients cope with the trauma of their diagnosis and treatment and are able to move on from the experience without lasting negative emotional effects. It's common, however, for breast cancer survivors to experience episodes of anxiety and depression related to fear of recurrence. In a Q&A in the New York Times, renowned trauma expert Francine Shapiro stated that "in a study of 244 breast cancer survivors five-to- nine years post-diagnosis, published in the journal Oncology Nursing Forum, researchers found that fears of recurrence were frequent. The most commonly reported experiences that triggered fear included yearly follow-up appointments, doctors' appointments, hearing of another's cancer, physical symptoms or pain, news reports about breast cancer, and the anniversary of the diagnosis."
http://consults.blogs.nytimes.com/2012/03/16/expert-answers-on-e-m-d-r/

In my understanding of trauma, the complex physical and emotional reactions to a traumatic event can become stuck in our nervous system, thus ensuring we are continually re-traumatized when triggered by an event that reminds us of the original trauma. The fear associated with the moment of a cancer diagnosis can be triggered repeatedly, not just during treatment but long after it ends.

Think of a person traumatized by a life-threatening car accident who re-experiences the terror of the event when triggered by a very loud noise. She might feel as if she is back in the moment of the collision, with the same anxiety and fear for her life. It can be the same for breast cancer survivors: getting a mammogram six months after having a cancerous tumor removed from the breast can be an intensely stressful event, causing anxiety even several weeks before the exam. Even if her chance of recurrence is statistically low, returning for a mammogram recreates the scene, sometimes exactly. Because trauma that is stuck in our nervous system can be impossible to "think" our way out of, these types of events can confuse us to the point where we feel as if we've been transported back to the original trauma, or that we'll re-experience a similar trauma.

Today, we are lucky to have therapeutic interventions for trauma such as EMDR (www.emdr.com) and Somatic Experiencing (www.traumahealing.com), both of which are different from traditional talk therapy because they incorporate "body memories" of the event. These therapies incorporate the mind-body connection to help people process and heal from traumatic memories.

Aside from fearing for her life, breast cancer can also be traumatic for a woman who loses part or all of one or both breasts, as her sense of womanhood can be deeply affected. As a society we place huge value on breasts as a symbol of femininity and sexuality. Permanent changes in a breast or the loss of breasts, in addition to adjusting to reconstructed breasts can threaten a woman's ability to feel feminine and sexual. In turn, this can affect self-esteem and intimate relationships.

Moreover, the psychological effects of breast cancer often extend into other aspects of a woman's relationships. Husbands or partners, parents, other family members, and friends experience their own fears and feelings of helplessness and stress.

The effects on children of mothers with breast cancer are especially complex, and vary depending on the age of the child. Young children rely on parents and others close to them for a sense of safety and meaning as they navigate the world. Living with a mother undergoing breast cancer treatment can be a profoundly confusing experience for young kids. Not only are they keenly aware of the shift in family dynamics that results when a parent is under a great deal of stress or unable to follow through with normal parenting activities, they often believe that stressful changes in the family are their fault. Older children who understand what cancer is often struggle with fear and worry, as well as changes in routine. It's helpful for kids in this situation if parents explain to them what is happening (age-appropriate tips are in the links below), assure them that they didn't cause it to happen, encourage them to express their feelings, and use a support system to help them maintain a sense of "normal life" and stability.

http://www.cancer.org/treatment/childrenandcancer/helpingchildrenwhenafamilymemberhascancer/dealingwithdiagnosis/dealing-with-diagnosis-how-to-tell-children

http://www2.mdanderson.org/cancerwise/2013/04/when-a-parent-has-cancer-helping-teens-and-kids-cope.html

Psychological effects that extend to friends include shock, fear for their friend's life, and fear that they might find themselves in a similar predicament. It's common for friends to feel helpless. People wonder what to say and what not to say. They wonder when to reach out, when to give space, and how to help in practical ways. There are many resources online that offer suggestions for friends of breast cancer patients. I've included one below.

http://www.cancer.org/cancer/news/when-your-friend-has-breast-cancer

After talking about all of the challenging aspects of breast cancer trauma, I want to come back to the idea that healing from it can be transformational. Many women talk about cancer helping them understand what they want to prioritize, and they go on to live more meaningful lives as a result. That's certainly what happened to me.

My Story

The day I was diagnosed with breast cancer, my husband was in Manhattan for work. Nobody, including two doctors, were worried about the lumps in my left breast. One said I probably had fibrocystic breasts, and another said I was "young for breast cancer." So there I was, alone with a radiologist doing an ultrasound and declaring (after I begged her to give me her honest opinion) she was "99 percent certain" I had breast cancer. That was my initial moment of trauma; I thought I was going to die and leave my two toddlers without a mother.

Like other animals, when we experience a real or perceived life-threatening event, we go into "fight, flight or freeze" mode. It's an instinct that dates back to the beginning of time and helped us survive in the days when our biggest fear was being attacked by a wild animal. Fight, flight or freeze is an automatic response that fills us with adrenaline to react to real or perceived danger. There I was on the ultrasound table, pulsing with that adrenaline as I shook uncontrollably. My heart beat fast and my breathing became shallow.

What happened next was a crucial turning point. The radiologist took one look at me panicking on the table and said, "You're going to be okay."

At that moment, I developed a deep understanding about hope. There were a few doctors and nurses who said something similar to me along the way. Of course, they didn't know if I would be okay. But, prior to being diagnosed I knew very little about breast cancer; I certainly didn't know that so many women survive an early-stage diagnosis. As soon as the radiologist opened my mind to the *possibility* that I could survive, I was able to refocus and set my sights on getting through treatment.

Propelled by an instinct to survive and armed with hope, I hit the ground running. I began 14 months of intensive treatment, including chemotherapy, a double mastectomy, radiation, 52 weekly infusions of a drug targeting my aggressive type of cancer, and reconstructive surgery.

Now that treatment is over, I look back on the experience and feel astounded by the positive attitude I maintained throughout a very difficult time. I was full of adrenaline and a desire to fight. For me, fighting cancer meant many things. It meant holding my head high when I lost my hair and started wearing head scarves. It meant driving my son to and from school every day, even when I was exhausted and my mother could have done it for me. It meant taking the time to prepare fresh food, even when the last thing I wanted to do was chop vegetables. It meant developing a positive relationship with the tedious and often painful processes of treatment and surgery. I learned to breathe a certain way when the nurse put the needle in my port, and to imagine the toxic liquid flowing through my veins zapping rogue cancer cells in my body. Fighting cancer meant surrendering on the days I was so sick and drained that I couldn't get out of bed, knowing that as soon as I felt better I would hit the ground running again.

I think there was an aspect, too, of feeling strong and wanting to portray that. One of the worst feelings for me was pity. I hated it when people felt sorry for me, and I think part of my enthusiasm throughout the process was an attempt to curb that – to prove to everyone that even though I was skinny and bald and losing my breasts, I was okay.

The truth is, I *was* okay. I was incredibly happy to be alive. I had a tremendous support system of family, friends, acquaintances, and even strangers who checked in with me often. I realized how helpless they felt and that allowing them to help me, even in small ways, was important. It isn't easy to ask others for assistance, but once I did I discovered its value, both for me and for the helpers. In a crisis, everyone wants to feel as if they are doing something about it. Asking a friend to bring me a meal was a relief for both of us – I didn't have to cook and my friend felt helpful and grateful to relieve some of my stress.

My kids were also a driving force in my determination to maintain a good attitude. Even though they were just one and three years old, I knew that they relied on me for a sense of self, safety, and well-being, and I fought to be strong for them. I did everything I could to keep things as normal as possible. In the end that was a tremendous motivating factor for me. Maintaining the routines of toddlerhood kept me occupied, active, and focused, much like continuing to work does for many women going through treatment.

My husband and I learned the meaning of the vows we took on our wedding day to remain a team through sickness and health. He is an upbeat, friendly, and funny man who is also incredibly loving, supportive, and loyal. I look back at photos we took while waiting for doctors or surgeries and observe that we were always laughing. We laughed about the decor in a surgeon's office that reminded us of a spaceship. We laughed about the puffy suit I wore in the hospital to stay warm before surgery. We often joked with doctors and nurses. Of course we took the situation seriously, too, and had moments of fear and tears, but we also maintained the sense of humor that forms a foundation of our relationship.

However, cancer did push our partnership into stressful territory. Before it came into our lives, my husband and I focused on many things together: our kids, my work, his work, social issues, our friends and families. One recent evening, we watched an episode of 'Parenthood', a TV show in which one of the characters deals with breast cancer. When her treatment was over, that character's husband remarked about how relieved he was that didn't have to "share" her with cancer anymore. My husband said that he could truly relate to that sentiment; I was so wrapped up in appointments, research, hope, and fear that cancer was always the first thing we focused on, and it dominated most of our conversations.

Although I felt well during chemo, I was certainly more easily fatigued and had predictable bad days after each round. Whenever I was lagging behind, my husband picked up the slack; during these periods it was exhausting for him to take care of everything with the kids and the house because we normally shared these responsibilities.

One of the most interesting aspects of my cancer experience, which I've learned is not uncommon, is that the hardest part came when treatment ended. When treatment began to slow down after chemotherapy, surgery, and radiation, I began to feel anxious and depressed.

I was still full of adrenaline, but I didn't know where to aim it anymore. It wasn't the type of energy I'd felt before – it was *fighting-cancer* energy, and it was much too big for the "normal" life I was supposed to go back to. Cancer had dominated my life for over a year, dictating my schedule and monopolizing my conversations with other people. You would think I'd be ecstatic for it to be over, but like so many things in life, cancer had become familiar. I'd grown accustomed to the appointments, doctors, nurses, and treatment rituals. I felt comforted knowing that I was being proactive and closely monitored. When treatment was over I felt like I was leaving the mother ship, floating away in a little dinghy, wondering if I would be okay.

I felt a sort of identity crisis. I could no longer identify with the woman I was before cancer. I didn't think the same way. I didn't eat, drink, love, or pray the same way. I didn't even look like her; I was boney and bald with fake plastic boobs. I still wanted to talk about cancer all the time, but I knew that I had to start focusing on other things again. And at the center of it all was that fear – the feeling that I was in the dinghy leaving the ship, wondering if I was going to make it on my own.

Today, I am well into reconciling all of that. The most profound lesson I have learned is to embrace my fear. I learned about a Buddhist nun and teacher, Pema Chodron, through a couple of girlfriends who devoured her books. I began to read her teachings, listen to her archived talks, and practice mindfulness meditation. Pema teaches that running away from fear only fuels it. As a therapist I learned and taught many ways to "cope" with fear, but I'd never faced it head-on. It's a tricky thing to embrace fear, because you're at risk of drowning in it. What I've learned is to stay with the *feeling* and let go of the *story.* When I'm triggered and start to worry about my cancer recurring, I notice how I'm feeling, let go of the story, and sit with it for a little while. Meditation is a powerful tool, because it teaches you how to let go of the words in your head. I have learned that when I am afraid and I say, *I feel you and I know you're there, but I'm not listening to your story,* it loses its power, and I'm free to turn my attention where I want it to be.

Today, my attention is on living a mindful life in which I am open and receptive to whatever is happening. Brene Brown, who writes and lectures on the value of being vulnerable, talks about how until we open ourselves up to the dark spaces in our lives, we are never fully able to access the light. In remaining open to all of the dark parts of cancer, I have experienced intense light. Having gone through periods of not being able to get out of bed because of chemo or surgery, I relish in feeling well and being able to exercise. I live with gratitude and focus on creating a healthy and vibrant life, being kind to myself and others, and laughing often. Cancer scared me to the point where I finally learned what is actually important in my life, and I feel extraordinarily alive.

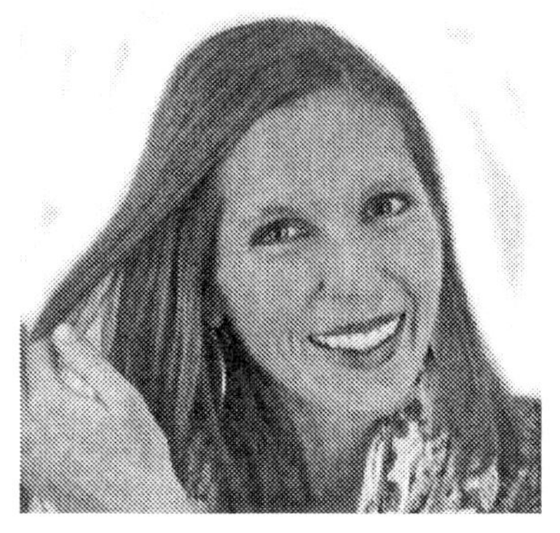

Mary Darling Montero, Ph.D.

worked as a photojournalist in Boston before moving to Miami and earning a Master's Degree in Social Work. She then moved to Los Angeles, where she earned the title of Licensed Clinical Social Worker, applying her knowledge and skills in various settings as a therapist, including a private practice where she focused on resolving trauma. Several of her articles and essays have been published online, in well-known websites like The Huffington Post. Mary is currently back in Miami, focusing on her two young children, working on writing projects, and living life to the fullest after cancer.

Chapter 23

Breast Cancer and Its Treatment: Effects on Sex and Sexuality

Cristina Pozo-Kaderman, Ph.D.

Introduction

Sex and sexuality are vitally important aspects of being a woman but both are dynamic and change, evolve and are redefined throughout a woman's life and throughout and after her treatment for breast cancer. For a woman with breast cancer, the initial focus of the healthcare team is appropriately on issues related to diagnosis, treatment and management of side effects. The woman herself may be besieged by anxiety and concerns about her survival, her family and many other issues. Sex and sexuality will almost inevitably be affected by breast cancer and its treatments (Table 1) but are frequently not discussed early on. Survivors and women undergoing active treatment are encouraged to seek information and express concerns about their sexuality regardless of age, changes brought upon by treatment or their prognosis. Women are treated, not just their cancers, and attention should be given to the whole person.

Sex and women's sexuality are complex and this chapter is not intended to be a comprehensive or exhaustive resource. Rather the aim is to provide information and suggestions based upon concerns often expressed by women with breast cancer.

Table 1. Factors Influencing Sexual Functioning	
• Cancer Treatment — Surgery — Chemotherapy — Radiation Therapy • Other medications • Fatigue • Stress	• Pain • Changes in body image • Relationship factors • Psychological factors — Anxiety — Depression

The following will provide a starting point to understand how treatment may affect the sexual aspect of a woman's life (Table 2) and recommendations that may be helpful in adapting to or ameliorating some of these changes.

Table 2. Factors Affecting Sex and Sexuality During Diagnosis, Treatment and Survivorship	
Event	**Effect**
Pre-diagnosis/Diagnosis	Anxiety*, depression
Surgery	Self-image • Loss or disfigurement of breast • Scarring

	Diminished sensation in breast Numbness in breast Pain
Radiation Therapy	Changes in skin color Changes in skin texture
Systemic Therapy	Fatigue Alopecia Weight gain Nausea Menopausal changes • Vaginal dryness • Mood changes • Sleep difficulties • Hot flashes
Post-Treatment	Uncertainty Body image Menopausal changes Fatigue Weight gain
*Emotional reactions such as anxiety, may exist to varying degrees throughout and beyond treatment but will generally resolve.	

Defining Terms

Sex and sexuality are distinct but closely inter-related. *Sexuality* is a *perception of self* – an identification of one's self as a sexual being and as a woman. It may be expressed in the way a woman talks, dresses, moves and who or what she considers sexually attractive or arousing. *Sex* is an *act* that may have many functions: Reproduction, reinforcing relationship bonds and many other outcomes including simply pleasure. Sex may involve a partner or not and can be expressed by touching, kissing, oral sex, intercourse, masturbation and other activities. Women usually experience phases of the sexual response cycle which is comprised of desire (libido), arousal, orgasm and resolution.

Desire is comprised of sexual thoughts and images. In the general population 1 out of 3 women report low sexual desire and 40% of women who go through natural menopause report decreased libido. Desire is partly mediated by the hormone testosterone. Women produce testosterone in the ovaries and adrenal glands. During menopause there is a reduction in the production of testosterone which may in part impact desire. Arousal or excitement results from sexual thoughts, fantasies and physical touching and stroking. During excitement a woman's heart rate, blood pressure and breathing may increase and there is increased blood flow to the genital areas. The vagina becomes moist, flexible and open, and the body may feel very warm. Arousal is effected in part by psychological, physical, relationship and hormonal variables. For example, hormonal changes during menopause may result in decreased estrogen levels which may cause vaginal dryness and atrophy. This can cause painful sexual intercourse. With enough arousal some, but not all women may reach orgasm during a sexual encounter. Most women need some experience in learning to have an orgasm. Orgasm results in intense pleasure in the genitals as the muscles contract and the nervous system sends waves of pleasure throughout the body. During resolution the body relaxes and gradually your heart and breathing rate decrease. Importantly, it is not necessary for all women to go through all phases to enjoy sexual intimacy.

Sex and Sexuality during Diagnosis Treatment and Survivorship

Pre-Diagnosis and Diagnosis

When a breast abnormality is identified during a self-exam or mammogram, anxiety is expected and normal. Upon diagnosis of breast cancer women often report being emotionally "overwhelmed." Despite this internal turmoil, a woman will need to process a significant amount of often confusing and threatening information and incorporate medical appointments to their already busy lives. Anxiety and fatigue are not uncommon as a woman attempts to balance new stressors with demands from relationships, work and oftentimes children. During this period of time, sex, sexuality and numerous other basic aspects of daily life will likely be disrupted but are not necessarily the focus. Survival is the focus. For those women in relationships, it will also impact their partners.

Local-Regional Treatments

Surgery – whether lumpectomy (partial removal of breast) or mastectomy (complete removal of one or both breasts) – is the primary treatment of early-stage breast cancer. A woman's breasts may have been central to her sense of sexuality/attractiveness and for many women a source of pleasure during sex. A woman may experience post-operative pain/discomfort, scarring and changes in her body image. After complete removal of one or more breast(s) a woman may have loss of sensation or numbness on the chest wall at the mastectomy site. While reconstructive surgery may rebuild the shape and size of the breast, the pleasure from caressing the breast and nipple is likely to be changed, diminished or absent. Over time, women may experience a return of sensation in the reconstructed breast but will not likely be the same as before surgery.

For women undergoing lumpectomy, temporary pain, discomfort or numbness typically resolves over time and typically no long-term effects on sensation are evident. For women undergoing lumpectomy, radiation therapy may also be included as a part of local treatment. As a consequence there may be breast tenderness or pain during treatment which diminishes over time. Some women report a change or decrease in sensitivity. Additionally, there may also be changes in the color and/or texture of the skin and hardening of surgical scars in the irradiated area. While women who preserve their breast may have better body image, they do not have better or more sex. Now and throughout treatment, communication with partners will be important and can serve to further reinforce the relationship.

Systemic Therapy

Systemic therapy basically refers to drugs taken orally or received via an infusion at the oncologist's office or cancer center and compromise different types of medicine (Table 3).

Table 3. Types of Systemic Therapy for the Treatment of Cancers

Type of Therapy	**Function**	**Brand (generic) Examples**
Chemotherapy	Kills tumor cells	Adriamycin (doxorubicin), Cytoxan (cyclophosphamide), Taxol (paclitaxel), Taxotere (docetaxel)
Hormonal therapy	Blocks estrogen receptors on tumor cells or decreases	Nolvadex (tamoxifen), Arimidex (anastrozole), Femara (letrozole), Aromasin (exemestane), Faslodex

	estrogen levels	(fulvestrant)
Biologics	Interferes with biologic processes of cells	Ibrance (palbociclib)
Targeted therapy	Affects specific targets believed to drive cancers	Herceptin (trastuzumab), Perjeta (pertuzumab), Kadcyla (T-DM1)

Table 5. Activities to Reduce Fatigue

- Use a diary to track energy levels
- Prioritize demands
- Enlist others to help with daily tasks
- Pacing yourself in daily activities
- Exercise
- Relaxation
  — Meditation/imagery
- Music

While fatigue is one of the most frequently reported side effects of treatment, perhaps the most direct and significant effect of systemic therapy on sexual functioning is due to changes in the hormonal milieu resulting in menopause or a menopause-like state. At menopause, women experience a decline in estrogen which is a natural change for all women and is gradual occurring over several years the average age being 52. Menopause may be associated with a number of changes (Table 6) including weight gain, hot flashes, night sweats, moodiness and vaginal dryness which can impact sexual functioning. Women will also experience a decline in the "male hormone" testosterone which may be associated with a reduction in libido.

Table 6. Menopausal Symptoms

- Vaginal dryness and decreased elasticity
- Hot flashes
- Sleep difficulties
- Fatigue
- Changes in mood
- Weight gain
- Decreased libido (sexual desire)

In younger women with hormonally sensitive breast cancer medical or surgical treatments that suppress or remove the ovaries will result in an abrupt shift to menopause which may be more difficult than naturally-occurring menopause. Additionally, treatment with certain chemotherapeutic agents particularly alkylating agents like cyclophosphamide may also result in premature menopause. This risk varies based upon the age of the woman at treatment, wherein the risk of premature menopause is 25-40% in women under 40 years old and 76-90% in those over 40. Postmenopausal women receiving hormone replacement (HRT) will be asked to discontinue HRT once diagnosed if their breast cancers are "hormonally driven." Often this will result in a return of some menopausal symptoms. Postmenopausal women are also often treated with aromatase inhibitors (i.e., Arimidex, Femara, and Aromasin) which will further decrease circulating estrogen levels.

Among the changes associated with menopause, by far the most important predictor of sexual dissatisfaction is vaginal dryness which may result in pain and even bleeding during intercourse. Several over-the-counter, non-hormonal vaginal moisturizers and lubricants are readily available and if used properly, have been highly successful in countering this particular side effect (Table 7). The first step in combating vaginal dryness is to use a vaginal moisturizer regularly every other night prior to bedtime so the moisturizer can be absorbed while you sleep. The moisturizer is to be used regardless of sexual activity. Even if a woman is not currently in a sexual relationship, vaginal health is important and by using a vaginal moisturizer the vagina stays moist and flexible. There are several moisturizers available and the most common and easily available is polycarbophil or Replens. Some women report that Replens, if used regularly can be as effective as estrogen cream. When sexually active, before penetration a woman needs to use a vaginal lubricant. Common lubricants are Astroglide and K-Y Jelly. It is best for the lubricants to be water-based and to avoid those with perfumes, flavors or parabens which can cause irritation. The lubricant needs to be applied not just inside the vagina but also on the vulva. Women may use the application of lubricant as part of foreplay and include their partner. If vaginal penetration continues more than a few minutes, lubricant may need to be reapplied. Vaginal suppositories which will melt inside the vagina are also good options for some women and can be applied prior to sexual activity. Petroleum jelly, skin lotions and oil-based lubricants are not good choices compared to vaginal lubricants as they can raise the risk for yeast infections.

Finally it is worthwhile noting that in addition to systemic treatments for breast cancer, a number of other commonly taken medications may also contribute to or exacerbate sexual problems. For example, allergy medications may help dry up nasal membranes but also exacerbate vaginal dryness. Women should check with their physician to determine if any medications they are presently taking have sexual side effects.

Table 7. Interventions for Vaginal Dryness

Nonhormonal and Over-the-Counter

- **Vaginal Moisturizer**
  - — Use every other night
  - — Use prior to bedtime
  - — Use regardless of sexual activity or relationship status
  - — Commonly used products include Replens (polycarbophil), Luvena, hyaluronic acid

- **Vaginal Lubricant**
  - — Use prior to penetration and during sexual activity
    - o Apply inside the vagina as well as on the vulva
  - — Avoid perfumes, flavors and parabens which may cause irritation
  - — Commonly used products include: Astroglide, K-Y Jelly or vaginal suppositories

---

Enhancing Your Sexual Life During and After Breast Cancer Treatment

---

Table 8. Tips to Enhance Your Sexual Life During and After Breast Cancer Treatment

- Be patient with yourself and your partner

- Communicate with your partner
  - — Share what you have learned about how cancer may affect your sex life
  - — Share your feelings and listen to your partner's fears and concerns
  - — Discuss your preferences and ask about his/hers

- Emphasize intimacy and pleasure over performance
  - — Bathing together

  - Sensual touching or massage
  - Erotic literature or movies
  - Extra time for foreplay

- Keep an open mind to alternative ways to experience pleasure
  - Sexual positions
  - Oral and manual stimulation
  - Adult toys

- Exercise
- Kegel exercises

Conclusions

The diagnosis, treatment and survival of breast cancer present numerous physical, psychological and social challenges to a woman. While the primary concerns of survival and quality-of-life are often center stage, it will be important for many women to maintain or reclaim their sense of sexuality and to continue a satisfying sexual life throughout treatment and beyond. Many sexual side effects are completely reversible after completion of treatment and others may be effectively addressed through relatively straightforward activities of the individual woman, her partner and her healthcare team.

Helpful Resources

1. Sexuality for the Woman with Cancer

http://www.cancer.org/treatment/treatmentsandsideeffects/physicalsideeffects/sexualsideeffectsinwomen/sexualityforthewoman/sexuality-for-the-woman-with-cancer-toc

2. Look Good...Feel Better

1-800-395-LOOK, or visit www.lookgoodfeelbetter.org

3. International Society for the Study of Women's Sexual Health (ISSWSH)

http://www.isswsh.org/

4. American Association of Sexuality Educators, Counselors and Therapists (AASECT)

http://aasect.org/

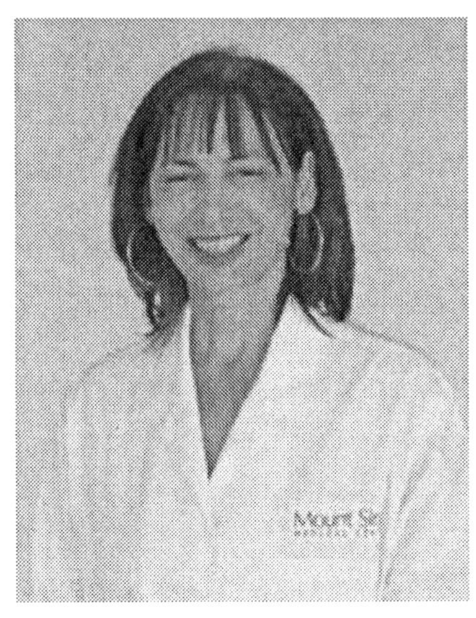

Cristina Pozo-Kaderman, Ph.D.

received her Ph.D. in clinical psychology at the University of Miami. She completed her internship at Cornell Medical College at New York Hospital and followed with a fellowship in Psycho-Oncology at Memorial Sloan Kettering Cancer Center Psychiatry Department. She started and was the Director of the Psychosocial Oncology Program at the Mount Sinai Cancer Center for 18 years and was also the Administrative Director of Psychosocial Oncology Courtelis Center, Assistant Professor in Psychiatry, at the University of Miami for 2 years. She has been actively involved in training doctoral students in psychosocial oncology. She has published articles in peer reviewed journals primarily in the area of breast cancer. She is a certified sex therapist. She now works part-time at the Mount Sinai Comprehensive Cancer Center and is adjunct faculty at the University of Miami, Department of Psychology.

Chapter 24

Peace of Mind Planning – The Legal Side of Things

Jonathan David, Esquire

Why the need for planning? (a/k/a "If you don't tell them, they won't know.)

[1] You knew you were going to see it, and so here it is... the legal disclaimer! Despite the great info and guidance in this chapter, the author strongly recommends that you seek the counsel of a competent attorney specializing in estate planning to draft legal documents referred to in this chapter, and to understand your needs. For some convincing in this regard, see the sections entitled "Cautionary Tales" [or "War Stories" – haven't decided – JD].

Your planning for a future eventuality is all about *speaking now*, in anticipation of a time in the future when you may not be able to speak for yourself. Without wanting to sound too much like the author of a sci-fi novel, think of your planning documents as letters to the people of the future, to be read at a time when necessary.

With whom in this future time are you communicating? Anyone! Doctors, judges, family, friends... And what are you saying to them? Anything! (just about).

Telling people around you what you want them to do (or know) includes:

- Advising doctors what to do/not to do to you while you're undergoing treatment;
- Appointing a trusted person to manage your affairs in case you can't;
- Telling a judge whom you want to be in charge of your *estate*[9];
- Advising your family/estate executor whether you want to donate organs, the kind of funeral or memorial service you'd like to have (including disposition of your remains);
- Telling the judge whom you want to take care of your minor children (if the co-parent is not fulfilling that role) and whom you want to have your possessions;
- Passing the baton on obligations, maintenance of your home and/or business, and other projects, for as-smooth-as-possible continuation: What do your successors need to know? Have you planned for

[9] Defined later in this chapter.

continuing payment of your home mortgage? Do you run a business?

Summary:

There might be a lot more to take care of than you realize (a lot more of a mess than you think, that needs to be cleaned up after you). Creating adequate planning documents will minimize problems and uncertainty for those managing your affairs when you are unable to do so. Whether the intended objects of your planning documents are family members, friends, business associates, doctors, or a probate judge, making a clear record of what you want to be done will save a lot of wondering, guessing, bickering and problems.

Further along in this chapter, I'll explain what the *probate* process is, and define the words "probate", "guardianship," etc., but first, let me list and describe some common planning documents:

Planning Documents:

It's helpful to be acquainted with the basic planning vehicles. Here are the most used documents, with a brief explanation of each:

Power of Attorney: This is a document in which you (the "principal," in legal nomenclature) designate a person who can act for you – in your place – to do various things, while you are alive. The person to whom you designate the authority to act for you is known as your "attorney-in-fact". This person doesn't have to be a lawyer. The word "attorney" in this phrase simply means someone authorized to speak and act on your behalf.

Common examples of possible uses for a power of attorney might be:

- My mother signs a power of attorney giving me the power to withdraw money from her bank account. In the event that she becomes incapacitated and her home bills need to get paid, I can do that for her;
- I know that I will be traveling out of the country on the day of closing on the sale of a house I own, so I sign a

power of attorney specifically giving a friend of mine the authority to sell my house – to sign any deed, bill of sale, closing/settlement statement, etc., and deposit the money into my account.

So, if there are things you think might need to get done (without court intervention), and you know of a trusted relative or friend who might be able to take care of those things, a power of attorney is a vehicle that can accomplish that.

A *durable* power of attorney refers to a power of attorney that specifically has a clause declaring that it should stay in force even if the person who signed it becomes incapacitated – something like this: "[THE EFFECTIVENESS OF] THIS DURABLE POWER OF ATTORNEY IS NOT AFFECTED BY THE SUBSEQUENT INCAPACITY OF THE PRINCIPAL, EXCEPT AS PROVIDED BY APPLICABLE LAW." This clause ensures that whoever is relying on the Power of Attorney knows that it remains effective even if the person who gave it is undergoing treatment in the hospital, unconscious, or unable to act for some other reason (other than death! See next section entitled "CAUTION").

CAUTION: A power of attorney loses its power upon the death of the person who gives it! For that reason, it can't be a substitute for a Law Will & Testament. It won't even allow the designated attorney-in-fact to withdraw money from a bank account after the death of the principal.

CAUTION #2: A power of attorney can be abused by the person to whom it is granted. Of course, it is illegal for the designated "attorney-in-fact" to use the power of attorney for his own benefit and/or to the detriment of the principal, but, sadly, it is not uncommon. Make sure that person you designate is trustworthy. Some people keep the power of attorney in a "safe" place at home, and tell the attorney-in-fact where it can be found in the event of the incapacity of the principal. As long as the attorney-in-fact has access to the principal's home when the time comes, this is a safe and effective approach.

Living Will:

"Living Will" is the common name for an Advanced Healthcare Directive. It's a document that instructs doctors and health care providers about what you do and don't want done to you in the event that you become incapacitated and cannot give the instructions directly. Common examples are: requesting (or requesting that the doctors withhold) life-support measures such as feeding tubes and breathing tubes.

The form of the document can vary. Sometimes a Power of Attorney includes the designation of a "health care surrogate" – a person chosen to make medical decisions on the spot. If you know where you are most likely to be treated (the nearest hospital, or your regular physician(s), for instance) it is best to have a form that particular hospital recognizes. The legal departments of some hospitals are picky about the exact language that they require (possibly based upon recent local law that has evolved), although any institution should honor a validly executed power of attorney.

Last Will and Testament:

This is a document, *executed with the formalities that your state's law prescribes* (the proper number of witnesses, etc.), to tell a judge what to do with your property, and whom you want in charge of managing the collection, maintenance and distribution of your assets. It can also contain some instructions or statements of desire concerning non-property matters, such as designating who should take care of your minor children in a situation where the co-parent is not able to do so. It is intended to be a document formally processed ("probated") by the court system. In the absence of a *last will & testament*, each state has laws dictating which family members get what portion of your assets (called "laws of intestacy"). Such a law might say, "spouse gets half and children share the other half," or "if a person dies having no spouse or children, then the estate is shared by decedent's siblings."

Why you need a will:

- **For certainty**: Whenever a person dies without a will, one preliminary step is *making sure that there **isn't*** a will. That is, if a probate judge asks, "Are you sure that this person did not have a will?" the only way to be 100% sure is to rifle through all personal effects – shaking books, looking under mattresses – that kind of thing – until you can say for sure that "after diligent search, no known will could be found." When there is a signed, sealed and delivered document with "Last Will & Testament" on its face, the court has a clear starting place to begin its proceedings;

- **To designate the person or persons you wish to manage your affairs** and act as your executor. Family members could fight over who should be in charge of your estate/probate affairs;

- **Because law changes** from time to time, and if you rely on what you *think* the law governing intestacy[10] is, it may not be the same at the time of your death. But it's best not to leave it to a law that could change with every sitting of your state's legislature.

- **Designation of a guardian for your minor child(ren)**: Making sure that the decision of who should raise your kid(s) is not left up to a court hearing where two sides of the family (the in-laws!) sling mud to convince a judge that they are the better surrogate parents than those unbearable people on the other side of the courtroom;[11]

---

[10] "Intestacy" is the legalese word meaning "having no last will".

[11] Caveat: If you are a parent of a minor child and live separately from the co-parent, you have to face the fact that the co-parent has parental rights that will probably trump whatever desires you express about who should raise your child and how.

- **To communicate any special desires:** for your pets, for your funeral, etc. In such cases, your statements of desire may not be practically legally enforceable, but you can let them be known. For example, you may communicate how you wish your funeral to be conducted, but by the time the matter gets to court, your funeral would probably have already been conducted. To the extent that pets are considered "possessions" ("chattel" in legalese), you can devise (or bequeath or convey) them in your will, but you can't necessarily make sure that the person who inherits them take care of them.

THE PROBATE PROCESS:

What is *probate* and how is it handled?

We've all watched the classic scene in a movie: the family gathers around in the family lawyer's office and listens as the lawyer reads the loved one's will aloud. In real life this happens very rarely. Usually when the time comes, the decedent's will is quietly filed with the court, and a proceeding (known as "probate") is begun. The word "probate" is from the Latin *probatum*, which means "a thing proved" (referring to the will itself, which is proved up in court). The steps include:

1. Presenting papers to the court;
2. Establishing who is entitled to notifications of court goings-on;
3. Appointment of the most appropriate person to act as executor (also sometimes called the "personal representative") to manage the estate case. This executor has to report to the court with an inventory of the decedent's assets, and will be in charge of collecting or paying debts, gathering ("marshaling") the assets of the decedent, selling property, etc.

4. Determining who gets paid what;
5. Actually distributing the assets to the appropriate people.

Even though it may be notarized and look about as official as a document can get, a beneficiary can't simply go to a 3rd party and present the will to receive his inheritance. Ask any bank officer if he or she has ever had a person (heir) come into the bank with a relative's last will & testament, present it to the bank officer and demand the money they are entitled to under the will. The bank has to turn the heir away, declaring, "We can't just acknowledge this will as dispositive (the final word). We need a court order directing us to give you the money."

Exceptions: Not everything needs a judge's involvement to transfer ownership

All of the above having been said, there are lots of assets that pass "outside the estate" – without the need for probate.

Some things are not considered estate assets: some assets pass directly, either by operation of law or by private contract, to other people, upon the happening of certain contingencies. Some examples are:

- bank accounts that specifically designate a "pay on death" beneficiary or accounts which are held jointly with another person with rights of survivorship;
- life insurance policies that name a specific beneficiary, who, by contract, is paid the benefit directly (not through the court);
- real property (house or land) owned by spouses (sometimes, whether the deed says to or not), or real property held with title (deed) designating a survivor owner;
- "homestead" (usually the primary home of a person) and other property with very specific local laws about who inherits it automatically, and may even prevent a person from disposing of it through a will.

If a life insurance policy names no one as the beneficiary (or designates only the person whose life is insured as the beneficiary), the matter must go through probate. Since the payee beneficiary (the very person whose life was insured) is now gone, how can the insurance company send them a check for the life insurance proceeds? In this case, the life insurance benefit goes into a special estate account, and is dealt with as part of the total assets of the decedent. The court either follows instructions in the last will and testament or local laws of intestacy to determine who should get that life insurance money.

What's all the hullabaloo about TRUSTS?

It's true that the probate process (going through all court procedures) can take a long time, even years in many cases. It can also be costly in terms of attorney's fees. For this reason, people try to devise ways to avoid the probate process and the court system altogether. One of those methods is a trust.

A trust is a device (usually a written agreement) through which one person holds property for the benefit of another person, with a set of instructions for what to do with that property. For example, the title to your house could be transferred (signed over, or "deeded") over to a *trustee*. Even though the trustee's name is now on the deed to your house, it is understood and agreed, in this scenario, that the trustee is only holding the property for you. The instructions to the trustee may be along the lines of: "If something happens to me, sell the house and distribute the proceeds equally between my nieces and nephews." Since the title-holder to the property (the trustee) is alive and empowered to sell the house, it can be done without delay that a court proceeding can occasion.

Wow. That sounds great. Why doesn't everyone do a trust?

Yes, a trust can prevent certain delays posed by the court process. But here's the reality: everything is a double-edged sword. For the flexibility one gains by not going through probate, one loses the court oversight and the transparency that a court proceeding gives. Also, there can be snags, if one is not careful. If the trust agreement (the document itself) is lost, then the family could end up with a situation where a trustee is holding property but doesn't know what he is supposed to do with it. And the trust has to be *funded* – that is, the title to assets must be changed to name the trust/trustee as the new owner. Often enough, people pay an attorney to draft a trust, but then the person creating the trust forgets to transfer assets into it. And lastly, but not least: if your trustee turns out to be untrustworthy, you may end up in court after all, when it is too late to prevent some loss.

GUARDIANSHIP: The law's formalities for taking care of those who can't take care of themselves.

If you were to find yourself unable to manage your affairs and you didn't have a designated attorney-in-fact (through a power of attorney, described above), nor a health care surrogate to make decisions for you, you could find yourself in a position where the court must appoint a *guardian* to manage your personal (physical) affairs and finances. Your guardian acts kind of like a parent, making sure you have what you need, and in some ways stands in your shoes, since your guardian (with court approval) can transact business and make decisions that you would if you could.

The legal process for accomplishing the appointment of a guardian is, very generally stated, the filing of the appropriate papers with the court, and a hearing in court (after notifications to all interested persons) where it is determined whether or not the prospective *ward* (the person to be protected or cared for) needs a guardian. If it is determined that a guardian is needed, the court will try to choose the most appropriate person or professional caregiving company to fill that role. A guardianship may be very limited in scope, or the court may declare that a person is completely in need of care (lacks the capacity to act for herself in any degree), in the areas of personal physical care and/or management of financial matters. In those cases where a guardian is appointed, the court requires the guardian to file periodic reports to ensure that the ward is being taken care of, and that any powers given to the guardian (including financial management powers) are not being abused.

Some jurisdictions have a procedure established for declaring a "pre-need guardian." This is accomplished through a written document which clarifies your preference for a guardian to manage your affairs if you should become incapacitated (we used to say "incompetent" but that word is frowned upon now). It is a formal statement (observe any legal formalities required!) and is filed with the Clerk of Court in your county of residence. You can then have some peace of mind knowing that if you become incapacitated, someone you know and trust will take care of you.

MAKING AN INVENTORY:

In this section, I list some of the main things you may want to consider, just as a starting point for formal planning, and maybe for your attorney to use to help in drafting any documents. The idea is to evaluate what you own, and to ask yourself what you envision doing with it. Once you have completed this task of creating a list, it important to let someone trusted know about it! Your family and friends could overlook something if they are unaware of its existence.

Assets: All physical (personal property and real estate) and intangible (stocks, accounts, insurance) things you own.

Real estate: Making sure you don't lose it for failure to make the mortgage payments, and deciding what you want to do with it

Life insurance: Making sure it does not lapse; Designating the most appropriate beneficiary(ies).

Business Interests: Making a plan for operation in your absence or succession.

Jewelry

Intellectual Property?

What to do with each item:

Sell?

Give away while living (*inter vivos* transfer?

Devise? (that is, provide for in will?)

Donate organs?

Debts:

Passing on the responsibility for making mortgage payments (or having family member re-finance). It's a pity when a house goes into foreclosure because no one steps up to take care of that.

Taxes

Don't forfeit your home for failure to pay real estate taxes.

IRS? Information that would be needed for a final tax return.

Funeral/Burial Plans:

Preferred funeral home?
Preferred method of disposition?

Who's paying? When?

Notification: Who should be notified about your death (many times, the loved one's family doesn't know the names of old friends)?

Charity donations in lieu of flowers?

What information should be included in the obituary?

War stories from a practitioner:

In my years of practicing law, I've come across some doozies – stories I keep in my mental files and re-tell to make valid points. Here are a few of the general narratives to give you a sense of some potential pitfalls:

Lost Estate Documents

If no one around you can find your estate-planning documents, then they do no good! There are cases where the family finds a will in a hiding place at a time when it is too late – when the probate case is already long over and done with. There are also cases, as briefly alluded to above, where some property/asset is put into the name of a trust, but then later no one can find the Trust Agreement setting out what was to be done with the trust's property.

Some people assume that the attorney who drafts the estate documents will keep an original or copy of the papers – somehow committing to act as a depository -- but this is not necessarily the case. And anything can happen even to a lawyer's papers: destruction in a fire, files getting moldy in a storage facility, etc. Therefore, you will want to find a safe place for your documents, or make/keep multiple originals to share with trusted family members.

If you have a safe deposit box, that is a good place for your important documents, but don't forget to *tell someone* close to you that the safe deposit box exists, and at what bank branch. In one of my probate cases, long after it was determined that the last will could not be found, a piece of mail arrived from a bank – an invoice for annual renewal of a safe deposit box that the next of kin knew nothing about. A court order authorizing the opening of the safe deposit box in front of witnesses (to take an inventory of the contents) yielded the discovery that there was, in fact a will in the box. Luckily it was not too late in that case.

Do-it-yourself Last Will & Testament

One of my favorites is the occasional phone call from someone saying, "I've just written and signed a will. Can you look at it and tell me if it's OK?" Do I need to tell you that *after* signing is not the time to be getting an attorney's opinion about a document that has legal effect?! Although there is nothing necessarily invalid about a will that you have drafted on your own, there are enough lawyers around, and it is easy enough to avoid a lamentable outcome.

Minors Getting Their Hands on Big Money at a Young Age

In my practice, I have been involved in a guardianship cases in which the minor child receives a substantial sum, whether through life insurance from a parent, settlement of a personal injury lawsuit, or inheritance. In such cases, the court monitors and protects the minor's money, keeping it in a court-restricted account, and requiring annual reporting to the court that the money is still there, safe and sound. *But these guardianship cases terminate when the minor reaches age 18*, and the court, by law, has to turn the money over to the young minor-turned-adult, who can then do with it whatever he or she pleases.

In all too many of these instances, an 18 year-old comes into an amount of money he or she really doesn't know how to manage. The young adult often blows through the money frivolously in short order – on expensive cars (sometimes later wrecking them, without insurance in place), loans to friends, bad investments, or living an unsustainable lifestyle .

To prevent something like that from happening to, say, the life insurance benefit that may be paid to your minor beneficiary or beneficiaries, a *trust* is a useful tool. Instead of naming a minor beneficiary on your life insurance policy, you name **the trust** as the beneficiary. You can then have a trust agreement which instructs your trustee to make payments to your beneficiaries over time, with any schedule you can envision and establish, such as:

Trustee shall pay to Beneficiary:

- $3,000 per month while Beneficiary is in college
- $10,000 upon graduation from college
- $35,000 upon reaching age 23
- $50,000 upon Beneficiary reaching age28
- The balance of any remaining funds upon Beneficiary reaching a certain age

The trust could also have discretionary terms (things left up to the trustee) and could provide for payments to third parties for health and education of the beneficiary.

War Story: Trusting a Family Member to Distribute Funds

Sometimes a client will tell me that he or she intends to leave a life insurance policy to one child, and *that* child will share (divide and distribute) it amongst his or her siblings. This works fine if the child really *does* it (setting aside any possible tax consequences to the child who receives the funds). But how can you know if it will really be done? I have had cases where family members come to me claiming that the sibling who was supposed to share what he or she was given is not doing so. In such cases, it is an uphill battle to sue the recalcitrant sibling for refusal to share.

CONCLUSION: Gazing Into the Future

Wouldn't it be great if we all had a crystal ball? One that could accurately predict the future and tells us in specific terms exactly what's going to happen, what we need to worry about, and what will resolve itself?

Unfortunately, none of us has an all-knowing crystal ball; therefore, we must plan ahead. Regardless of the apparent urgency of the situation, creating a plan now is the way to ensure that as much of your affairs and wishes as possible become effectuated, and that the complications and uncertainty are minimized.

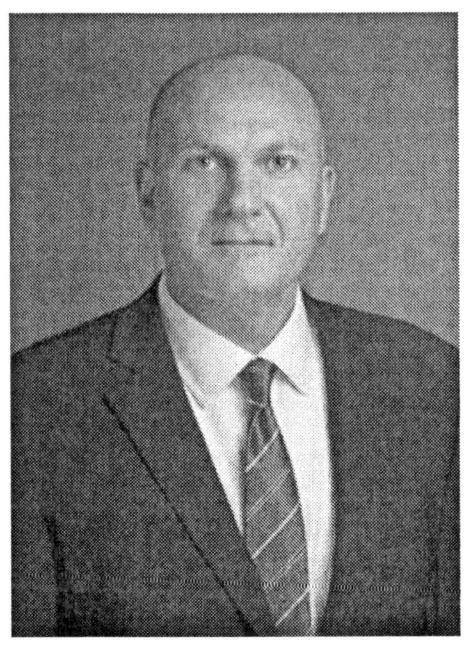

Jonathan Noble David

is a Miami-based attorney and mediator specializing in estate planning and inheritance matters. A native of Coral Gables and a graduate of Duke University (bachelors) and University of Miami School of Law, Mr. David has been practicing for over 20 years, and prides himself on being conscientious, practical, and possessing the ability to convey concepts to his clients without the using more legalese than necessary, and focusing on a more human approach to legal questions. He can be reached at jdavd@southmiamilegal.com. His law firm's web address is www.southmiamilegal.com

Chapter 25

Palliative Care – It's Never Too Early

Khin M. Zaw, M.D. and Mariana Khawand, M.D.

"Palliative Care."

Quite often – and incorrectly – these words are associated with "giving up" in the medical world. When they hear the words, "palliative care," people feel sadness. They become scared and uncomfortable, and in many cases, shut down emotionally, refusing to listening to any further on the subject.

But this is all a big misunderstanding!

The simplest definition and purpose of palliative care? Improving the quality of life for individuals with serious illnesses.

As palliative care physicians, we typically spend a great deal of time explaining its meaning to patients and colleagues, with an emphasis on how it can help anyone coping with a serious or chronic medical condition, regardless of prognosis and whether or not it's curable.

But before we discuss what palliative care is, it's important to note what palliative care is NOT:

- Palliative care is not just for dying patients;
- Palliative care is not the inevitable outcome when doctors have determined there's "no hope," or that they "have done everything they can;
- Palliative care is not the same as hospice care;
- Palliative care is not just about administering strong pain medications to sick patients;
- Palliative care is not physician-assisted suicide or euthanasia;
- Palliative care is not only for patients with incurable illnesses or for whom curative treatment has failed.

What is Palliative Care?

Palliative care is the name given for treatment of the discomfort, symptoms, and stress of serious illnesses like cancer, COPD, and heart failure. The palliative care approach takes more than just a patient's disease into consideration; it also addresses his or her spirituality, life goals, family dynamics, functionality, and even financial concerns.

This comprehensive approach to patient care allows palliative care teams to fully understand a person's core values and what is most important to them during their journey through life with a chronic illness. Palliative care teams often help patients and their families digest the influx of medical information coming at them from various specialties and devise a plan of care that is most appropriate for their individual values and goals.

Although palliative care is still a growing field, its role in cancer care has been well-established for many years now. Both cancer and its treatments often lead to undesirable symptoms including:

- Pain
- Fatigue
- Nausea
- Loss of appetite

- Insomnia

Of course, we could add many more to that list.

Sometimes the symptoms a patient experiences are so unpleasant and overwhelming that they interfere with and interrupt treatment plans. One common example is chemotherapy, when side effects like nausea and fatigue simply become too severe for the patient to continue. Palliative care teams help cancer patients cope with the side effects of treatment as well as the impact cancer and cancer treatment impose on their lives in general. Late on in this chapter, we will discuss the many benefits of early palliative care in diseases like cancer.

While many doctors across the varied specialties treat symptoms of serious illness, a palliative care specialist brings special training and expertise in pain management and symptom control for chronic illnesses to his practice. Furthermore, palliative care physicians work in an interdisciplinary team that includes palliative care nurses, psychologists, social workers, and chaplains. This team may also include nutritionists, pharmacists, physical therapists, recreational therapists, and other valuable members who can provide a holistic approach to patients with cancer and other serious illnesses.

Palliative care teams help patients not only with medical management of symptoms and side effects, but also with patient and family stress revolving around sickness, fears about the future, and guidance in choosing treatment options aligned with a patient's overall goals of care. One of a palliative care physician's many roles is to discuss treatment options and help patients navigate through their journey.

You may hear the phrase "quality of life" employed by many in the medical setting. The palliative care team is essentially a task force dedicated to maximizing this very aspect of taking care of YOU: the quality of *your* life as *you* define it.

How Does the Palliative Care Team Provide This Support?

Palliative care physicians most commonly see patients when

they are hospitalized. Generally, a palliative care "consultation" is requested by your primary doctor in the hospital. Often, the purpose of this consultation is to serve the purpose of managing difficult symptoms and/or discussing your "goals of care" to help guide you through tough medical decisions.

Unfortunately, palliative care teams are often consulted at the later stage of illness, or when symptoms are too difficult to control with standard management. This is a regrettable byproduct of the common misperception surrounding palliative care: that it is exclusively for the end of someone's life. But let us assure you, it is not.

Palliative care can help countless people with many years yet to live!

In the hospital setting, one of the most commons symptoms addressed by palliative care specialists is pain. Pain management using strong medications called "opioids" requires a specific set of skills for which palliative care specialists receive training. This training includes a thorough understanding of what kinds of pain will respond to what kinds of medication, along with their possible side effects and safe usage.

Palliative care physicians also address and work to alleviate nausea, vomiting, constipation, diarrhea, depression, anxiety, insomnia, fatigue, lack of concentration, problems with walking or performing daily activities, and the emotional and social stress that accompanies being diagnosed with a serious or chronic disease.

Aside from recommending medications for pain and other symptoms in the hospital, palliative care teams are also asked to help when patients and families face difficult decisions about how to proceed with treatment; they also assist in discussions about *advance directives* – the name given to your wishes in the event you're unable to express yourself at the time of medical decision-making. This is accomplished through a careful review of your medical records, consultations with the multiple specialists involved in your care, and most importantly, conversations with *you*.

The members of the palliative care team, including the

doctors, will spend a lot of time speaking with you in order to understand and determine what is most important to you. The types of questions posed by palliative care specialists are:

- What do you understand about your illness?
- How do you prefer to hear medical information – are you a "big picture" person, or do you prefer to know all the details?
- What brings you joy in life?
- How has your illness affected your ability to enjoy your life or do what you need to do?
- Who is closest to you? Who would make decisions on your behalf if you were unable?
- What is your faith or belief system?
- Do you consider yourself spiritual or religious?
- What things do you believe in that give meaning to your life?
- How important is your faith or belief system? What influence does it have on how you take care of yourself?
- How have your beliefs influenced your behavior during this illness? What role do they play in regaining your health?
- Are you a part of a spiritual or religious community? Is this of support to you? How? Is there an individual or a group of people you really love, or who are of utmost importance to you?
- As your healthcare provider, how would you like me to address these issues in your healthcare?

Through the process of spending time getting to know you, reviewing your medical history, and discussing your care with all of your specialists, palliative care doctors and team members can help you navigate through decision-making as it pertains to your medical care by discussing options and providing medical opinion. After palliative care consultation, patients tend to have a deeper sense of what's most dear to them over the course of their illness.

In some hospitals, palliative care teams are automatically notified of any patients entering the hospital who have a past or current diagnosis of cancer; advanced heart, lung, or liver disease; or other chronic illnesses. Consequently, someone from the palliative care team will meet with these patients. From there, they can help determine whether or not the patient will benefit from seeing a palliative care specialist outside of the hospital. The team can also help patients define their goals and prioritize them in the context of their illnesses. This "reflex palliative care consultation" is becoming more and more popular as this medical specialty continues to grow.

Thus far, we've only discussed palliative care in the hospital.

Though still an evolving and expanding part of the field, outpatient palliative care practices are beginning to emerge throughout the county, especially at large cancer centers.

Going to an outpatient palliative care practice means that aside from seeing your primary care doctor, oncologist, radiation oncologist, and any other specialists, you'll have additional support for your pain and symptom management. Although it may seem daunting to add yet another specialist to your list of doctors, most people enjoy their visits to palliative care practices, due to the focus on well-being and big-picture type considerations.

These office visits often consist of chronic pain management, discussion and management of other distressing symptoms, and conversations about advance care planning and care goals. During each visit, your palliative care practitioner will work closely with you to ensure you still have good quality of life while undergoing treatment for your cancer – or even for years afterward – in order to address the residual side effects or symptoms of cancer treatment.

Outpatient palliative care practices often network with supportive care services. These include outpatient psychologists, psychiatrists, integrative medicine specialists, and interventional pain specialists. Integrative medicine specialists are medical doctors who focus on lifestyle and nutrition. Thus, they can offer some alternative options for patients including acupuncture and herbal and plant-based medicine.

Interventional pain specialists treat pain with intricate

procedures including pain management pump placement, injections called "nerve blocks," and multiple other procedures to alleviate pain that is not well controlled by medications. Your palliative care specialist will involve these other specialties to give you a comprehensive approach to a good quality of life. Your palliative care physician will also keep in touch with your primary care physician as well as any other specialists involved in your care – from oncologists who provide medical treatment for cancer to surgeons, to radiation oncologists who specialize in the use of radiation for cancer treatment.

Besides focusing on quality of life through management of symptoms, palliative care specialists address who you are as a person – not just your medical history. Many initial visits last well over an hour, both in the hospital and in the office setting.

Why?

Palliative care physicians want to know who you are, what is important to you, and how you cope with adversity. Combined with medical knowledge, this information allows palliative care physicians to guide you through complicated medical decisions.

Finally, your outpatient palliative care team will assist you with "advance care planning." This involves discussion about your preferences in your medical care, should you become unable to communicate. This process works most efficiently when it includes the people closest to you, so they are fully aware of your wishes. Palliative care physicians and other providers can help you put these wishes into writing. As your health status changes, your palliative care doctor will revisit the topic and update your documents as necessary.

An Example of Palliative Care in Action

To paint a fuller picture of what it's like to receive help from a palliative care team, let us tell you the story of Jane – a fictional patient whom we'll use to illustrate what a palliative care team does.

Jane Smith is a 45 year-old woman with breast cancer who is currently at the Saint Elsewhere Cancer Center receiving an infusion of chemotherapy. While at chemotherapy, she experiences nausea and vomiting, then faints. She is then transferred to the hospital for rehydration and observation. During her hospitalization, Jane continues to have very severe nausea and vomiting. She reports to her doctors that she also has a lot of pain and tingling in both of her feet, and that the pain meds she takes at home no longer work for her.

The palliative care team is called upon for help with managing Jane's nausea and vomiting as well as her pain.

Dr. Kay, a palliative care physician, meets with Jane to discuss these undesirable symptoms and side effects. Through this conversation, Dr. Kay also discovers that Kay has been very unhappy lately because her foot pain has been preventing her from participating in her favorite activity – dancing. Jane also confides to Dr. Kay that she's worried about her children, who rely on her for help with homework. She also admits that since her cancer diagnosis, she's been struggling with insomnia, a poor appetite, and a general lack of motivation.

In response, Dr. Kay administers stronger medications for nausea, vomiting, and pain. While Jane is in the hospital, Dr. Kay and her team visit her every day. In three days, Jane improves and is ready to return home.

Before she leaves the hospital however, Dr. Kay and the palliative care team work together to ensure that Jane's concerning issues are being addressed. Together, Dr. Kay and Jane create a list of Jane's most important goals:

- She wants her pain under control so she can resume her dance classes
- She wants to be awake and alert enough to help her kids with their homework
- She wants to stop losing weight
- She wants to maintain her strength
- She wants to continue chemotherapy and live as long as possible so she can be around for her kids

- She wants to feel happier

Dr. Kay, with the help of the palliative care pharmacists, recommends a stronger set of medicines for Jane. The team also suggests a medication to help with concentration and energy on those days when she's feeling tired or requiring more of the pain medications that make her sleepy.

The social worker and nurse then meet with Jane to ensure she's able to get her new prescriptions and that her insurance will cover them.

The team nutritionist talks with Jane about foods that are more palatable to her, offering recommendations on which ones will help her maintain her weight and reduce nausea.

The psychologist speaks with Jane about her issues with moodiness and recommends an outpatient therapist who can continue to guide her through this very difficult period of her life. At this time, Jane is not interested in taking depression or anxiety medications.

On the first day they met, Dr. Kay asked Jane about her spirituality. Jane shared that she'd been raised Catholic and that previously, her faith had been source of comfort. However, now she's not so sure if her religion can help her. She'd agreed to meet with the team's chaplain, who helped her seek silent meditation and create a space to reconnect with her spirituality.

Finally, the team communicated with Jane's oncologist and primary doctor to apprise them of the plan moving forward, including her new medications. Dr. Kay advises Jane to follow up at her palliative care office on a monthly basis to monitor her pain management and other symptoms.

During her one-month follow-up, Jane reports she's feeling better and tolerating the chemotherapy much better, thanks to her new nausea medications. Although she still has pain in her feet, it is somewhat improved. While it's not possible for her to tolerate dance classes yet, she feels she's moving closer to that goal.

She continues to see Dr. Kay at the office to help her with her symptoms. At one point Dr. Kaye refers Jane to the integrative medicine doctor, who helps Jane with her sleeping habits and offers acupuncture for her anxiety.

Over the course of her visits, Jane talks with Dr. Kay about her wishes in the event she should become too sick to make medical decisions on her own. She designates her husband as her "surrogate decision maker" and completes advance directive paperwork – so that if does become sick in the future her family will have some guidance in how to proceed.

In the beginning, these conversations made Jane and her husband uncomfortable, but now they are grateful to have completed this step in planning their future. Doing so has given Jane a feeling of control over her cancer. Additionally, this will be extremely helpful in guiding Jane's husband and family should she ever become severely ill. Now they have a deeper understanding about her preferences, so that instead of feeling forced to make tough decisions without any guidance, they'll have a clearers sense of what to do.

Jane's cancer responds very well to chemotherapy and she continues to follow up with Dr. Kay to manage her foot pain.

Jane's story is just one simplified example of how a palliative care team can help a patient through many of the challenges of sickness, even in non-life-threatening situations. Thanks to Jane's time spent with Dr. Kay and her team in the hospital and at the office, she now has an improved quality of life and a deeper understanding of her health.

When Should I Ask About Palliative Care?

The truth is, it's never too early to involve a palliative care team once a patient has been diagnosed with a serious illness. The medical condition does *not* have to be incurable or life-limiting.
Palliative care services are often underutilized because many patients – and even doctors – unfortunately equate "palliative care" with "end-of-life care." We often overhear our well-meaning colleagues in the medical field stating, "there is nothing else we can do; let's just switch to palliative care."

We urge our colleagues and patients to see it in a different light. Palliative care should be provided ALONGSIDE all other care – not as an alternative or last resort. The medical team does not have to "switch" to palliative care; they can add palliative care to the total care of a patient to improve the patient's quality of life. So, if you are diagnosed with cancer or any other chronic or serious illness, and you have pain or other symptoms, palliative care can be of service. If you're faced with a difficult medical decision and need guidance, palliative can help. If you're having difficulty coping with the impact of a serious illness, palliative care is there for you.

Surely not everyone needs every aspect of palliative care, but everyone can benefit from reflecting upon what's important to them as a person, not just a patient. Conversations with palliative care teams are almost always guaranteed to help patients – whether by gaining a better understanding of their illness, reflecting more deeply upon the goals of care, or by alleviating distressing symptoms.

The most important thing to remember is that the core purpose of palliative care as a specialty is to improve quality of life in the setting of the illness. We do this through pain and symptom management, addressing you as a whole person, gaining a fuller understanding of your core values and goals, and guiding you in your journey through life with a serious illness. This holistic approach to patient care forms the very foundation of palliative care.

A Brief Overview of Hospice Care – Palliative Care at the End of Life

Oftentimes, palliative care is confused with hospice care – the name for palliative care given at the end of life. Hospice care always includes palliative care, but palliative care does not always include hospice care.

Hospice is a set of services and benefits offered to patients at the end of life. It can be delivered at home, at a nursing home or assisted living facility, or in an inpatient hospice unit in a hospital or other facility. In-hospital hospice care is usually reserved for patients who need specialized care such as intravenous (IV) medications, .or for patients who have symptoms difficult to manage at home.

Once enrolled in hospice, a hospice organization provides many services to maximize patients' quality of life. Home oxygen tanks, a hospital bed for the home, and other medical equipment are all provided by the hospice benefit. Patients receive daily visits from home attendants to help with bathing (if necessary) and other daily needs. A nurse comes to visit the patient at home at least once a week – sometimes more often – to check vital signs, arrange medications, and perform other medical tasks such as wound care. A hospice physician will come and visit once a month or more frequently as needed, to take care of prescriptions and examine the patient.

When patients become ill or have uncontrolled symptoms, the hospice nurse will notify the hospice organization and that the patient can be put on "continuous care." This means there will be health aides at the house 24 hours a day, a nurse will visit daily, and the doctors will visit up to once a day if needed. It's basically like having hospital-level care and supervision without the patient ever having to leave the comfort of home.

Home hospice allows patients to avoid admittance to the hospital and maximize comfort toward the end of life. Many people who enroll in hospice actually live longer than expected! There are many explanations for this, including the fact that being at home and experiencing such focused care prevents more setbacks and returns to the hospital.

If however, the patient requires IV medications, special procedures, or any service or intervention that cannot be delivered at home, he or she can go to an inpatient hospice unit. These units can be located inside a hospital or in a separate building. Inpatient hospice units are equipped with nurse and staff trained to care for hospice patients. A hospice/palliative care physician will see the patient daily while they are in the inpatient hospice unit receiving treatments.

When patients do reach the end of life, many prefer to pass

away at home, while others prefer to be under the care of doctors and nurses in a hospice unit. Hospice teams honor patients' wishes and provide support for patients and their families during these difficult times. Bereavement services, more commonly known as grief counseling services, are often included in the hospice benefit after a loved one has passed away.

In addition, hospice teams have social workers, psychologists, chaplains, and other trained specialists who help patients and families cope with the dying process. These team members are available both in the home hospice setting (including nursing homes and assisted living facilities) as well as in the inpatient hospice units.

The focus in hospice is patient comfort. Generally, at this stage of a patient's illness there are no attempts at curing the disease because no curative options exist; because the patient cannot tolerate the curative treatments; or because the patient and family decline curative treatments, due to their personal wishes and in order to maintain quality of life.

It's important to realize however, that hospice does not mean "do not treat." Routinely, patients under the hospice benefit are still given antibiotics for infections, blood transfusions for symptoms of low blood counts, and other treatments for other illnesses that arise. Patients on hospice continue their routine medications for their other medical conditions. For example, in the case of someone receiving the hospice benefit because of metastatic lung cancer, that person continues their routine diabetes, blood pressure, and cholesterol medications.

Another important misconception about hospice that must be addressed is the belief that hospice doctors "just give you medicine to help you die faster." This could not be further from the truth!

Hospice teams focus on comfort, and in the final days of life morphine is a great tool employed to treat pain and shortness of breath. The doses of morphine used are safe and effective for treating symptoms, but not high enough to cause death.

Any physician or palliative care team can discuss hospice and whether or not it is appropriate for you or someone you love.

The hospice approach to patients is 100% palliative care – patient-centered, comfort-oriented care that takes into consideration the physical, emotional, social, and spiritual aspects of a person's life.

While hospice care is only appropriate in specific situations, palliative care is appropriate for any age, for any diagnosis, at any stage of a serious illness. It's provided together with curative and life-prolonging treatments.

RESOURCES FOR HOSPICE AND PALLIATIVE CARE

Information on advance directives: www.caringinfo.org

National Hospice and Palliative Care Organization: www.nhpco.org

Palliative Care Provider Resource: www.getpalliativecare.org

National Institutes of Health Resources for Patients and Providers on Symptom Management and Other Issues in Palliative Care: www.nlm.nih.gov/medlineplus/palliativecare.html

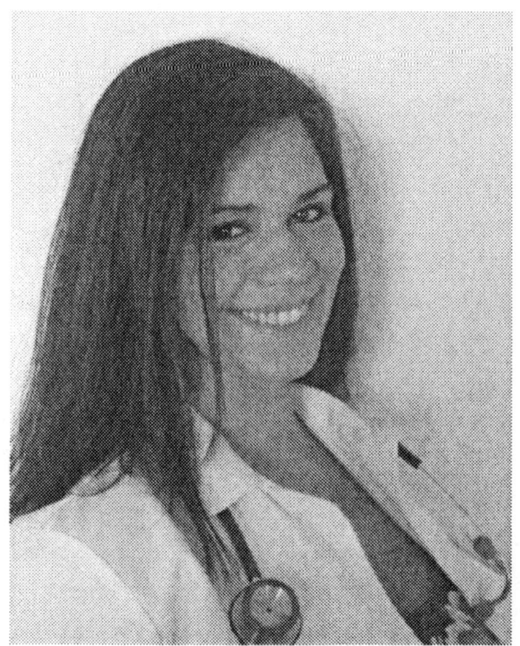

Mariana Khawand-Azoulai , M.D

was born in Beirut Lebanon. Shortly thereafter, her parents moved to Miami Florida, where she spent her entire youth. She minored in mathematics and earned a Bachelor's degree in Microbiology and Immunology, and a B.A. in Chemistry from the University of Miami. Dr. Khawand-Azoulai also holds a Master's in Physiology from Georgetown University, which she followed up with four years of medical school at the University of Florida in Gainesville. After completing her residency in Family Medicine at Columbia/New York Presbyterian Hospital, she's now training in a one-year fellowship in Hospice and Palliative Medicine at the University of Miami/Jackson Hospital healthcare system. She currently resides in Miami with her husband Yoni, an Emergency Medicine Physician at the University of Miami Hospital, and their two daughters.

Contact Dr. Mariana Khawand-Azoulai at Dr.Khawand@gmail.com.

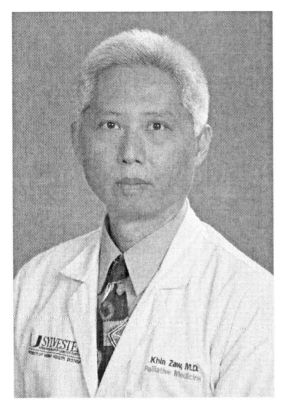

Khin Maung Zaw, M.D.

was born in Moulmein, Burma (Myanmar). He received his medical degree from Institute of Medicine (2), Rangoon, Burma and practiced general medicine in rural and urban settings before immigrating to the United States in 1992. He completed his internal medicine residency at St. Barnabas Hospital in Bronx, New York before starting a successful VA career including Fargo VA and Buffalo VA. He completed his VA Interprofessional Palliative Care Fellowship at Palo Alto VAMC in 2004 and the Geriatric Medicine Fellowship at Montefiore Medical Center, Bronx, New York in 2005. He is boarded in Internal Medicine, Geriatric Medicine, and Hospice and Palliative Medicine. During his career as palliative care physician at the Miami VA from 2005 to 2012, he founded a comprehensive palliative care program with a grant from the VA Central Office. As a full-time faculty member at the University of Miami, Dr. Zaw is responsible for the growth of the palliative care program, including the establishment of the outpatient palliative care clinic at Sylvester Comprehensive Cancer Center. He is the founding director of the Hospice and Palliative Medicine Fellowship program; ACGME accredited in 2014. He currently resides in Miami Florida with his family.

Contact Dr. Khin Maung Zaw at kzaw@med.miami.edu.

Chapter 26

Joy is the Choice

Patricia San Pedro

We're *supposed* to be happy. What a concept. Yet, it's what I believe....that we are placed on this earth to live a fulfilled, passionate, love-embraced, laughter-filled, healthy life. The reality however, isn't always that picture perfect utopia. Stuff happens. Sometimes it's divorce, other times it's financial, the passing of a loved one, betrayal, on and on and on. Then, sometimes....it's all about our health.

What happens when you hear the words "You have cancer"? I can tell you what happened to me: my whole world started to spin in slow motion. I heard nothing after that....at least for an hour. My brain replayed the life and passing of my young mom to the same disease 20 years prior. I felt a deep sadness but it was more about her than me. Very strange.

Funny how different personality traits pop up at a time like this. Sure I was scared and could easily have sunk into fear or depression. But I did not. I've always been a positive person and somehow that aspect of my personality surfaced quickly in me. I've always said that *joy is a choice.* The situation is what it is. We can't control that, but we CAN control how we respond to it and what we do with it.

You were diagnosed with cancer? Then celebrate being alive today and figure out what you need to do to heal. In the midst of it...grove to every song that plays on the radio, laugh to every comedy on TV, love every single special person in your life and live every delicious moment to the fullest. Right now as you read these words, you ARE alive and sucking oxygen. None of us know what tomorrow will bring. Be grateful for today.

What did cancer bring me? Amazing new friends. Renewed purpose and meaning. Greater wisdom, deeper compassion and more laughter. The blessings are too many to mention.

This book is one of those blessings. Paying it forward and helping others has given true importance to my life. I have no children of my own...so I've become a "mom" to strangers when they are diagnosed. This is why I'm thrilled to introduce this book to you. It is filled with stories and information written by experts, cancer survivors and thrivers, healers and a bunch of really smart and compassionate people that will guide you through and to healing.

I'm honored that co-authors Cindy and Sabrina asked me to write the first chapter. I met Cindy six years ago at the premier of a musical based on *Dish & Tell*, a book I wrote with a few girlfriends. We called ourselves the Miami Bombshells, not because we looked like bombshells, but because every time we gathered over wine and chocolate we dropped bombshells about our life. The book turned into a stage production called *Bombshell, The Musical* and that's where I met Cindy. I was in the midst of chemo and had less than an inch of hair on opening night but could not have been happier. Our Friends and Family Opening benefited a breast cancer organization that Cindy was involved with and that's where our paths first crossed.

Though if I'm to be totally honest, I don't remember her. There were hundreds of people there and the night was one glorious whirlwind. Plus I suffer from what I call Facial Dysplasia. Can't remember faces let alone names.

A few months later, I got a call from Cindy. She reintroduces herself to me and tells me that she is releasing her book *The Empty Cup Runneth Over*. She invited me to attend her book launch. I wanted to go but my life was nuts; finally, again I had PR clients and I was overworked, trying to make up for lost time and revenue and trying to pay off medical bills. There weren't enough hours in the day so I told her I would try. Little did I know then, what I know now. Cindy is OCD. Really. She proceeded to call me probably 20 times. Emailing me, leaving me messages on my cell, at my office, texting, through FB. Omg...ok. I will go!!!! Today I tell her she was a pain in my tushie. But I'm happy she was.

Otherwise we never would have connected. But some things never change; she still leaves me a thousand messages through every means of communication until I respond. But at least now I know what to expect.

Yes I went to her reading and the rest is history. I invited Cindy into my breast cancer support group and of course she immediately became an integral force in it. Since then her and I have grown closer and closer. As I write this, I am flying back home from a little getaway in North Carolina to be the Maid of Honor at her wedding. Cindy is sweet, kind and loving. She is giving and compassionate and would do anything for anyone. She has taught me to never judge a book by its persistent cover.

I'm going to share a little bit of my story with you now, with the hope that it will encourage and inspire you through your own dance with cancer. Some of these are excerpts from my book called *The Cancer Dancer: Healing One Step at a Time.*

My Story

On April 10th, 2008 I was diagnosed with breast cancer. As you would assume, the diagnosis shook my foundation and brought my very busy life to a screeching halt. I was sitting at "Books & Books" grabbing a bite with my friend Lydia when the phone rang. It was my breast doctor telling me I had cancer. Sadness took over every cell in my body. Yet there was something about this that did not surprise me. Maybe I had always known since my mom Daisy had passed away from breast cancer when she was only 59.

Driving back home with my friend, I looked up to the sky and it was a bright and sunny day. The world had no clue what I had just learned. Everything seemed normal. I didn't understand. I had always been an over-the-top positive person but how could I see this glass as half-full?

I arrived home knowing that five girlfriends were on their way to see me. We had called them on the way. My initial desire when I got home was to walk my dog Merlot. I guess I was trying to do something "normal". As I thought about my life, I began to view it from a 30,000 foot level, way above my every day perspective. What I "saw" was that every past experience, every trail and tribulation, every difficulty, was just a blip on the radar screen of my life now. So I could either let this moment swallow me whole and drag me into a dark abyss, or I could make a very conscious decision to focus as much as possible on the positive aspects of my breast cancer experience and avoid going into a self-pity destructive mode. What can I gain from this journey? Bigger breasts. That's the first comical thing that popped into my mind. Spending more time with friends and family? I was pretty sure that was about to happen. Learn more about myself and find deeper purpose for my life? Made sense. Help others through the lessons I would learn in the midst of healing? Possibly. Hopefully.

By the time my girlfriends arrived four hours later, I had talked myself into choosing joy in the midst of turmoil. I had no control over the "end result" but I did have power over how I would spend my days. I decided to turn my healing journey into a celebration of life.

We popped open two bottles of champagne. My instinct to be of service and my life in the media compelled me to pick up my camera and start videotaping. It felt right. My girlfriends and I didn't stop recording for an entire year: through my double mastectomy, 17 sessions of chemo (which I call Sacred Juice) and several reconstruction surgeries. We taped tips and advice to help, educate, encourage and empower others diagnosed with breast cancer. I recorded personal diary entries day and night hoping to take some fear of the unknown away for those facing treatments like mine. I had an overwhelming passion to be of service to others through my own dance with cancer. It actually gave me purpose and helped me heal.

It hasn't always been easy, but when I move past the difficult moments I am able to see that the blessings continue to pile up. My joy for living and my celebration of life escalates with each passing day.

My breast cancer gave birth to Positively Pat, a health and wellness community that touches people's lives every day. My book, *The Cancer Dancer* guides women and their caretakers through their journey, and the hundreds of video hours I shot during my own year of treatment became a documentary that I co-produced with Discovery, also called *The Cancer Dancer*. It's become my passion and mission; continuing to carry this care and compassion into the world to help others heal and thrive while encouraging them to flip that switch to the positive side and find joy even in the midst of turmoil.

One of my most rewarding "babies" from breast cancer is *The Link of Hope Sistas* which is the Positively Pat support group that helps women around the world. We have about 100 women that have gone through cancer or are newly diagnosed. We support one another, inspire, encourage and give hope. The group's doors are open as we welcome newly diagnosed women all the time. They are amazing, courageous and I am humbled by them, their strength and compassion.

I'm thrilled that there is one other project in the works right now for Cindy and me. A movie; yep, a big time movie that will be in a theatre near you soon. The working title is *Where it Once Was.* It's the story of Cindy's life, our friendship and our breast cancer journeys. It will be poignant and hysterical. Yes, laughter is healing and plays a role in all that we do.

Dive into this book with an open mind and let it fill you with the support, love, encouragement and vital information you will need to make your journey to health more joyful, graceful and successful.

This is the beginning of a new life. Remember, *Joy is the Choice*. You'll thank us later.

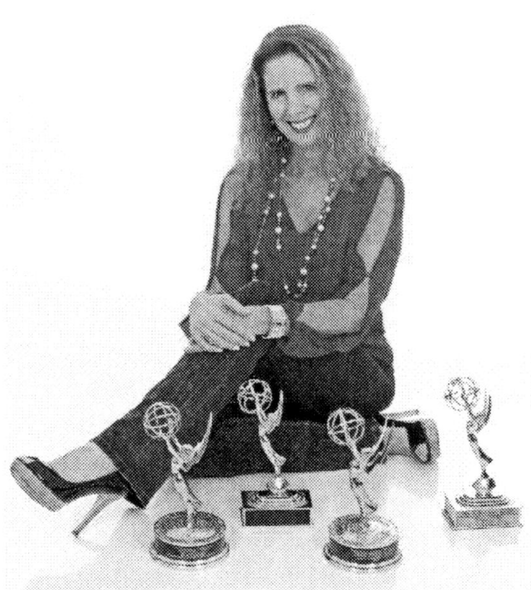

www.SanPedroProductions.com.

Patricia San Pedro

is a four time Emmy award winning TV producer, author, photographer, writer, PR/media expert and breast cancer survivor and advocate.
www.PositivelyPat.com

Chapter 27

Interview with a Survivor/Advocate

Astrid Justine Nicastri

She slips home with waves
that glint silver in the sun
before dispelling into
depths of shadow
in which tears fall
and emotions ache to find
comfort with her sisters
in regard to stony rejection
The sea cries for the utter
solitude in which their
sworn and loyal protectors
and fierce guardians live
rushing continually to lavish
loving caresses upon them
for undying service
ever trying to express gratitude
and bring peace at last
to compassionless hearts

Astrid Justine Nicastri

This is an interview between Astrid Nicastri and Laura Tan Nicastri (Astrid's stepmom) conducted over a period of days in April 2015.

Laura: You had survived 2 previous cancers; a meduloblastoma (brain tumor) in 1989 as a 12 year old, then another (benign) brain tumor in 2006 while you were a college student, both of which were life altering and sidelined you for long periods of time. By 2007 you had recovered and were moving on with your life. You were employed as a paraprofessional, in particular working with special needs children. Because your outlook on life has been so open and positive despite your health challenges and setbacks, you were also called upon to be a "Motivational Speaker" at several Fundraisers for cancer. What was that like for you?

Astrid: I was 12 years old and my life went from light to dark overnight, literally. I was diagnosed with medulloblastoma that was quite advanced. I was not expected to live. I went into surgery with all the hopes and dreams of any little girl. I came out of surgery not being able to see, talk or control my body. The condition wasn't permanent but nothing came back fully except for my ability to talk (I'm sure people who know me consider that a mixed blessing). When I had recovered from the surgery sufficiently, I underwent radiation from my head to the bottom of my spine, cranial-spinal radiation. When a child's brain is radiated, a lot is lost. I have difficulty with a lot of things both physically and intellectually. But for some reason unknown to anyone, my verbal skills have remained at a functional level.

Laura: How many years of formal education did you eventually complete?

Astrid: I have a college degree in expressive art therapy and was working on a master's degree in special education when the second brain tumor hit. That was that as far as schooling.

Laura: Despite all that, things were going well for you until January of 2007 when you began to feel a bit off. What physical symptoms were you experiencing that led you to seek medical advice before you knew you had breast cancer?

Astrid: I noticed at the very beginning of that year that I had developed a hard lump under my left armpit.

Laura: What doctors did you see about swelling in armpit?

Astrid: I first went to my primary care physician, Karen Raben who was and is a really caring and demanding doctor. Of course with my history I was immediately sent to have it biopsied. But before I could have it biopsied, I had to drink a horrible drink that I could hardly get down. I really didn't think I could finish it without gagging. While I was struggling with this, an infectious disease doctor was sent for. He said he was 80% sure it was an infection that developed as a result of shaving my underarms.

Laura: So what happened then?

Astrid: Not wanting to finish the horrible drink, I jumped on that idea and did not have a biopsy. I left with a prescription for antibiotics in my hand to the horror of my father who was there me. And even though my parents kept urging me on and off for months to have the biopsy and get it checked, I continued to stall. "I was an adult" and couldn't be forced to do so. Remember, this follows my childhood which was changed by cancer and guided by the decisions of all of the most caring and well-informed adults in my life: parents, doctors, family and friends.

Laura: Did you also see an oncologist at this time for a consultation?

Astrid: Everyone advised me to make follow up appointments with my oncologist but I never did. *It is here that I have to say, I had made a "beyond huge" mistake. My breast cancer could have been found months earlier if only I had finished the drink and done the* *biopsy.* With my history how could I have made the decision I made?

In the end I finally realized that my behavior was just selfish and stupid. Please don't ever make a mistake like that. *Get things checked out no matter what!* Then decide if you want to live or die.

Laura: So would you say *fear* was factoring pretty significantly in your decision-making at this time and or "denial?"

Astrid: I pretty much knew I was in denial. So I did not have the biopsy and I was given a Z-pack of antibiotics to take instead and the problem and the lump went away.

I can't blame everything on not wanting to finish the drink. The truth is I had already gone through so much with the brain tumors that I couldn't face going through it again. Part of me was willing to die and part of me was very afraid.

Laura: What would you tell someone today if they were in your position at that time?

Astrid: I would tell them not to let fear overtake you. You are the one in control. I know it is hard but you have to believe in yourself and be strong. Move fear out of your way. You don't have time for it!

Laura: What caused you to seek your primary care physician's advice again?

Astrid: A few months before Christmas, the hard lump developed under my arm again. I did not take care of it right away thinking I would just need another Z-pack. However the next morning I woke up to find red stripes running down my left side from under my left armpit almost to my waist.

Laura: What did your PCP, Dr. Raben say when she saw the red stripes?

Astrid: She took one look told me to go straight to the emergency room or to see an oncologist that day.

Dr. Raben didn't scold or yell at me for not attending to this even though she reminded me regularly. I have always found and continue to find her encouraging and supportive. She really cares.

Laura: So what did you find out?

Astrid: I went back to the oncologist that I had had one consultation with months earlier who had also told me to get it biopsied but who I never followed up with. When I lifted up my shirt, she took one look and said "You needed chemotherapy three months ago. You have a severe breast cancer. We are going to remove your breasts, your uterus, and your lymph nodes".

Laura: What went through your mind when she told you all this?

Astrid: I was completely and beyond devastated. I could not deal with the thought that I would have to go through cancer all over again and all the pain and horrors that went with it. I was terrified of having to sacrifice so much of my body. Would I feel less like a woman? What would happen to me if all those parts were gone? It was all just too terrifying and overwhelming.

Laura: How did you deal with it?

Astrid: Hey, I thought I had been doing pretty well up till now and had found a way to roll with the punches, but enough was enough already. This is where my optimism failed and I was pretty much ready to give up and let cancer have me. I was so tired of fighting and wanted to just let go, not care about anything and just melt into nothing.

I was so depressed I couldn't bring myself to act. Things were already so bad but I could not help it; I was letting things get worse. But there was some part deep inside me that wouldn't let me just give up. The support and encouragement I got from family and friends really helped me to hold onto that part in me.

Laura: So support communities were really important too, in helping to bring you out of your depression?

Astrid: Yes. Optimism, hopeful encouragement and understanding were so important. Then out came the fighter again. "Cancer you better watch out; I am back." Out came the anger and the willingness to persevere. My mantra became "I am going to kick the cancer so hard out of my life that you will never find your way back. You have no permission to ever be in my body again. Alright, let's do this!"

Laura: What did you do next?

Astrid: I wanted a second opinion; there had to be some other way. It was not that I did not believe that this oncologist was a good doctor. I was just so scared of the results she gave me that I just had to find out if there were any other options available. I sought a second opinion and my family and I found breast oncologist, Dr. Marc Lippman and breast surgeon, Frederick L. Moffat at UM Sylvester. They were two very highly recommended and experienced doctors in this field. I made a choice to go to them instead.

Laura: What was their diagnosis?

Astrid: In October 2007 my breast cancer was termed estrogen positive and stage 3b to 4. It was a right-sided and locally advanced ER/PR positive and HER-2 negative breast cancer. It was treated as though it was a stage 4-breast cancer. I had to start accepting that I would have to have a mastectomy.

I was told to have the lymph nodes in my right arm tested to see how far the cancer had spread. Four or five of my lymph nodes came back positive.

Laura: Why did you decide to only have a single mastectomy?

Astrid: The doctors told me that it was my decision whether to have just the one breast removed or both in case a later cancer presented in my left breast. I wanted to keep my left breast. It was fine and I wanted to keep as many parts of me as possible.

Laura: What treatments did you eventually choose and receive?

Astrid: This time I followed the recommendations and had chemotherapy before surgery to hopefully first shrink the tumors and to see if my cancer would respond well to chemotherapy. My chemotherapy consisted of Adriamycin/Cytoxan for four cycles followed by Taxol for one cycle. I was then moved on to Taxotere for three cycles due to the fact that my liver enzymes were becoming elevated.

Laura: Did you do anything special to prepare for chemotherapy like change anything in terms of your diet, vitamins, eating habits, etc. to help you throughout the entire treatment process?

Astrid: Yes. My mother, Jeanne Nicastri, is a firm believer in alternative therapies and had found some additional ways to help me get through. She found doctor in Nevada who was willing to work with a doctor here that could give me infusions of the vitamin C preparation sent here from Nevada. I was driven a few times a week to receive a three-hour infusion of the vitamin C preparation either through my chemo port or in my hand or arm if they could not get it into the port.

She also found a nutritionist who kept me on what I called "the swamp drink": water, oil and minerals diet. Basically the diet consisted of juicing vegetables and taking minerals and oils. The goal was to get me to the best PH level my body could have to help me through the process and give my body the additional strength and support it needed.

Laura: Do you believe the Vitamin C infusions and nutritional drinks helped?

Astrid: They absolutely helped—very much so! They helped me maintain both strength and stamina during the entire process.

Laura: Did the chemotherapy work?

Astrid: It did and I was now ready and able to have surgery. On April 23, 2008 I had a single mastectomy and my right breast totally removed.

Laura: What was next on the list?

Astrid: Next on the list was radiation to the area where my right breast had been removed. Once the skin and other soft tissues had healed enough from the surgery, I had targeted radiation to that area.

Laura: How long did the radiation last?

Astrid: I had radiation therapy from February 18, 2008 to August 4, 2008. I do have to say that the entire recovery from surgery aside from the extra help I was getting in nutrition and vitamin C was a big, fat, pain in the ass.

Laura: How did you feel about your doctors and your care at this point?

Astrid: I had really gotten lucky with doctors. I had the most wonderful radiation doctor, Dr. Takita and staff at the hospital. Radiation was the least difficult of all the therapies to get through.

Laura: Next was “to do breast reconstruction or not” right?

Astrid: Yes. All the talk about breast reconstruction which had been going on for a while really started to escalate. Wait let me not get ahead of myself. I was cancer free at this point! Did I really want to go through another surgery I asked myself? I could just stop right here.

Laura: What do you think ultimately made you choose to go forward with reconstruction?

Astrid: I was really undecided. I was so tired from all the procedures and the mental and physical effort to get to this point.

Also part of the "urgency" to decide one way or another had to do with insurance coverage and my deductibles. There were copays and bills on top of everything else. It was just a financial reality. If I was going to have surgery, try to do it the year where my deductibles had already been met. But anyway I had begun going to a weekly local cancer support group, "The Wellness Center" (formerly the CCC-Cancer Caring Community) a wonderful group which had become like a second family to me. Issues like self-image, feeling feminine, the pros and cons of reconstruction, etc. were common topics of conversation there. Part of me missed my breast and I felt like I wanted to not only feel like a whole woman again but also "look" like one! I was lopsided and I missed my breast! Yet I knew I didn't want to have something "foreign" like implants in my body. It was just my personal thing: implants weren't for me.

Fortunately you have to wait quite a while after radiation before you can have anything done and it gave me the time to really ponder my options and think things through. The radiated tissue needs time to heal. I knew I was really adamant that I did not want an implant. People kept talking to me about it. The argument was that semblance of a new breast would make me feel like a woman again. I agreed to go and both see and hear out a few doctors on the issue of implants. But after meeting with all of them I was still not convinced. I did not want something artificial inside me to remind me that I had lost a breast because of cancer. I just wanted cancer gone from my life forever.

Laura: Why did you decide to do the BrAVA rather than the more frequently used flap/reconstruction?

Astrid: I attended a presentation by Dr. Khouri at the "Wellness Cancer Center." There he talked about a fat transfer method that gave you back your breast through moving your own tissue from one part of your body to another. It sounded right for me. I had already suffered the damage to my abilities from my brain tumors so healing myself from myself seemed like a much needed victory to me. For me, implants were just another concession to what I had lost. Implants were not for me. Needless to say, I signed up with Dr. Khouri that day.

Laura: So while you didn't really know what was involved in the treatment you signed up anyway?

Astrid: Yes I did. I just knew it was right for me.

Laura: As you learned more about the steps involved from wearing the device to the liposuction, did it give you pause?

Astrid: I just knew it was right for me. This new method of breast reconstruction certainly involved a lot of commitment. It would begin by wearing what I started to call the plastic breast vacuum which was the Brava System to create a new breast. I then would have to go through the liposuction to remove fat from one part of my body (mostly waist, hips and buttocks) and then multiple injections into the breast area.

Laura: Can you describe the experience?

Astrid: It is definitely not for everyone. Sleeping with the Brava System attached to you could be very cumbersome and clumsy; also the aftermath of each liposuction/injection session was definitely painful and messy with days of lingering discomfort.

Laura: Can you be more specific?

Astrid: All right, first I did not know what I was getting myself into when I signed up for this new form of reconstruction or the pretty big commitment that would be required to undergo this method of breast reconstruction. I was just so elated about creating my own natural breast that I did not stop to really think about everything that would be involved. It took a lot longer than the doctor first estimated it would take or that I had expected.

I had to be fitted for the device according to my body size and projected or estimated desired final size. Secondly, the fat-transfer procedure/Brava System was/is relatively new so unlike other breast reconstruction procedures, there was very little information on the Internet. For example, to help me understand fully the procedure and end result.

Every woman is blessed with her own body type and every breast is individual and in some ways unequal to the other. My left breast was pretty big. I was a triple D. The bigger the breast that you are trying to match the new breast with the longer it takes.

Laura: Was it uncomfortable or painful?

Astrid: Yes, it was both uncomfortable and painful. It was very uncomfortable sleeping every night for three weeks at a time with a large suction device over the area of my mastectomy. It was like wearing a big plastic dome-like breast over my skin. It took a few minutes to apply a cream you need to use to avoid skin irritation when attaching the dome. It was attached to a box by hose to a machine that when set would act as a vacuum and would suck and relax on and off during the night. Also I had to get used wearing the device making me have to sleep on my back which I didn't like. I also had to get used to the little whirring sound the box itself made. It took a long time to get used to it but I was finally able to sleep.

At the end of the three weeks, I would undergo the outpatient fat transfer procedure. Through liposuction fat was taken from some part of my body and then the procedure was reversed. Utilizing what seemed like a large hypodermic needle the fat was injected into the area that would eventually be my new breast.

Other women who had undergone this procedure said they just were in some discomfort and pain for the weekend and then back on their feet again. I was in pain for a week. I had to have lots of paper blankets under me in bed at home because there was so much fluid leakage from the areas where the liposuction had taken place. There was a poke every time fat was taken and every time it was injected. My breast area, butt, back and legs were like one huge pincushion.

Laura: Was it hard to move after each procedure?

Astrid: Moving around was the most painful part. I wore this constrictive white girdle stocking which was excruciating when doing things like attending to Mother Nature. It was terribly painful especially immediately following liposuction procedures. I learned that liposuction which was sourced lower down on your legs was much more painful than when fat was taken from my buttocks and back.

I owe so much credit to you, Laura for getting me through these post-surgery weeks. You were there for me every step of the way, especially when I knew I was behaving like a baby.

Laura: How many times did you ultimately have to go through this procedure?

Astrid: I went through about six of them before the right breast was achieved matching the other breast. This included a couple of additional fat removals from the new breast because it was too large.

Laura: Were you finished at this point?

Astrid: No. The breasts were still uneven and did not look or feel good.

Laura: So how did you and your doctor resolve that aesthetic, cosmetic issue?

Astrid: A basket was inserted beneath my existing breast in an attempt to lift it up in order to match my new one. However it didn't last or "take." After that we decided to do a breast-lift procedure to my left breast in order to match my new, reconstructed right breast.

Laura: The final "detail"...the nipple! Nipples as you learned along the way are also an aspect of reconstruction that is a very personal choice, and in many cases a creative solution: some women leave them off, some tattoo pigment or personal designs, some use skin to recreate them, etc. It's the final "to do or not to-do." What did you do?

Astrid: I had toyed with the idea of getting a nipple put on to my newly created breast. It would not make a really big difference but there would be two "points" that showed through my t-shirt not just one. At different seminars and breast cancer meetings I had seen many different possibilities. I could get a tattooed nipple; there were some nice 3D ones that I saw. I could also get a stick on nipple that I would wear when going out. I finally tried a procedure that took skin from the areola of my left breast and used it to make a nipple on my right breast. Unfortunately it also did not take and so now I am a "one-nippled" woman. I don't really mind. My fiancé still loves my breasts and it's not like you can really tell that a nipple is missing.

Laura: All in all, how long did the entire reconstruction process take?

Astrid: It took a year and a half to accomplish including many stressful setbacks, but I was thrilled with the results. Sometimes though I catch myself looking in the mirror to see if you can really tell in some of the tops I am wearing any difference in my physique. Overall I am elated and so happy and proud of my new breast. It was worth the commitment, the procedures and all the pain. After all as the saying goes, "no pain, no gain." My new breast was totally worth it and will be with me forever and my own.

Everything was worth it. I got my very own breast back. I love my new breast. Except for the difference between the nipples I am overjoyed all the time with how they turned out. I have to say I am very proud of my breast and not at all embarrassed to show them off in the proper context. For example a doctor I have seen for something else but still involving a physical exam will ask to show my reconstructed breast to someone. They think the way it was done and how breast reconstruction has evolved is amazing. I am not ashamed to say that I don't mind at all. In fact I am more than happy to further encourage this new way of breast reconstruction. So many people are amazed with the result. I know my fiancé definitely loves my breasts.

Laura: What is life like today, 8 years later?

Astrid: Until a few years ago I never had a real date. And yes, I actually have a fiancé now. I never thought it possible. I had always thought "Who would want me with all my disabilities?" I know that is a very negative way of looking at things but I could not help it. It was how I felt. When I reconnected through social media with a fellow cancer survivor whom I'd met at "cancer camp" when we were both 12 years old, it was instant friendship, chemistry and happiness. He, Ben Gibson is my fiancé now!

Laura: Do you have any advice for others who have shared or are about to share in your journey?

Astrid: Yes. If you are going to inspire anyone else, *you have to first inspire yourself*. I thought I was always going to be dependent on others during my life. But I have become independent now and with my own new breast to boot. I am living again and with a new freedom, definitely a cancer free one. I have a fiancé, a home and a daughter. She is a dog but she is my daughter and her name is Sassy.

I love and appreciate life so much despite the disabilities I have. I have found ways of turning my disabilities into positive forces and have created new ways of doing things. I have my own path to travel to success. I have total permission to win. I am doing well and even inspiring others. When life gets crazy, hectic and overwhelming, stop, step back and take time to reach inside to your inner self. Breathe and reclaim all the wonderful things about you; reclaim your inner warrior and you will be strong.

I have always believed in rainbows. In the darkest of storms there will be a beautiful rainbow above shining down hope. Make sure your rainbow armor is upon you as you step back into reality. I work on this all the time. I am a warrior in life in rainbow armor. Light pierces through darkness. I am still kicking and surviving. You too can do it. You can push the envelope.

I am a teacher again and have wonderful four and five year olds in my class whom I hope to give a helping hand in beginning their journey through life. The most important thing for me is that I am living my life and have the freedom to do so. I have the freedom to be happy and be myself, enjoy the dance, stopping to breathe in the flowers and look at all the beauty in life. One of my favorite quotes in life is "What would you attempt to do if you knew you could not fail". Think about that one and get back to me. Too often we are afraid to push the envelope to see how far things can go. I am telling you push it because however impossible our journey seems, we all have permission to overcome.

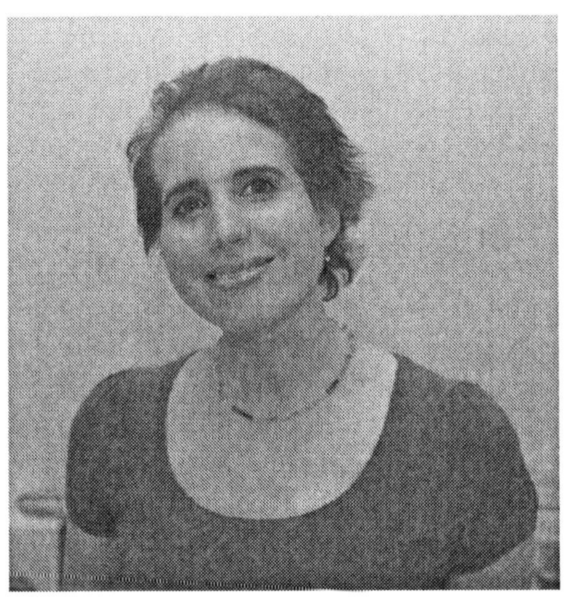

Astrid Justine Nicastri

Ms. Astrid Nicastri, age 38, is a three-time cancer survivor, beginning at the age of twelve.

She was the 2009 Recipient of the *"Champion of the Human Spirit Award,"* for the Wellness Community of Greater Miami's Annual Heart and Star Gala.

She has been a Motivational Speaker for various cancer support groups and organizations for many years, including the Children's Cancer Caring Center, Miami, FL.

She has been working as a Preschool teacher and Assistant teacher for Special needs children from 2009 to the present.

Astrid Nicastri is also a gifted poet, who currently resides in Vero Beach, FL, with her fiancé and their adorable dog, "Sassy."

Chapter 28

Angels in Disguise

Judy Garcia

They say all of us have angels who hover over us twenty-four hours a day, seven days a week. Heaven-sent angels, who guard and protect us. I believe this to be true. But more so, I know it to be true that God can also send angels in the form of people: that is exactly what He did for me the day I met Cindy Papale.

I had taken a break from running my personal business as a vocal coach and decided to work as a waitress in a restaurant for about four months. The truth is, the real reason why I took a break from my personal business was because I was going through a depression; I knew that being around people in a restaurant environment would snap me out of it. So I left the comfort of my studio to get back in the work force and help myself the only way I knew how: by being around people.

One day while on duty at the restaurant, the manager asked me to please work the bar area because he was short bartenders. Although I have never been a bartender and know nothing about tending bar, I still went over there without question and did as my manager requested.

The first guests I served at the bar that afternoon were a group of three women. These ladies seemed to have been celebrating something because they were ordering champagne. I was running around the whole day as guests constantly came in and out of the bar non-stop. Because I was so swamped, I barely had the time to speak with these three women in an effort to get to know them – something I would normally do.

These ladies were having such a great time laughing and toasting the whole afternoon until the sun came down. Other guests came and went but they were there for about three- to- four hours. Every time I passed by their table I overheard them talking to each other, saying things like, "The wedding is going to be beautiful," "How many people did you invite?" "When are you doing the book signing?"

When I walked up to them to ensure everything was going well and to see if they needed more drinks, one of the ladies began to ask me about myself. Right away – just by talking to her – I felt she was special. She made me feel so happy simply by speaking to me. I kept apologizing for not having enough time to check on them, but really I was just sorry that my busyness prevented me from spending more time chatting with them. Exuding positivity and happiness, they seemed to be enjoying themselves immensely – the kind of people everyone wants to be around.

"Tell me your name again sweetie," she said to me. "Judy, what's yours?" I asked. "Cindy Papale," she replied. I was automatically enchanted with her spirit and her joy. All I could do was smile because I knew then, in that moment, that I was in the presence of an angel.

Eventually the time came for them to leave. And that was when she approached me to explain she'd come to the bar to celebrate with her girlfriends because she'd be re-marrying her ex-husband in just a few months – right there in the restaurant where I worked. I immediately asked if she'd already booked a band for her wedding; I was hoping she hadn't because I wanted to be the one to sing at this joyous event. Since I have a band and we perform at weddings, this seemed only appropriate and perfect. Cindy told me she had not yet booked anyone to perform and expressed how awesome it would be if I could.

We spent about ten minutes standing there talking, astounded by the way God brings people into our lives so suddenly. I remember telling her "What a coincidence we met!" and will never forget her reply, "In life there are no coincidences my dear!"

And it was true. It was fate. Destiny. Sometimes I think and feel that perhaps one of the reasons God allowed me to work in the restaurant again after so many years was to meet this angel, Cindy.

She subsequently became my very good friend. I felt within the few minutes I spoke to her that I had known her my whole life. I respected her and admired her right away, but even more so when I discovered she was a breast cancer survivor. It made me admire her even more because in spite of having endured so much she still managed to be this upbeat, positive, energetic person; her character is heroic and admirable.

One day last October we were having lunch and chatting about the plans for her fast-approaching wedding. Our meeting was supposed to be exclusively about the ceremony and putting together the final touches on the songs she wanted me to sing. But out of nowhere she brought up the fact that it was breast-cancer awareness month and asked if I had already gone for my check-up.

I admitted I'd never had my breasts checked. As those words came out of my mouth, I thought about the lump I had been feeling in my left breast for the past six months. Cindy urged me get checked even if I didn't think it was necessary. I then confessed that for a few months I'd been feeling a small lump on my left breast but that I hadn't gone to see a doctor due to fear and a lack of health insurance. In a sudden motion, Cindy picked up the phone, called her doctor, and set up an appointment for me the very next day.

She stressed how important it was to get checked, told me I had to be proactive, and advised me that waiting wasn't the answer. She knew just what to say; she could see the fear in my eyes and expressed herself with the perfect blend of gentleness and firmness. I knew I *had* to go. In spite of my embarrassment about not seeing a doctor sooner, the matter had been resolved: I would see Cindy's doctor the following day – rain or shine.

The very next morning I walked into the clinic at ten, accompanied by my mom, whom I'd asked to come with me. Although she was just as nervous as I, she tried to be strong for me by cracking jokes and looking up funny videos on her phone. I filled out some paperwork and within the hour I was outside the waiting room for a sonogram, dressed in a white robe and sitting alongside about ten other women who were also waiting their turn. I was probably the youngest one there. I am 29 now. All of the women around me that day seemed to be in their 40's and over.

Some of them had worried looks on their faces, others were playing on their phones and/or laughing at a text. I felt like I just wanted to get it over with and find out what the lump was all about. In my head I played out two scenarios: 1.) The nurse examines me and announces I have nothing but fibrosis, and 2.) The obviously worried nurse immediately calls in more doctors for further review.

As I contemplated both possibilities, my thoughts were interrupted by the nurse who called out my name. It was my turn.

Upon entering the room, she told me to lay on the bed. Before we started she asked a few questions: "For how long have you been feeling the lump?" "Can you show me where you feel it?" I laid there and watched her do the sonogram on my left breast. She found the lump right away and then she found another lump in the bottom part of my breast. So it turned out I had two of them.

When she checked my right breast, she discovered that one didn't have any lumps at all. Then she called the doctor in to examine the sonogram and he scheduled a biopsy for the next day. He told me the only way of knowing if they were benign or not was to biopsy the lumps. Although he had this look on his face that concerned me, he assured me we didn't need to worry until we had to.

That night, I prayed like I had never prayed before in my whole life. Not because I was afraid of the biopsy, but because I was terrified to be sick. I was already thinking of chemo treatments and shaving my long blonde hair.

The next day I went in for the biopsy first thing in the morning. I was more at ease than I thought I would be. My mom came along. They called me into the waiting room and I experienced the same waiting process until it was time for the nurse to call my name again.

The nurse held my hand the whole time as the doctor biopsied the two lumps on my left breast. When he was done doing the procedure I got up and began to get dressed. I noticed his face when he was inspecting the samples he had obtained from the biopsy. The nurse looked at him with worry and as he looked back at her he pressed his lips. He closed the box where he had placed the samples and got them ready to send to the lab.

After seeing the look on his face, I asked, "Is it bad?" and he said, "We can't be sure until the results come back. We will know soon enough."

He told me that the clinic would call me with the results in four days. Needless to say, I was incredibly nervous as I waited for that phone call. I have never eaten so much chocolate ice-cream in my life!

And finally, it came. My cellphone rang and I picked it up to hear the nurse ask, "Hi, is this Judith Garcia? Your results came back negative. No cancerous cells were found. You will have to now go back to see your surgical oncologist to see whether her would like to remove the benign module or just repeat another mammogram in six to twelve months."

Thus far in my life, that was the best phone call I have ever received. I called Cindy right away to tell her the good news.

Prior to that biopsy, for about six months I walked around knowing I had a lump in my left breast. I felt it in the shower one day when I was self-examining the way a doctor had taught me once. I didn't tell anyone about it because I was scared to go to the doctor and still I knew deep inside that I had to. It's embarrassing to admit I was afraid to see a doctor, and in all honesty, if it wasn't for Cindy I probably still would have not gone. She gave me that courage.

I thank God every day for my health; more so when I think about all of the negative repercussions a cancer diagnosis at the age of 29 could have brought. Now, I have health insurance. I see my doctor regularly and in a few months I have a consult with my breast doctor to see if he will operate and take out the lumps.

I celebrated my life more than ever that day when I got the phone call. It felt like I was getting another chance. And my life has been different since that phone call. I am now more proactive about my health and wellbeing. After I told this story to my friends, many of them came forth and told me they have found lumps too and have been scared to go to the doctor.

I told them about my experience at the doctor's office and the clinic. It was helpful that the nurses and doctors had the best bedside manners and were wonderfully sensitive to my situation – especially because it was my first time at the women's center.

I have returned to my studio to teach my voice students and I have come back to local stages, singing and playing the saxophone with my band. Since I met Cindy my life has changed so much for the better. And I thank her for giving me the courage to face my fears with regard to the breast exam. I am incredibly thankful to God because I feel like I got another chance. Even though my prognosis wasn't breast cancer, I still feel like I have been blessed with the chance to stay healthy. That is something we all take for granted sometimes.

Through it all I learned a very valuable lesson: if my diagnosis had come back positive, I probably would have freaked out for a while but then I would have fought the cancer and beaten it. Cindy and her friends did. So could I. I realize now that fear is a lie. And as long as we get to live another day, wake up to another sunrise, and enjoy another sunset, then really we should feel more than blessed and highly favored.

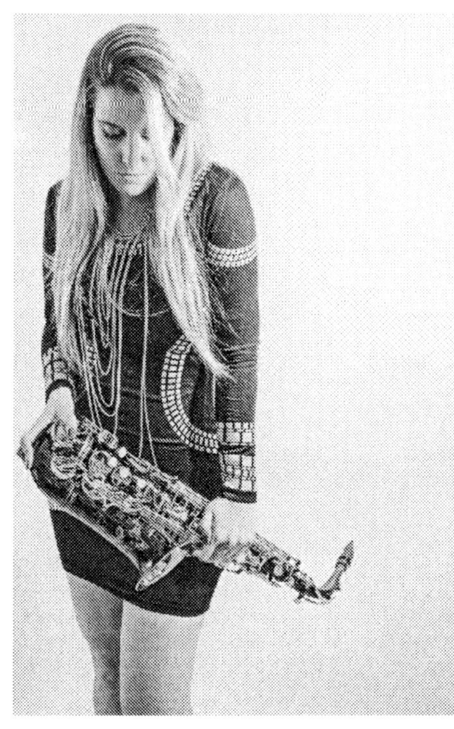

Judy Garcia

Cuban born singer/songwriter and saxophonist Judy Garcia began her musical journey by learning the saxophone. A proud brother of the National Music Honorary Fraternity Kappa Kappa Psi, she also had the privilege and honor of being one of FIU's Marching Golden Panther Band's Drum Majors in 2005.

Judy embarked upon her singing career seven years ago and to-date has had the privilege of playing saxophone and singing backup vocals for internationally renowned artists like Thalia, Gloria Estefan, Camilo Sesto, Leo Dan and Angela Carrasco. She currently performs nationally and internationally with her band, 30Vice, singing original music and Top 40 hits at private and public events.

This multi-talented young woman is also the CEO and Vocal Director for the Miami Florida-based Onstage Academy – which provides music instruction for aspiring singers, pianists, saxophonists, drummers, and guitar players.

For more information or to schedule an interview for lessons, please contact Onstage Academy at 786-262-3840 or visit Judy's website at www.judygarciaofficial.com.

Resources

Living Beyond Breast Cancer
10 East Atthes Avenue, Suite 204
Ardmore, PA 19003

Phone - 610-645-4567
FAX - 610-645-4573
http://www.lbbc.org

Living Beyond Breast Cancer, founded in 1991, is a national nonprofit organization dedicated to empowering all women affected by breast cancer to live as long as possible with the best quality of life. Programs and services include:

- Conferences;
- Teleconferences;
- Toll-free Survivor's Helpline (1-888-753-5222);
- Website lbbc.org;
- Free quarterly newsletters;
- Publications for African-American and Latina women;
- Recordings;
- Networking programs;
- Healthcare-provider trainings;
- and the Paula A Seidman Library and Resource Center.

The Susan G. Komen Breast Cancer Organization
http://www.komen.org

Young Survival Coalition (YSC)
Phone 646-257-3000 - toll free - 1-800-972-1011

LympheDIVAS, founded by RachelTroxell
http://www.lymphedivas.com

FORCE (Facing Our Risk Of Cancer Empowered)
FORCE's mission is to improve the lives of individuals and families affected by hereditary breast and ovarian cancer.
Debbie Setuain, South Florida Peer Support Coordinator
http://www.facingourrisk.org/index.php

Positively Pat – founder Patricia San Pedro
www.postivelypat.com

Facebook Link of Hope Sistas Support Group
www.facebook.com
Note: This is a private group; use the search feature on Facebook to look it up and request to join.

American Cancer Society
http://www.cancer.org

Beatriz Amendola, M.D.
Innovative Cancer Institute
http://www.innovativecancer.com/oncologist/beatriz-e-amendola-md-pa

Hummingwell Wellness Bar
Sabrina Hernandez-Cano, RDN, NC, CDE
http://hummingwell.com